tracey cox

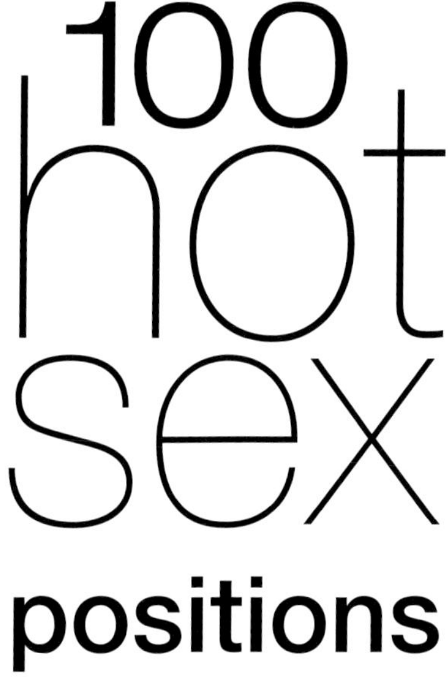

positions

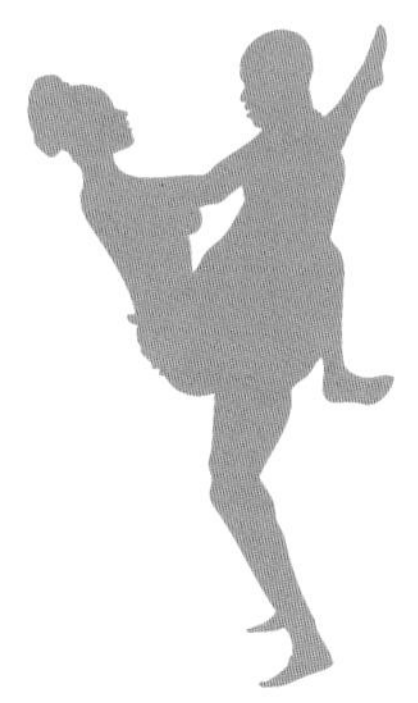

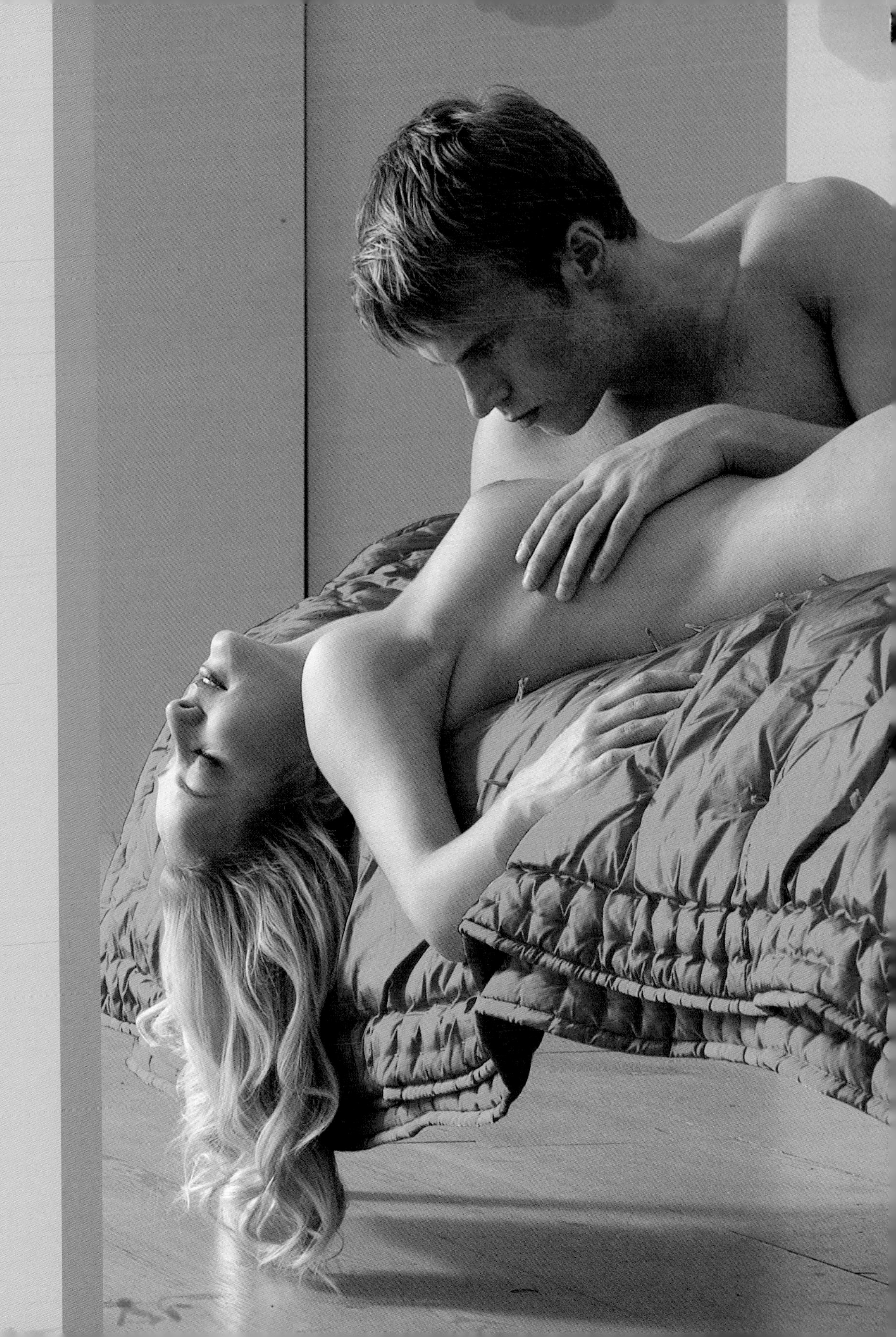

tracey cox

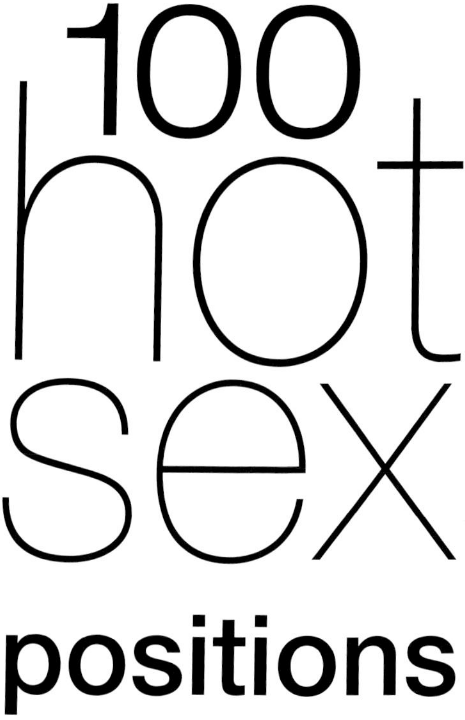

positions

Includes content previously published in *Kama Sutra*, *Supersex*, *Superhotsex*, *Quickies*, and *Secrets of a Supersexpert*.

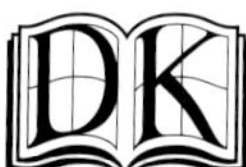

contents

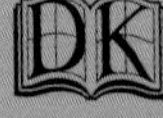

LONDON, NEW YORK, MELBOURNE,
MUNICH, AND DELHI

Project Editor: Daniel Mills
Senior Art Editor: Isabel de Cordova
US Editor: Shannon Beatty
Managing Editor: Penny Warren
Managing Art Editor: Glenda Fisher
Production Editor: Maria Elia
Senior Production Controller: Man Fai Lau
Creative Technical Support: Sonia Charbonnier
Art Director: Lisa Lanzarini
Publisher: Peggy Vance

Produced for DK by:
Project Editor: Dawn Bates
Designer: XAB Design
US Editor: Margaret Parrish

First American Edition, 2011
Published in the United States by
DK Publishing
375 Hudson Street, New York, New York 10014

11 12 13 10 9 8 7 6 5 4 3 2 1
001—178979—April/2011

Includes content previously published in: *Supersex*, *Superhotsex*, *Quickies*, *Kama Sutra*, *Secrets of a Supersexpert*.

Published in Great Britain by Dorling Kindersley Limited.
A catalog record for this book is available from the Library of Congress.
ISBN 978-0-7566-7157-0

DK books are available at special discounts when purchased in bulk for sales promotions, premiums, fund-raising, or educational use. For details, contact: DK Publishing Special Markets, 375 Hudson Street, New York, New York 10014 or SpecialSales@dk.com.

Color reproduction by Colourscan, Singapore
Printed and bound in Singapore by Tien Wah Press

Discover more at **www.dk.com**

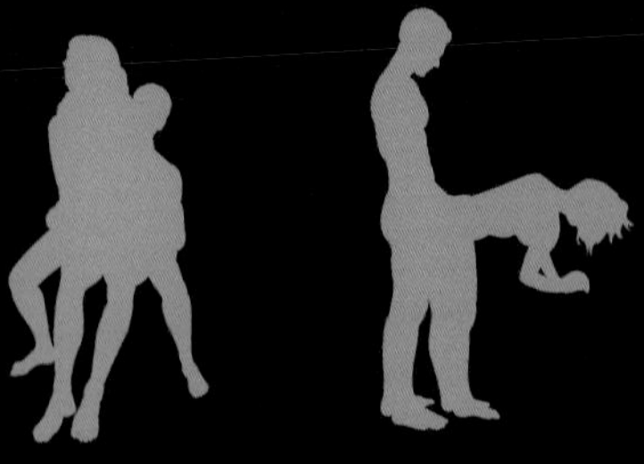

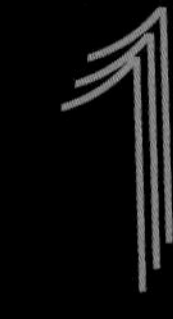

heartfelt

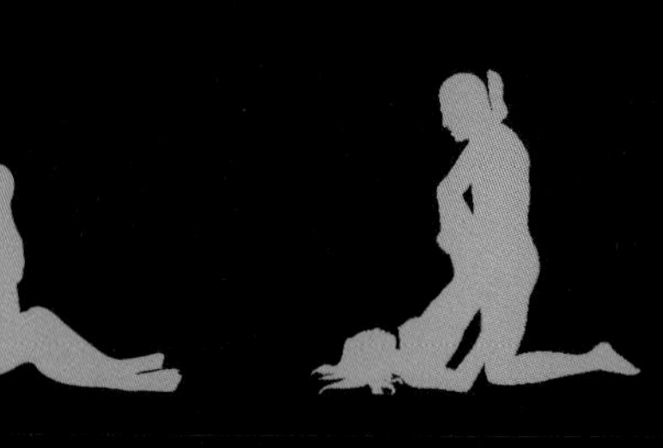
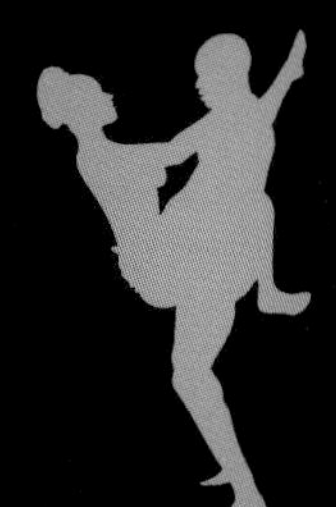
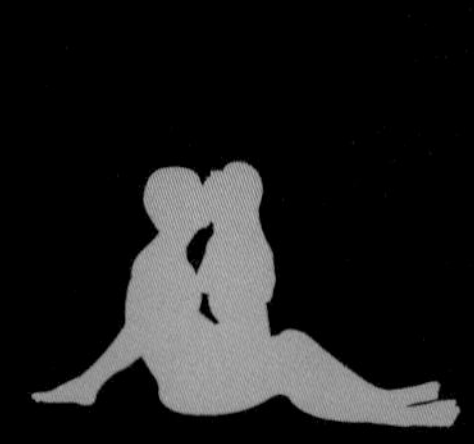
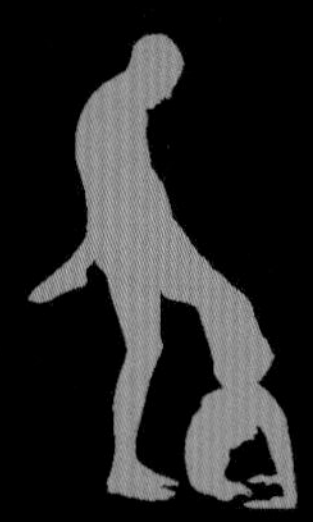

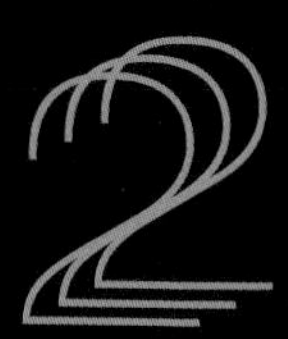

steamy

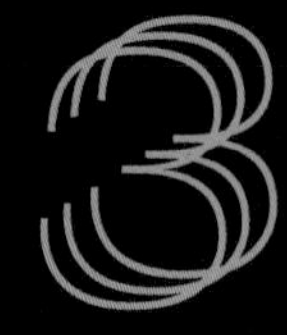

head games

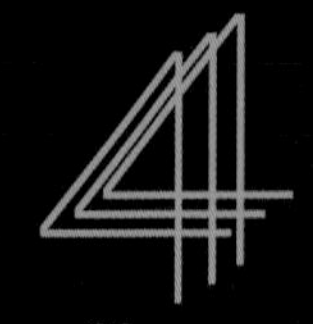

show off

ready to shake up your sex life?

Are you one of those couples who has two to three favorite sex positions and rarely deviates from them? Let me take a stab at what they are: If you're both a bit tired and in that guess-we'd-better-do-it-but-would-secretly-prefer-to-watch-TV mood, he rolls on top. If you've just come back from a fun, boozy night out and you're three sheets to the wind, she'll jump on top—or if you're feeling really adventurous, he'll take her from behind. How did I know? Take a closer look at that innocent-looking lamp, sitting on your bedside table—it's actually a sophisticated bugging device. Or it could be I knew because this is the routine pretty much all couples fall into when they've been together a while. We're all wildly experimental at the start when we're out to impress—happily locking our ankles behind our heads and dangling daringly upside-down without complaint. But it's a different story once you're both settled, all cuddly and nicely domesticated. You know you should try something new on the position front, something more dynamic, a bit bold and venturesome, but what? There are only five positions—side-by-side, standing, him on top, her on top, and from behind—and you've already chosen your favorites from that little line-up.

"You know you should try something new, something more dynamic, bold, and venturesome. But what? There are only five positions and you've already chosen your favorites from that little line-up."

But while there might be only five positions, by God, there are some deliciously tempting variations on each of them, and this book is going to make it sooooooo easy for you to choose from those variations that you'll want to try some (or all) of them! *100 Hot Sex Positions* is a saucy collection of all of my absolute favorites, handily organized into different chapters to suit all your different moods. Decide what you like, then flick to the section and style that suits you best—heartfelt, steamy, show off, or temptingly torrid. Alongside, you'll also find a good smattering of other stuff to tickle your fancy—tricks, tips, and talk pieces designed to intrigue you, inspire you, and up the orgasm quota for both of you.

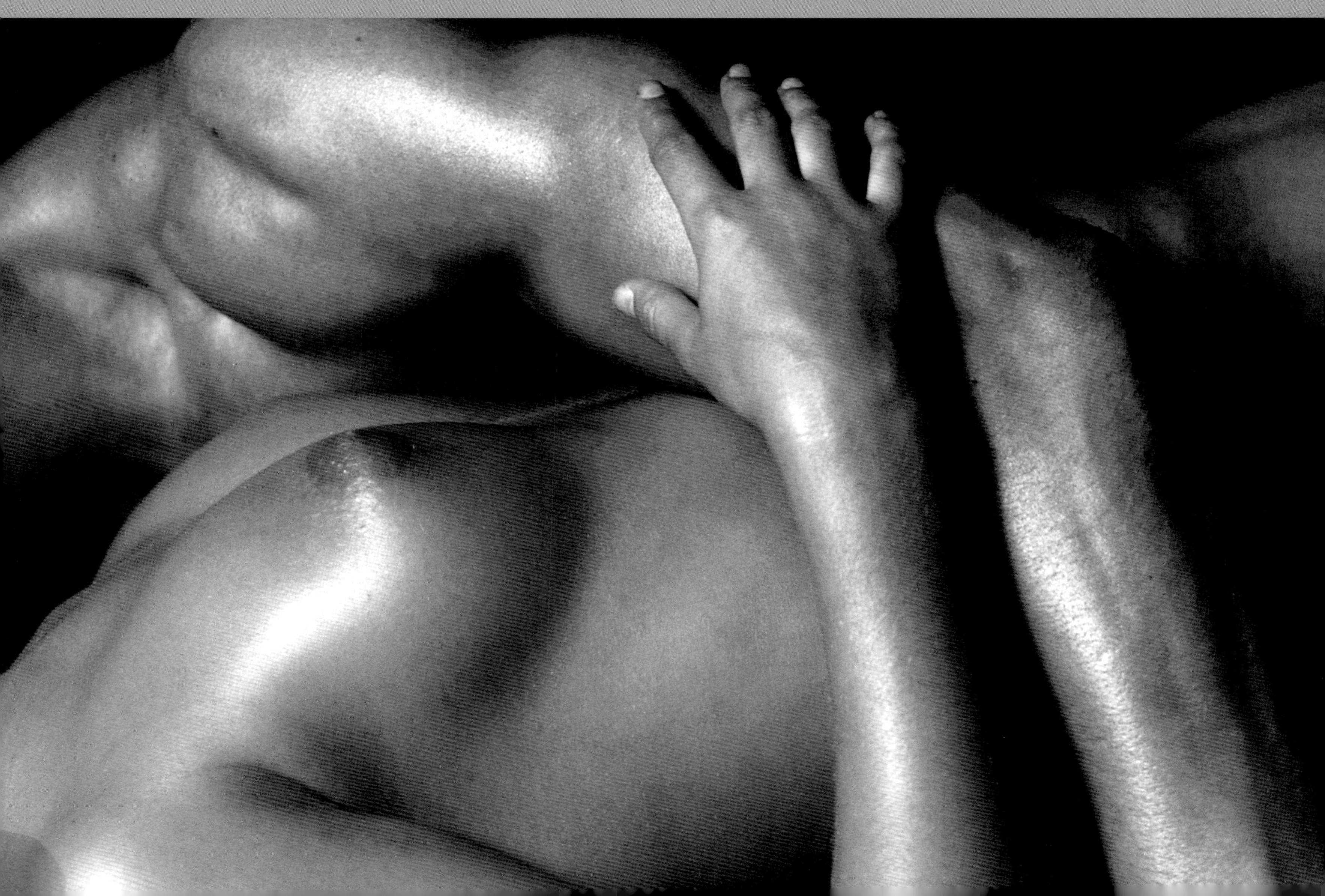

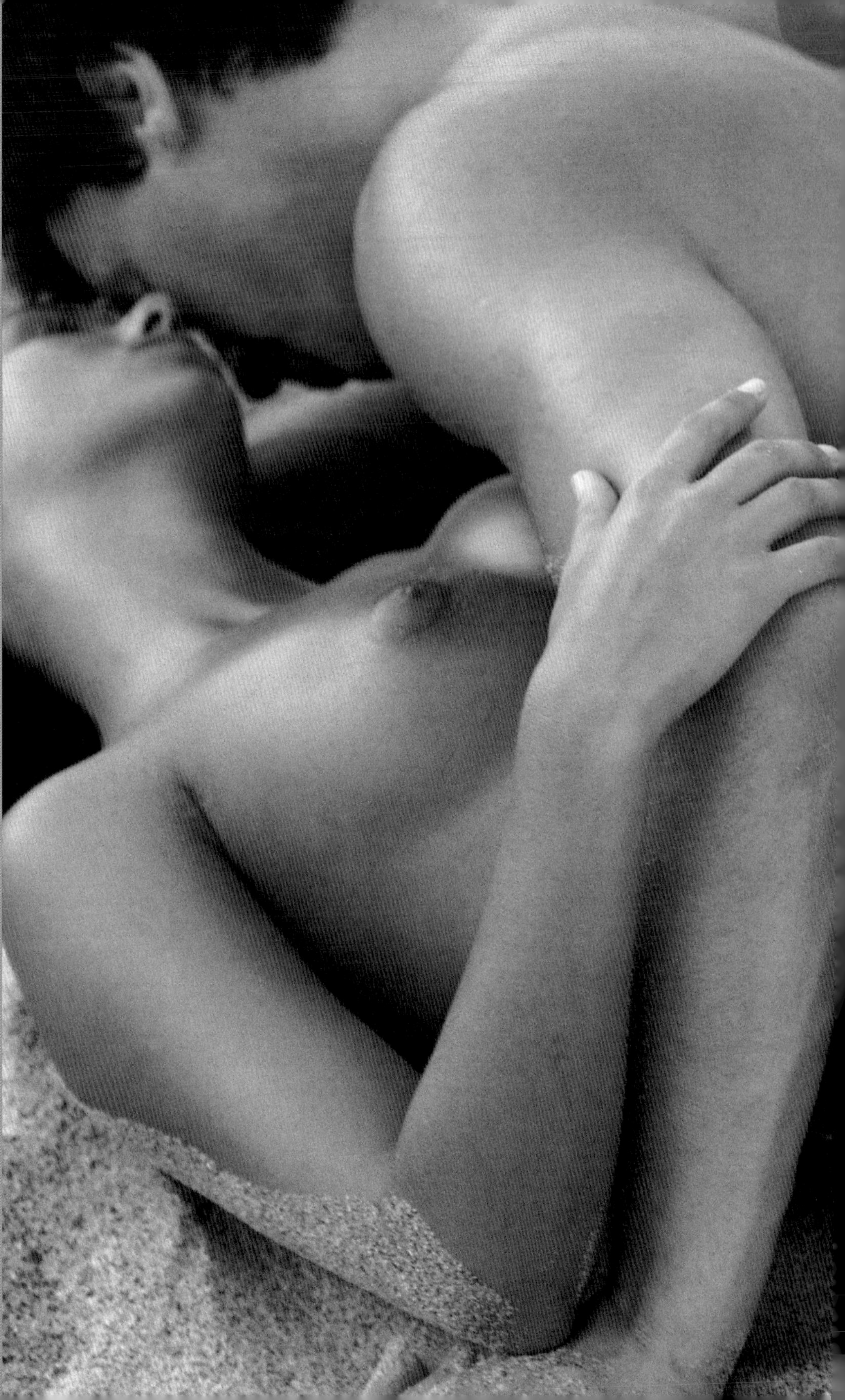

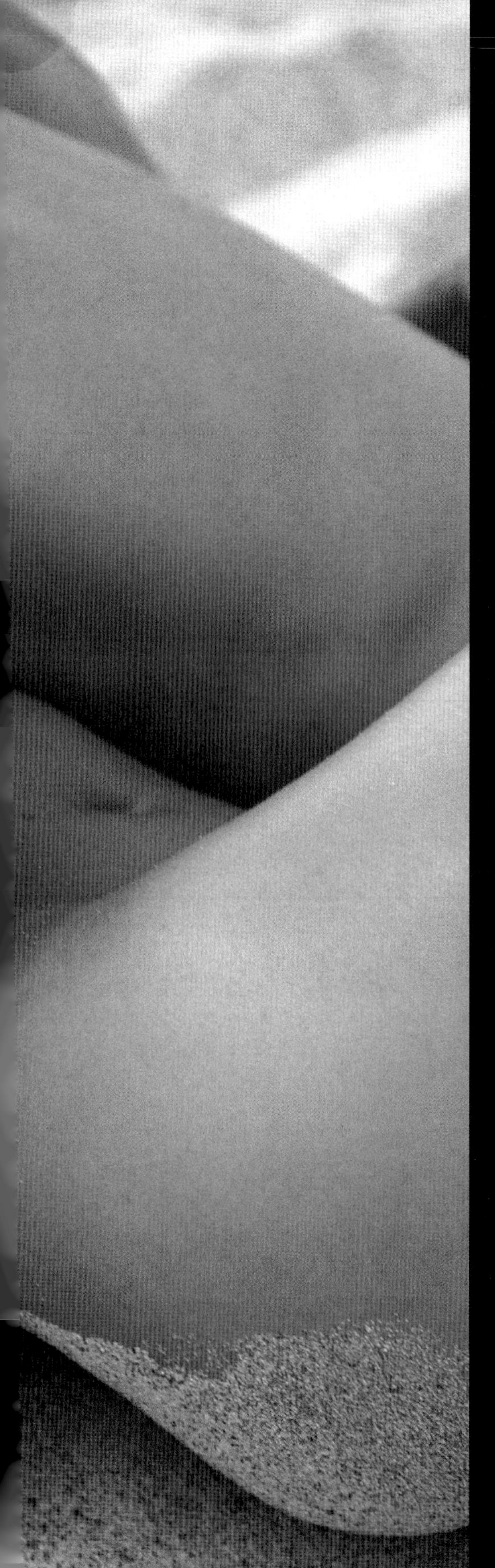

You can dip in and out of the book whenever the mood strikes you, but if you're both quite lazy little slugs (and who isn't?), make a point of trying one new position each week (yes, really!). Put a checkmark next to the positions you like on the handy checklist at the back (pages 188–9) and watch your list of favorites climb from a paltry two or three to double digits in no time! A healthier, happier sex life with minimum effort on your part. Now doesn't that sound appealing?

"A healthier, happier sex life with minimum effort on your part. Now doesn't that sound appealing?"

Tracey x

chapter

1

heartfelt

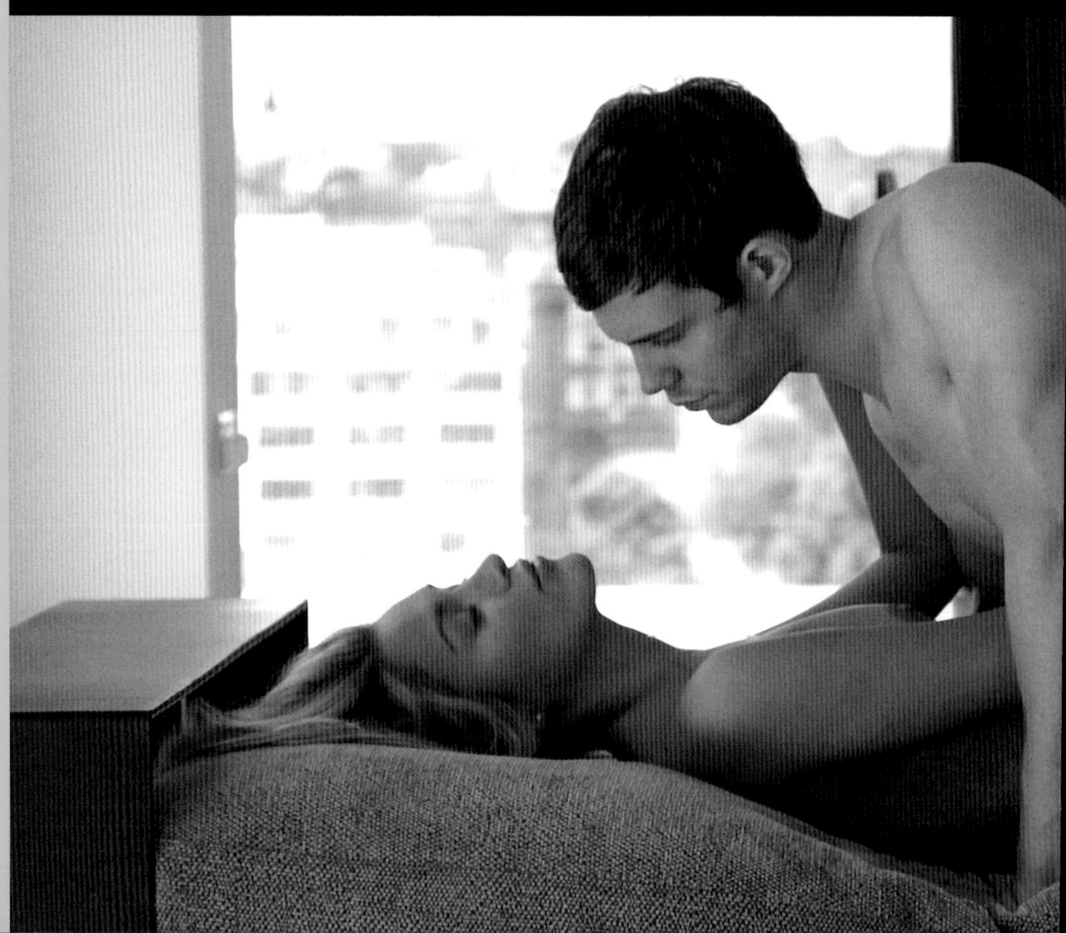

In the mood for dreamy, tender sex? Try these positions for lots of eye contact and for whispering sweet nothings.

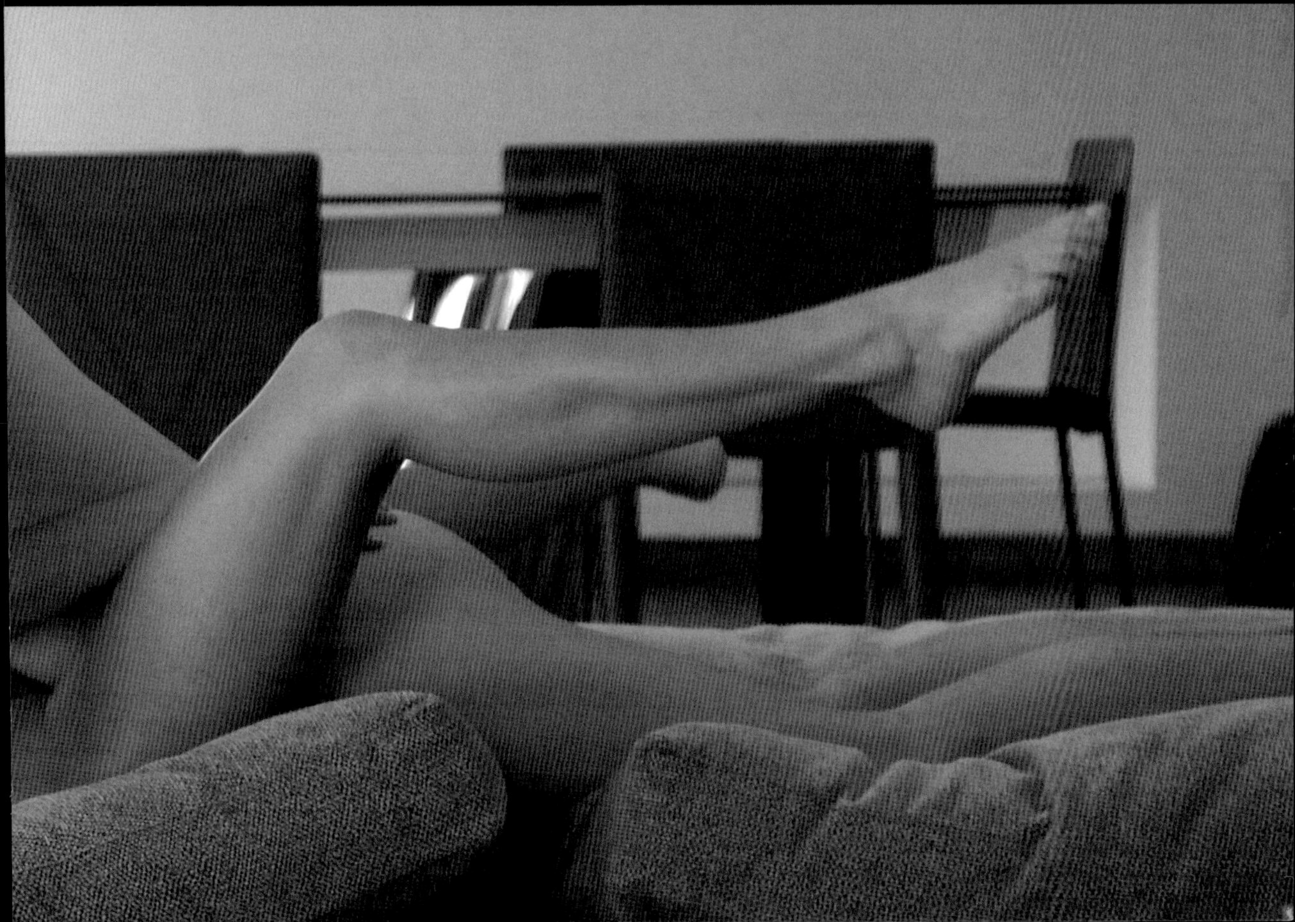

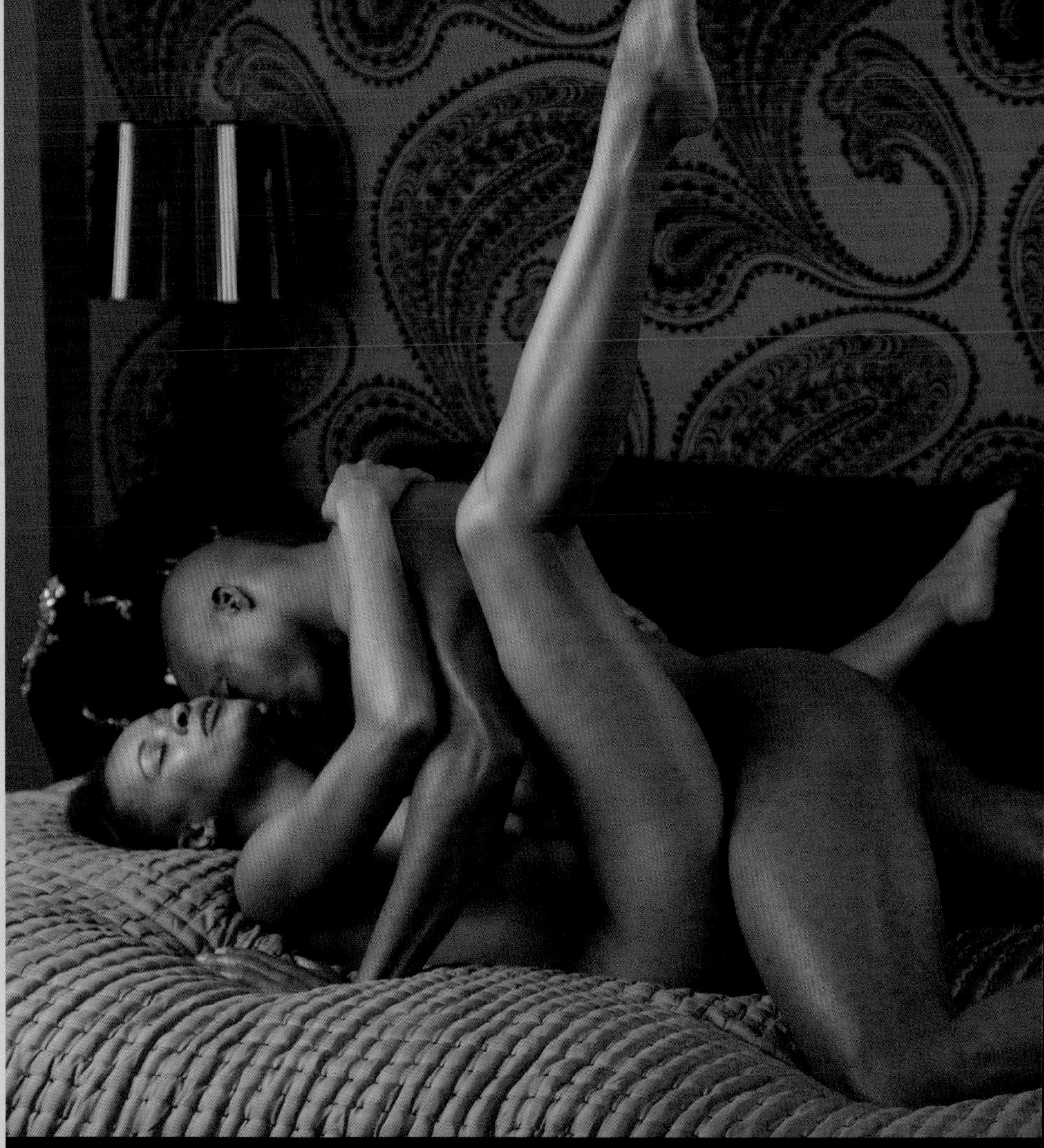

1 ballerina

She lies on her back and lifts her legs as high and as wide as possible—called "yawning" in the *Kama Sutra*. Try this position for profound penetration and to get a primitive buzz. It puts her in a vulnerable, submissive pose, while he looks all dominant and manly, leaning over her in a predatory fashion. Ballerina provides opportunities for lots of lovely face-to-face contact and kissing like teenagers, and makes the missionary position a tad more interesting.

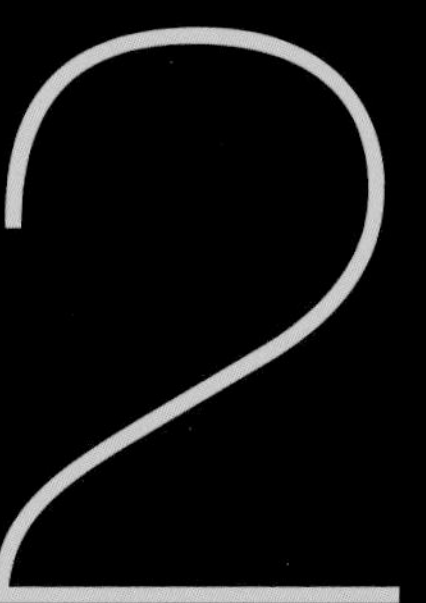

riding high

Move effortlessly from the elegant Ballerina position (see opposite) into a love triangle you'll enjoy, as she adjusts her legs to form a triangle shape. This allows him to position himself higher and penetrate more from the side, altering the stimulation so neither of you become desensitized. He's snuggled in more deeply, which feels more intimate. Even slightly repositioning the hips can make a huge difference in how intercourse feels for both of you, so alter your weight at regular intervals to keep stimulation fresh.

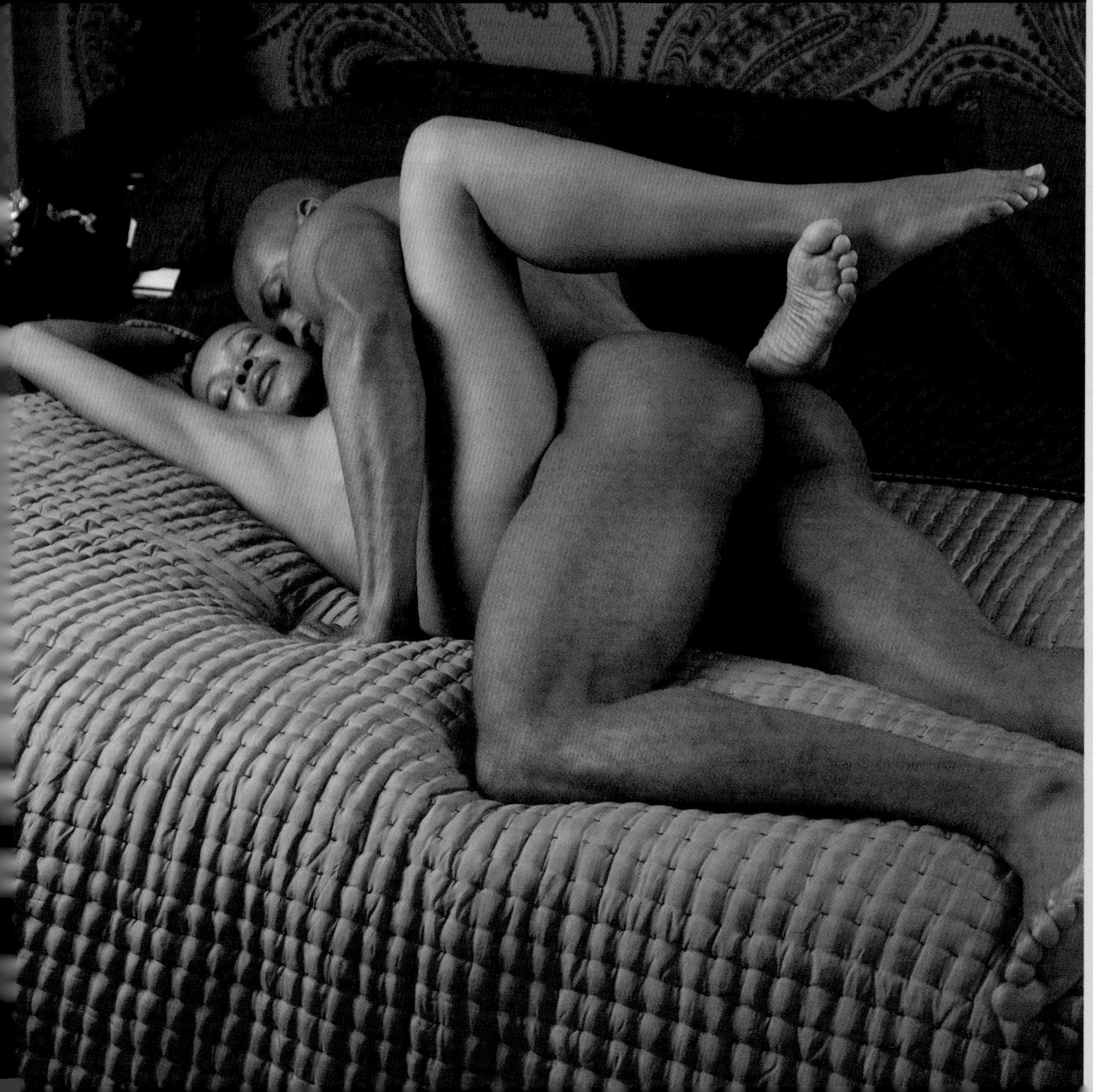

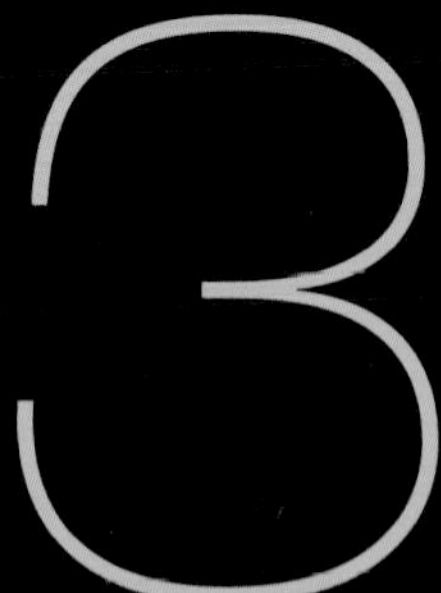

comfy sex

Face-to-face, intense eye contact, snuggled in each other's arms… this is more like an erotic cuddle than full-blown sex. Being side by side is a fantastic way to introduce a reluctant lover to spiritual sex, and this position is so easy to master.

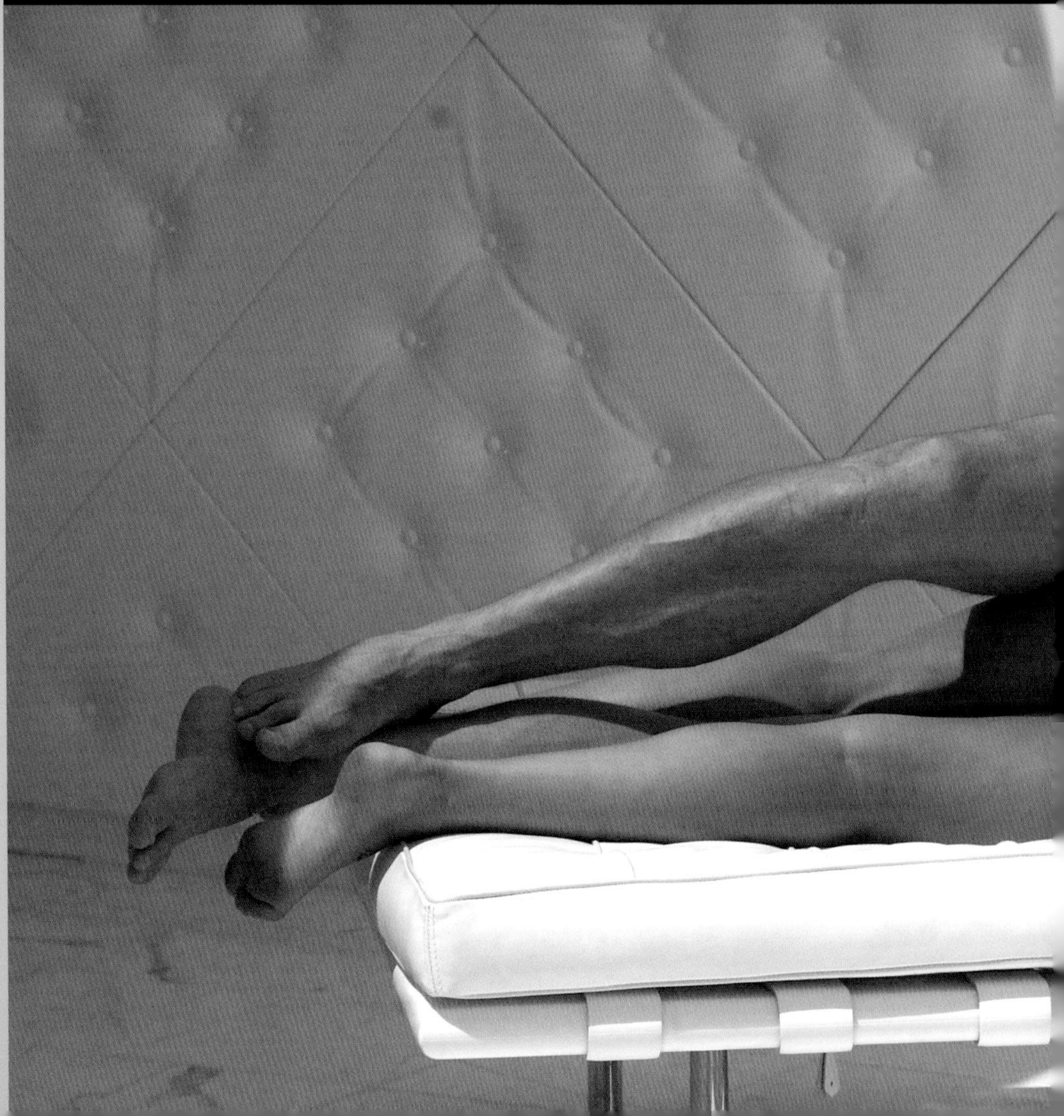

Start in the good old missionary position—him on top—then once he's penetrated, roll onto your sides, wrapping your arms around each other for support, his thigh straddling her hip. Don't attempt conventional thrusting here—instead, squeeze those pelvic floor muscles and enjoy more subtle thrusting movements. Her thighs are together, which makes her feel tantalizingly tight. And when you're done with the soulful stuff, this position is perfect for talking dirty face-to-face.

Side-by-side sex is perfect when you feel more languid than lusty. Had a rough day at the office? Or a three-course dinner that's left you feeling like cuddly, connective sex rather than ardent acrobatics? Positions like this are ridiculously easy to slip into—and surprisingly satisfying. (Enjoy the comfort while you can—I've got some interesting challenges ahead!)

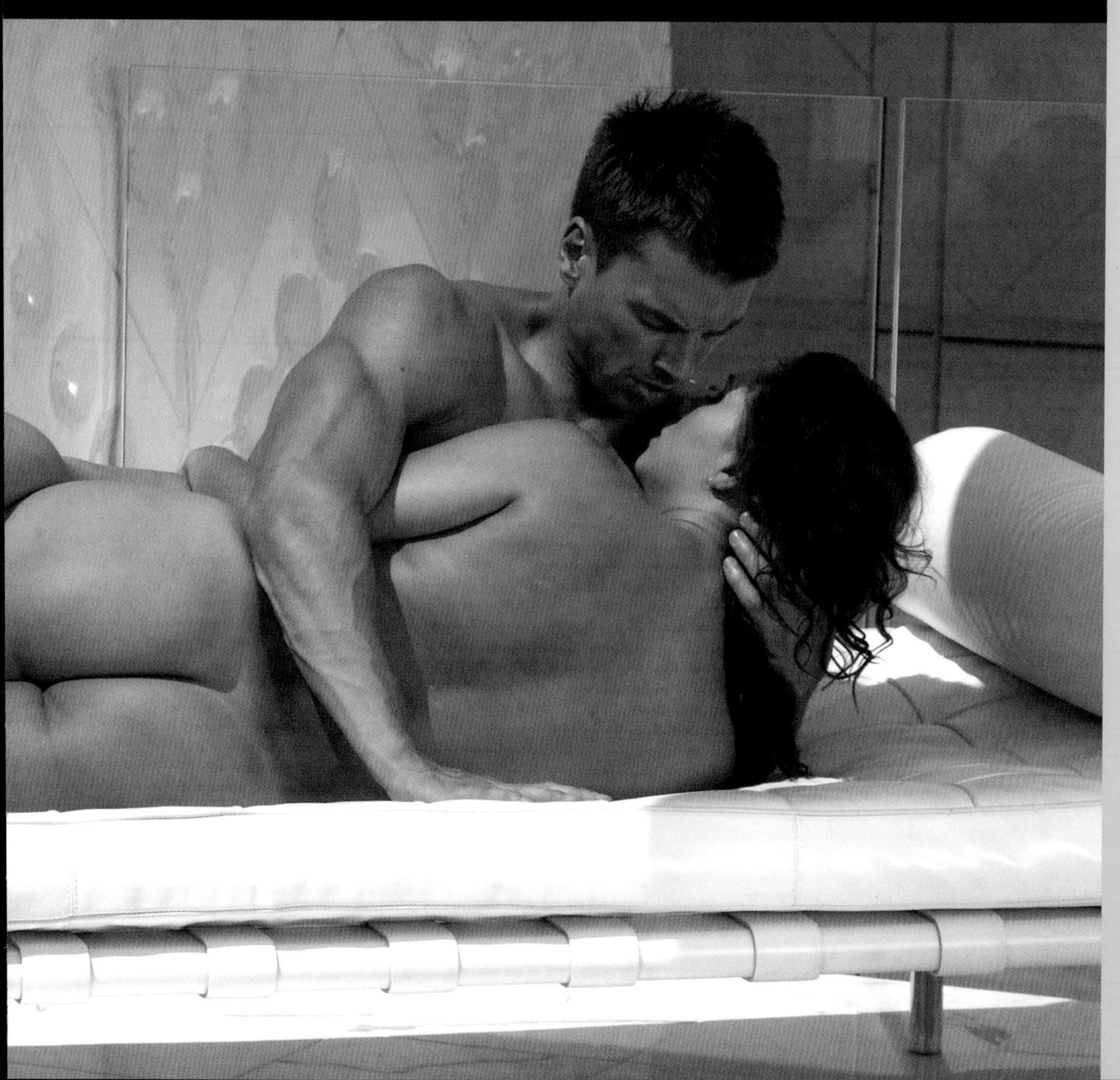

be a better boink

Don't believe the headline (it's a ploy to lure in the all-roads-lead-to-intercourse people), this is about everything BUT the boink. Want to have mind-blowing sex? It can't be done without memorable foreplay. Now, whether that involves dribbling cream all over her *derrière* or playing policewoman with the handcuffs, is up to you. But what it should do is whet your appetites, stimulate the senses, and give those stalled imaginations a bit of a jump-start.

touch Men, it's generally a good idea to start with her less sensitive parts. The genitals and other obvious hot spots get attention last, not first. Ask yourself "Where and how can I touch her in a way/place she's never been touched before?" Stand back so you can see her whole body. Then touch it slowly and reverently, like it's the very first time and it's something you never dreamed would be possible. Keep her at arm's length and let your eyes alternate between intense eye contact and gazing at the body part you're touching. Marvel at her body.

tease Girls, take him lingerie shopping and give him sneak previews as you're trying things on in the changing room. Then take him home, strip naked, take the shirt off his back and put it on yours, held together by one button only. Proceed to cook dinner, bending over a lot, while he chats to you. (Bet you burn the whole meal!)

Next time you undress for him, do it bit by bit. Slow everything down. Extend the torture by wearing sheer underwear: he can see the goods through the fabric but there's still a barrier between him and your flesh.

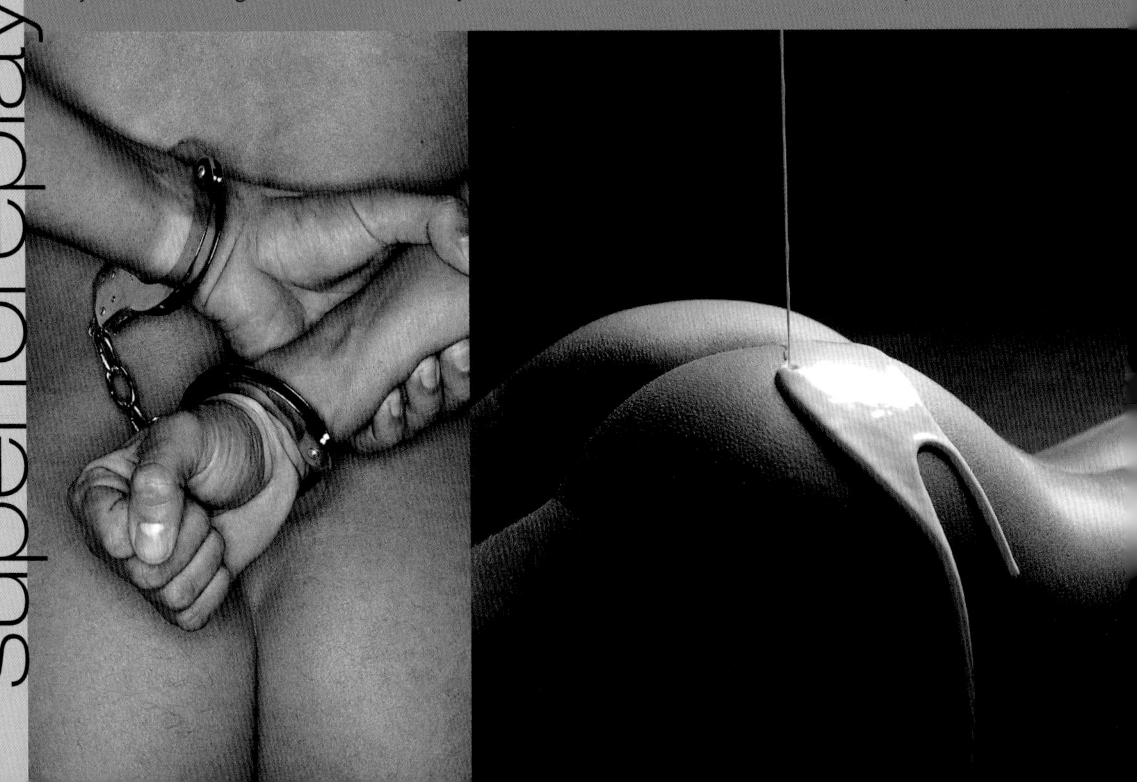

"Mind-blowing sex can't be had without memorable foreplay."

explore Stop seeing sex as a series of steps toward an end goal (intercourse/ orgasm). Stay focused on the here and now, not where you're going. Happiness is a means of traveling, and all that. Simple advice, but it'll make an extraordinary difference to satisfaction levels.

Vary the way she has orgasms by breaking out of the comfort zone. Most of us orgasm in the way that's easiest and ignore alternatives. She only orgasms through oral sex? Ban it for a month! Yes, she'll hate you. But not if you master other techniques. Her body will resist initially, but then respond with: "I'm not getting any tongue action here, so I might as well try to get used to his fingers instead." By varying her means to orgasm, you up the chances of her becoming multi-orgasmic.

excite Have phone sex during his lunch hour. Wait until the rest of the office steps out for a sandwich, then close your door and call him with creative carnal confessions.

Share a sexy food experience. Eat phallic-shaped foods (cucumbers, carrots) suggestively in front of him. Dip and smear the spreadable variety (chocolate mousse, cream, honey) all over his nipples, penis, and testicles. Try licking them off by running your tongue in a figure eight around his testicles.

play Jump on her just as you're both about to rush out the door, late for a party/ your mom's for dinner. Pause, with your hand on the doorknob, let your eyes travel over her body and say, "Does it matter if we're three minutes late?" Putting a time limit on things ups the tension and makes everything urgent. In all the right ways.

Break the routine. Do the opposite of what you did the last time you had sex. It was in the morning? Then do it at night. In the bedroom? Try the kitchen. You did it in missionary position? Tonight it's rear entry.

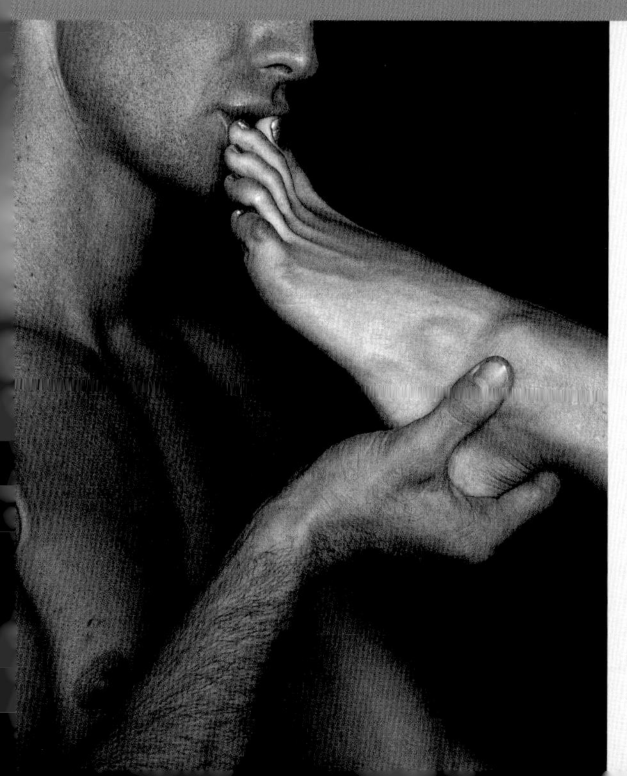

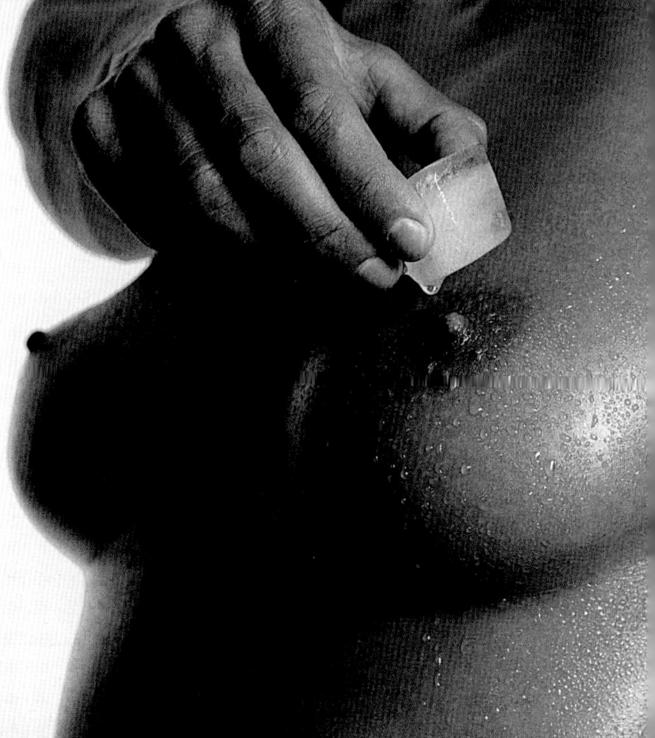

cocoon

1 Simply hug, breathing in unison and appreciating each other. This is a gentle "let's connect on a spiritual level" position, but you can heat things up through some sexy kissing and touching. Stay in the moment though, for a few minutes at least, before moving on to step two.

2 He kneels, she climbs on top, continuing to cuddle. He's now inside her, but there's no thrusting just yet! This is all about merging as one, so you both feel "cocooned" in your love for each other. Sappy, yes, but come on—there's penetration involved, so it's not that sappy! Stay still, be patient, and try your damnedest to stay in the moment. Yes, you can.

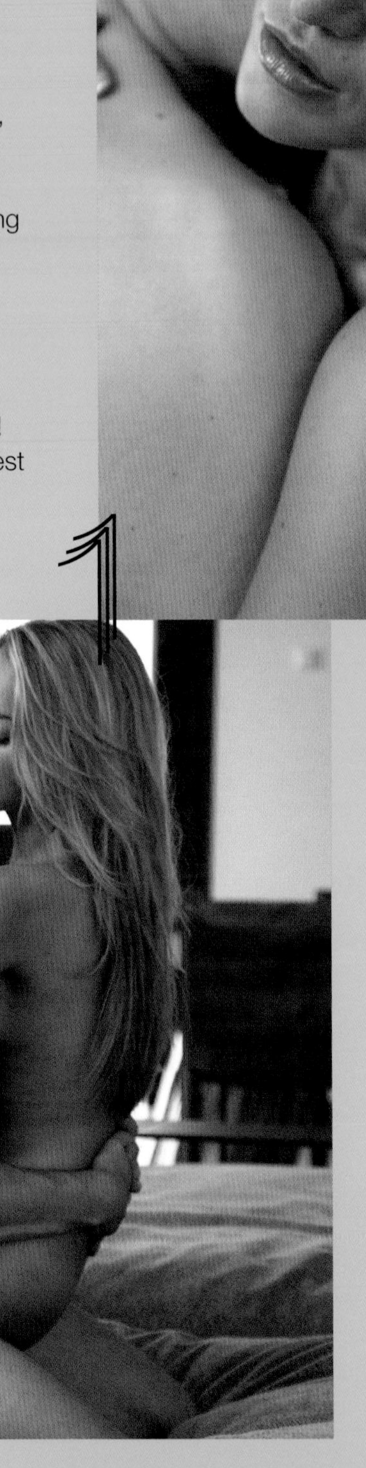

4

3 OK, now we're into the real action… She leans back and hangs on to his neck for support as he begins moving her back and forth to create some much-longed-for friction. Move in close again if you want to make out some more (and who doesn't?).

3

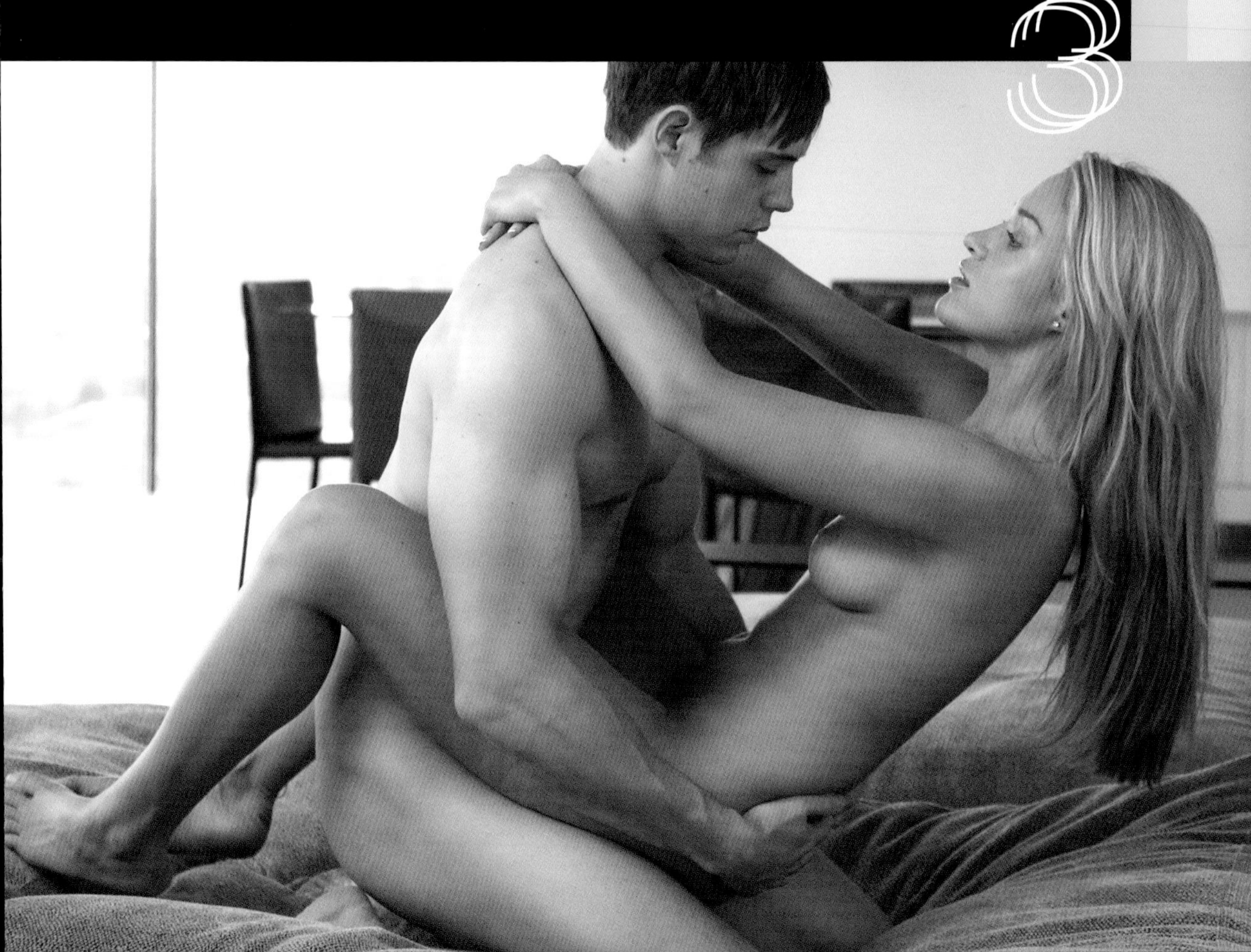

nice and tight

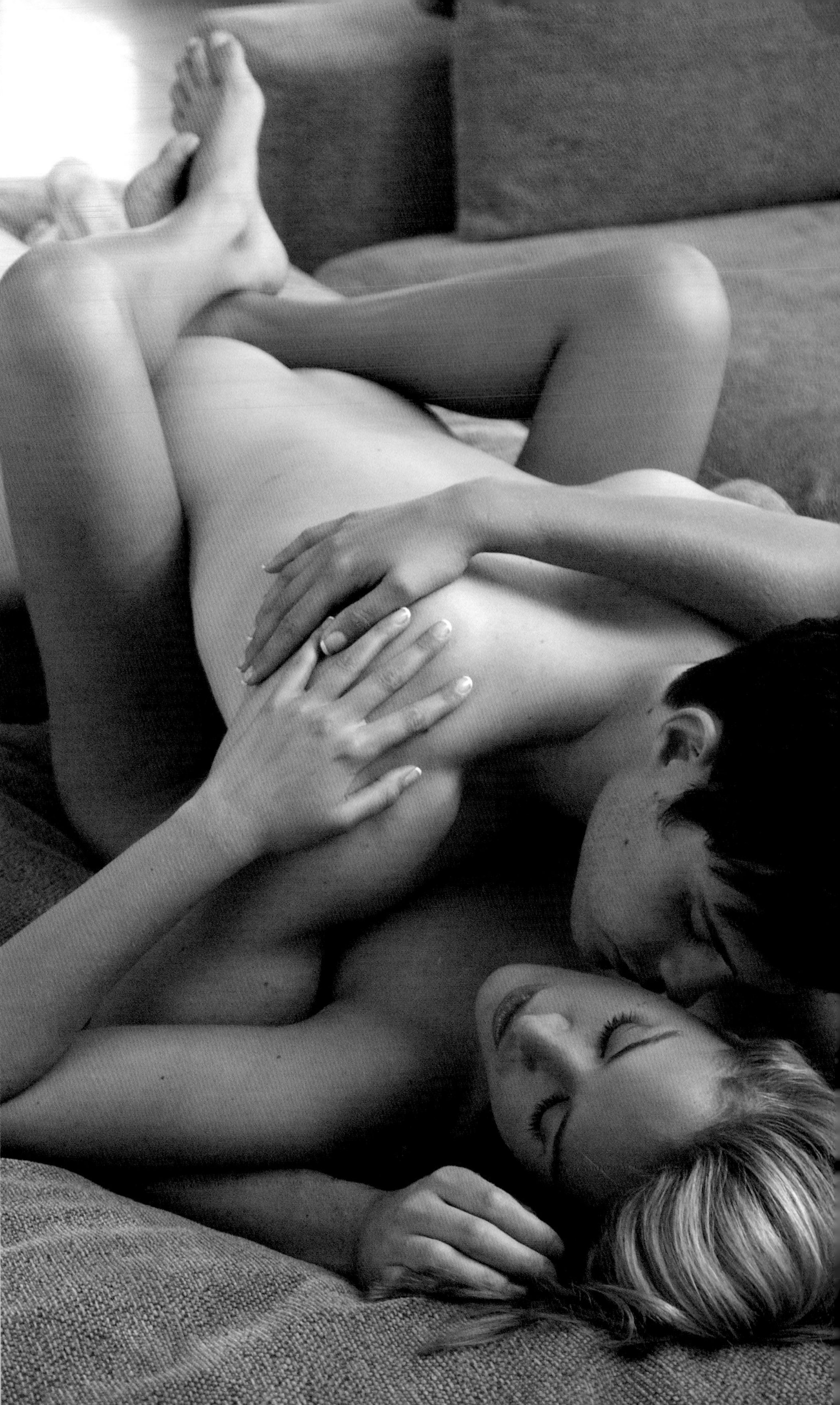

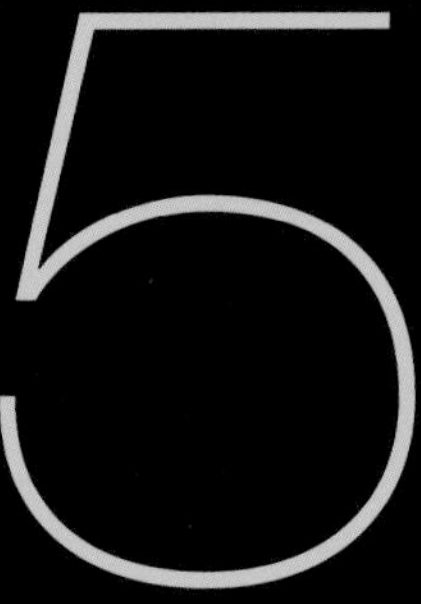

pressing

You both start in the standard missionary position, she then bends her legs and presses her thighs around his body. This one's all about the action of gripping with the thighs—rather than just wrapping them around him—which has the effect of tightening both her vaginal and pelvic muscles. It's easily done by resting her calves on his lower back, ankles crossed, but it also works with her feet flat on the bed. If her thigh muscles tire, she can squeeze and release her pelvic-floor muscles instead, "milking" his penis internally. It's a totally different sensation, since his penis is being squeezed rather than "pulled" up and down.

erection fix-its

The myth that says you'll always get an erection, on cue, and ejaculate the second you want to also says men get an erection at the start of sex and maintain a level of hardness all the way through. Bull!

keep calm, carry on

* Lost your erection? You don't stay at exactly the same level of excitement during a session, so it's logical your penis won't either. Don't panic when it happens. Instead, take a break, pleasure her to take the pressure off, and calm down. Then start again, focusing on the sensations you're feeling rather than how hard you are.
* Semi-erect? You don't have to be hard to have intercourse, even if the "putting it in" part is now referred to as (a rather undignified) "stuffing." Use lube and get in a side-by-side position. Get her to push the head of your penis inside her—the base naturally follows. Once you're inside, resist the urge to pump furiously. Simply stay inside, get her to clench and release her vaginal muscles, and you do the same with your PC (pubococcygeus) muscle. Focus on how it feels, relax, then start to thrust gently.

sneaky penis tricks

* Trim your pubes—your penis will look bigger and she'll find giving you oral easier.
* To last longer, put on a condom to reduce sensation or masturbate before the session.
* Hate condoms because you lose your erection? Try wearing a larger, thinner one with a vibrating penis ring to hold it in place.

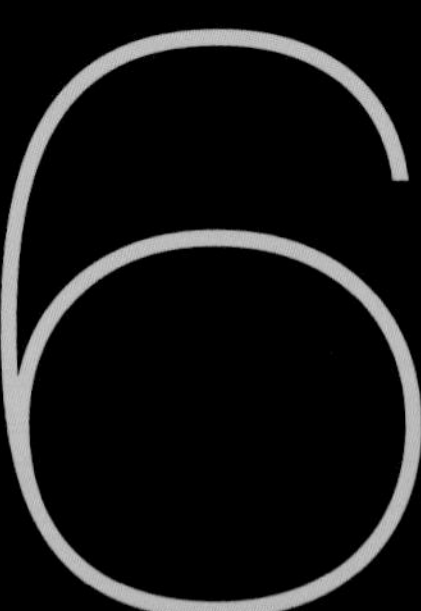

the chameleon

This is a gloriously sexy position that's both lusty and languorous, comfy and erotic—in short, it checks a lot of boxes for not that much effort on anyone's part! It's easy to do. He lies on his side; she lifts both her legs over his and wiggles around a bit to allow him to penetrate (or, if it's easier, he penetrates first, then she swings her legs over once he's inside).

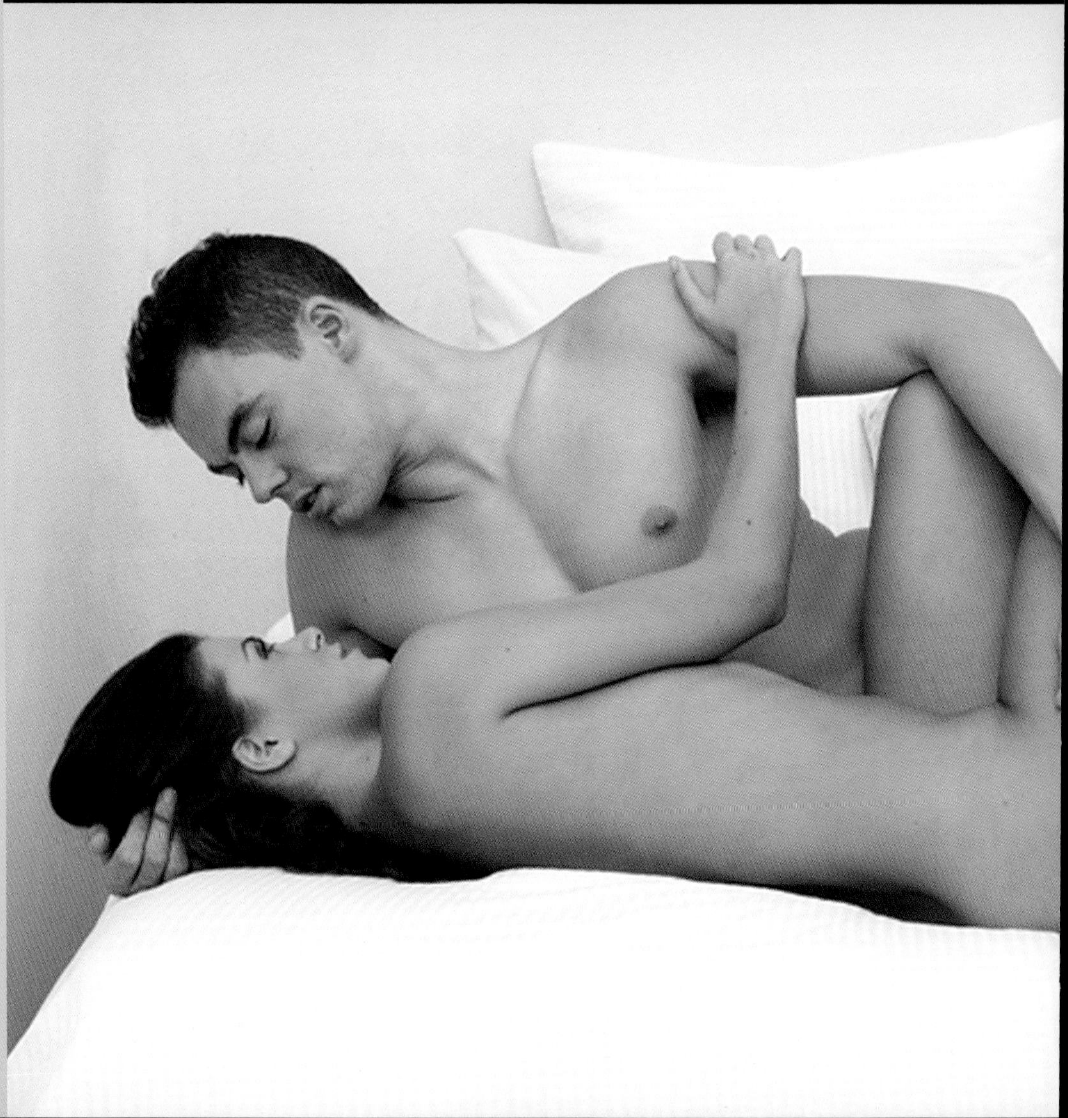

Then it's up to the two of you how energetic you want to be. This suits a slow, gentle style of thrusting for sweet sex, or, equally, he can take a firm hold of her buttocks and turn it into a feistier, smuttier session. As with all side-by-side positions, it works better if he's got a long penis—too short and it easily slips out. To mix things up a bit, alter the angle of her vagina and make him feel more tightly gripped by getting him to lift her legs higher.

The traditional name for this one is "Two Fishes" because the position imitates a pair of spawning fish bending their tails around each other. This will either titillate you or bore you silly, depending on how cuddly or carnal the two of you are feeling. Either way, try it—it's fab!

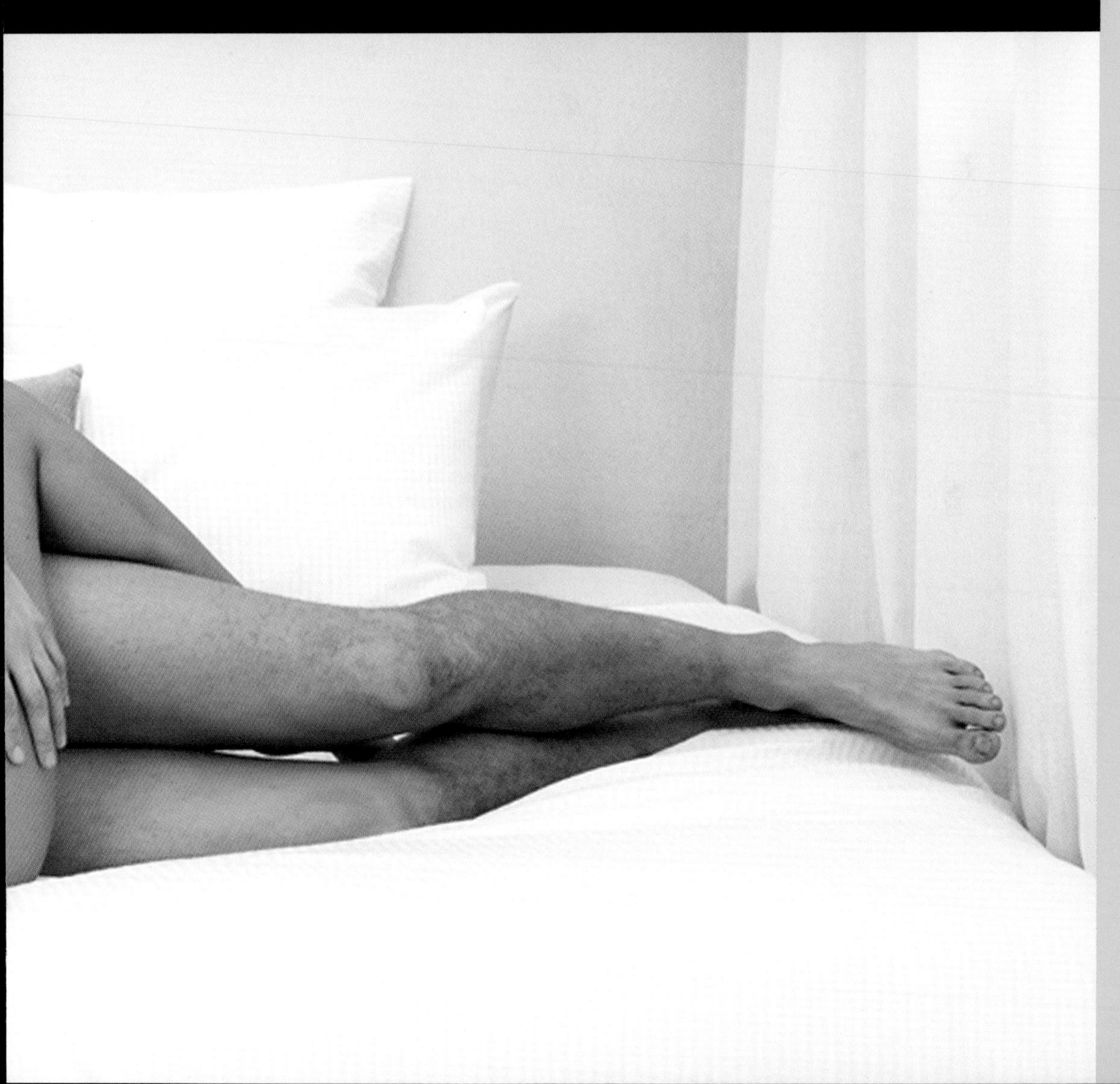

rock 'n' ride

1 He kneels with his legs tucked beneath him. She climbs on top, positioning herself high on his thighs so she's riding him. Both hug closely for balance and to keep him penetrated. She can experiment by moving higher or lower on his thighs until she hits the most sensitive spot on her vaginal wall. She's got several? Well who's a lucky girl, then?

1

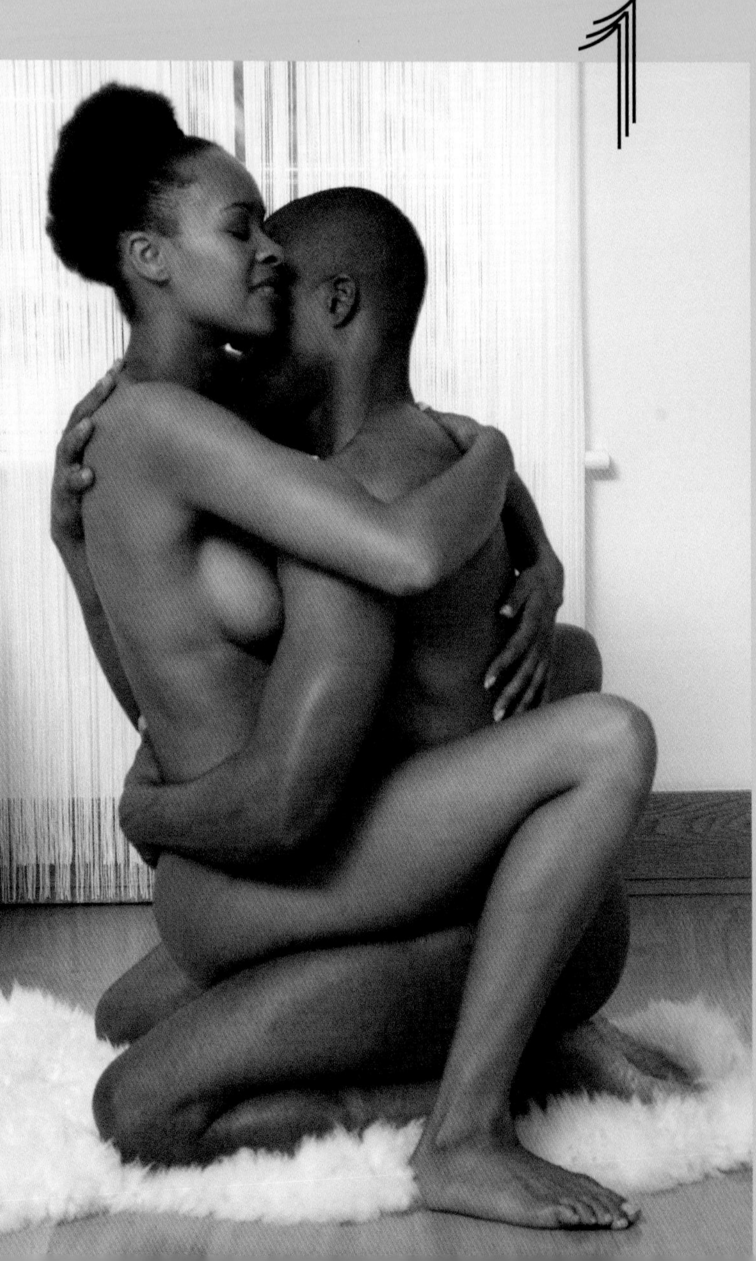

2 Move into a rocking motion to set off a subtle but exquisitely effective thrusting sensation. Her feet are flat on the floor, giving her something to push against. He lifts up with his thighs. It's way easier if he keeps his back erect and his stomach muscles turned on. (Yes, you can skip the gym tomorrow.) It's easy for her to keep him hard by squeezing her pelvic-floor muscles.

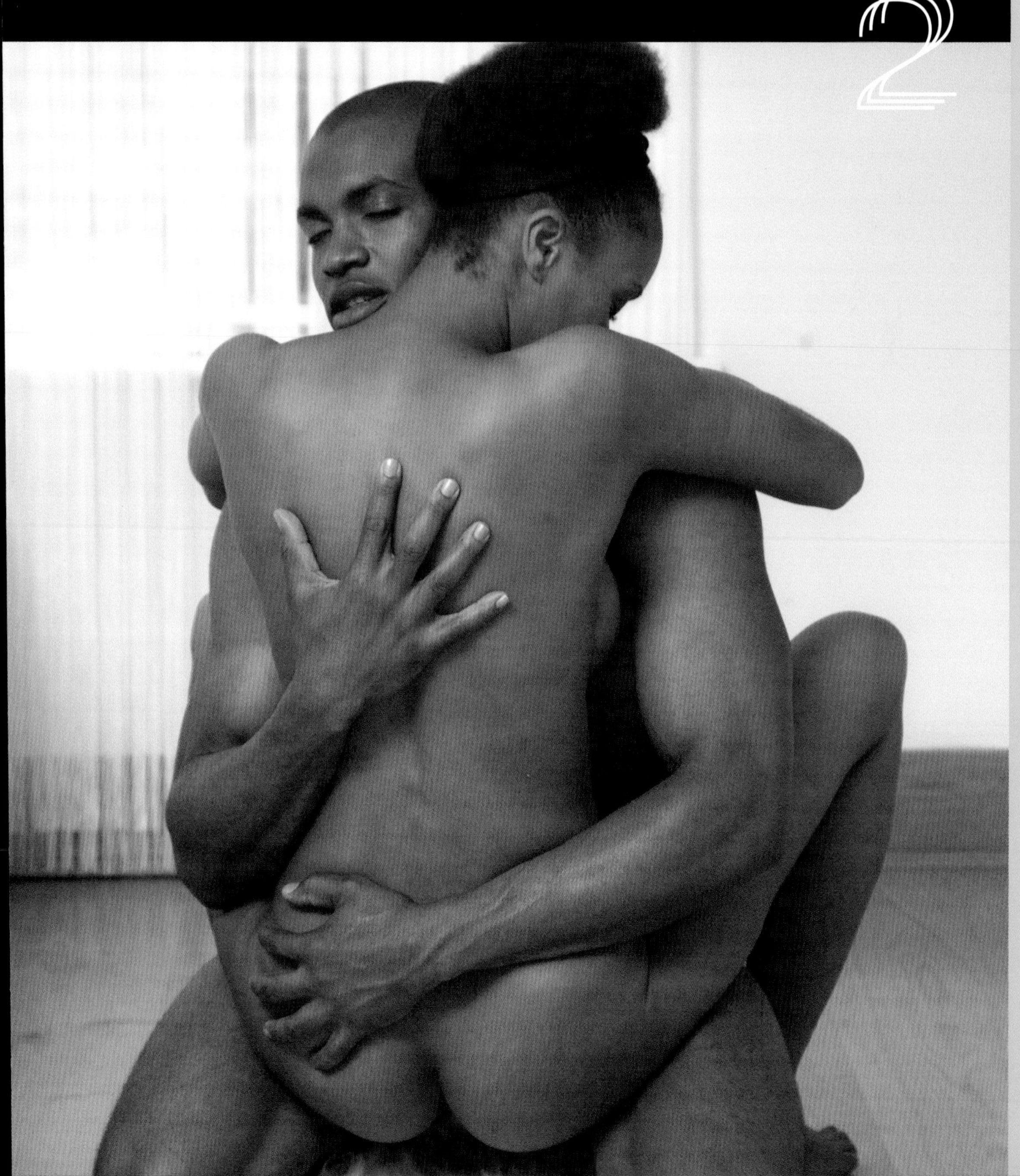

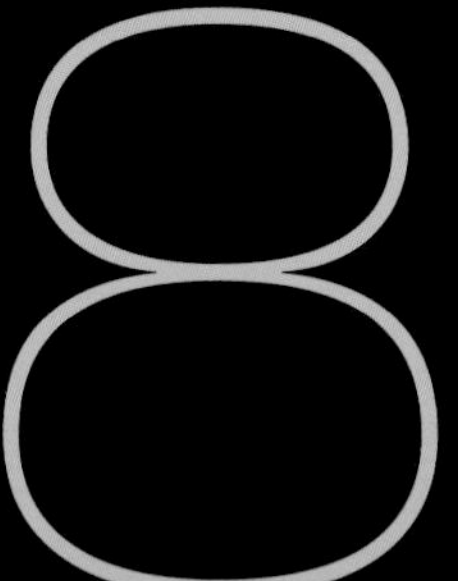

horizontal dancing

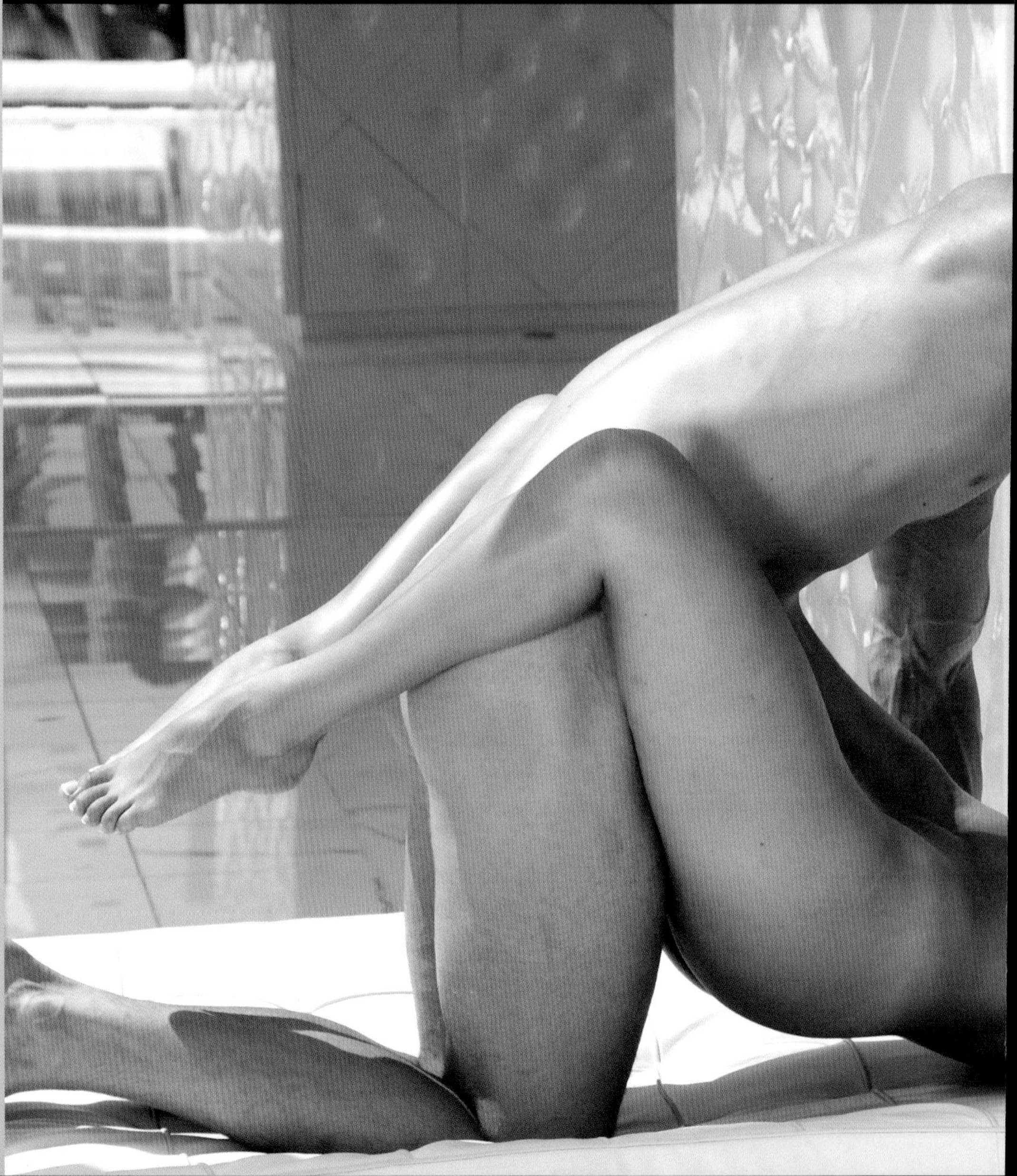

One question before we start: do you dance well together? If the answer is no, it's probably best you skip this because it's all about couple coordination. She lies back, legs parted, and grips the headboard with one hand. He kneels between her legs and penetrates, she grips her legs around his hips and allows herself to be pulled upward as he leans forward to also hold on to the

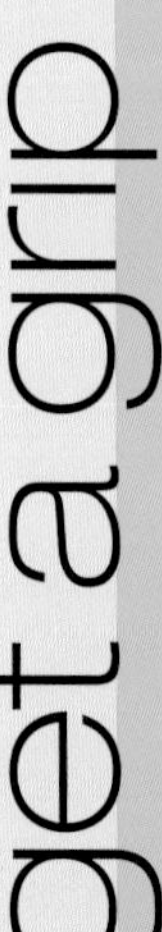

as he leans forward to also hold on to the headboard. You then move in a seesaw motion, using your hands to pull and push against the bedhead. Finding it all a bit too much like hard work? Cheat by putting two firm pillows underneath her bottom, or try it with her holding on to the headboard with both hands, while he takes a firm hold of her bottom.

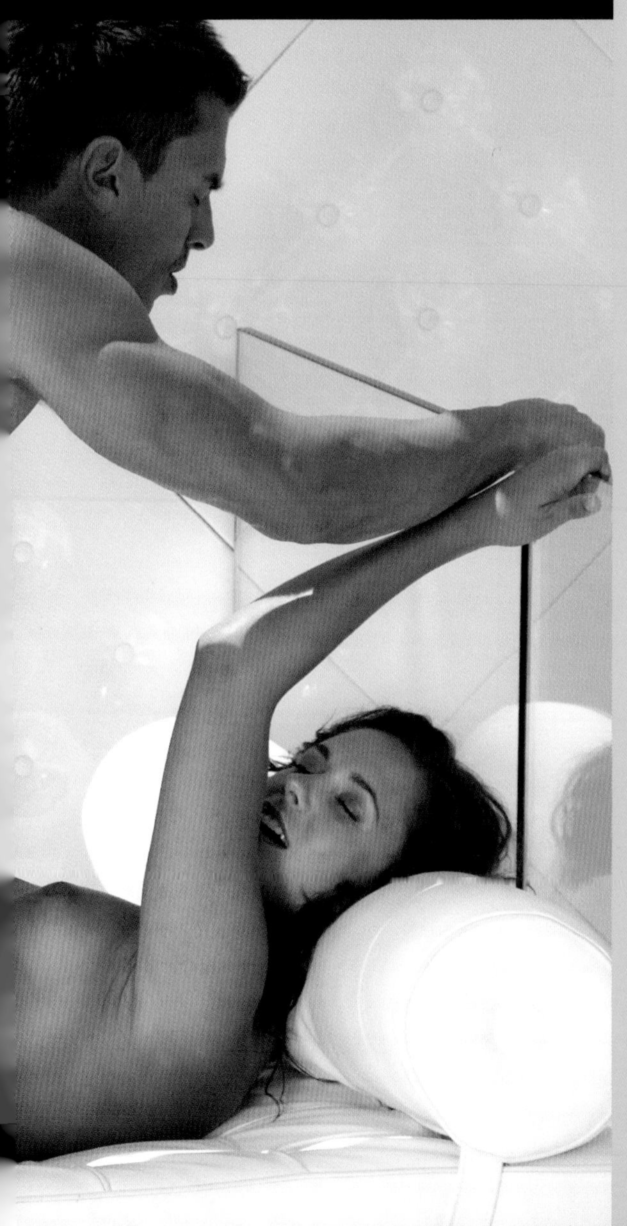

dirty talk

Talking dirty is so easy in the beginning. It's later, when you're friends, that talking dirty starts to feel wrong. Incestuous. You're not alone—it's normal to feel more embarrassed talking dirty as time goes on, rather than the reverse. Easily fixed though!

set the ground rules

* What kind of language do you want to use? Set limits if one of you doesn't like slang or swear words.
* Good discussion points: When should you do it? Just before orgasm or to get you in the mood? What sort of themes (you're a slut, virgin, goddess, etc.)? Do you want them to do it to you but for you not to have to answer? Do you want to take turns?
* What about talk that involves other people? Some people love pretending their partner's "sleeping" with someone else, others get all jealous, which destroys the mood in two minutes flat.

what to say

* Describe what they're doing to you—"You've got your hands on my breasts"—then add what that makes you feel, "... and it feels wonderful."
* Describe what you're doing or are about to do—"I'm going to take your penis in my mouth and suck it"—then add what that makes you feel, "... and it makes me feel powerful. Like you're in my control."
* Read out something sexy from a book or a magazine while your partner works on you with their fingers or tongue.

supersecret sex spots

Take a magical mystery tour to find supersecret sex spots you never dreamed existed. This is the quintessential kiss, lick, stroke, and nibble guide to touching naked flesh. Get to know their body even better than they do as you take a guided tour of their hottest sex spots.

his...

chest Not only does it make the perfect pillow to snuggle up on, but his chest also responds nicely to fingertip touches and strokes with your hand and tongue. If you've got long hair, use the ends of it to tickle him. Trail your fingertips up and down the sides of his torso, then brush your entire palm across his chest, ever so gently. Alternate with fingertip tickles, then (and only then) tweak his nipples between the thumb and third finger before more licks and light nibbles.

stomach His tummy is packed with pleasure points, particularly from his belly-button to his pubic bone. Follow that lovely trail of hair downward, stroking lightly with fingertips or tongue.

hips The V-shape that's formed from his groin to his hip bones is a favorite with lots of us girlies because it points to the number one body part. Which is why it's such a tease to trace it with fingers or tongue on the final run to home base. The hips are one of the most overtly erotic body parts, with jutting bones making subconscious allusions to his erection.

thigh The crease where his torso meets the front of the thigh is a hot zone. Use your tongue to lick upward until you hit the base of the penis where you... suddenly stop. Switch to kissing, licking, and nibbling your way up the outside of his thighs, then show mercy by doing the same on the inside.

buttocks The part where the top of his thighs meet his bottom doesn't just look good, it's extremely sensitive and a great tease zone because if you moved your fingers or tongue a fraction of an inch, you'd hit the perineum or scrotum. Use a light tickle on his buttocks to start, then move into a firm, circular, kneading motion. If you really want to make his day, lightly spank.

testicles Be gentle—the sensitivity that makes his testicles susceptible to pleasure makes them vulnerable to pain. Another ouch—moving both testicles in opposite directions. Instead, hold them between your fingers and thumb and roll gently, slowly, and lightly, using the pads of your fingertips.

penis Squeeze lubricant into your palms, rub them together until it heats up, then make a fist and grasp his penis firmly before sliding it up and down the shaft, closing your fist as you go up and over the head.

her...

face Facial stroking feels exquisite and, combined with lots of eye contact (and details of how you're going to pleasure her), is a shortcut to sexual arousal and intimacy.

lips Don't waste the erotic potential of this hot zone by planting a kiss smack-center with tongues flying. Instead, nibble, kiss, and lick the upper and lower lip separately. Plant little kisses around the edges of her mouth, and then move in for some nice, long, sexy kisses.

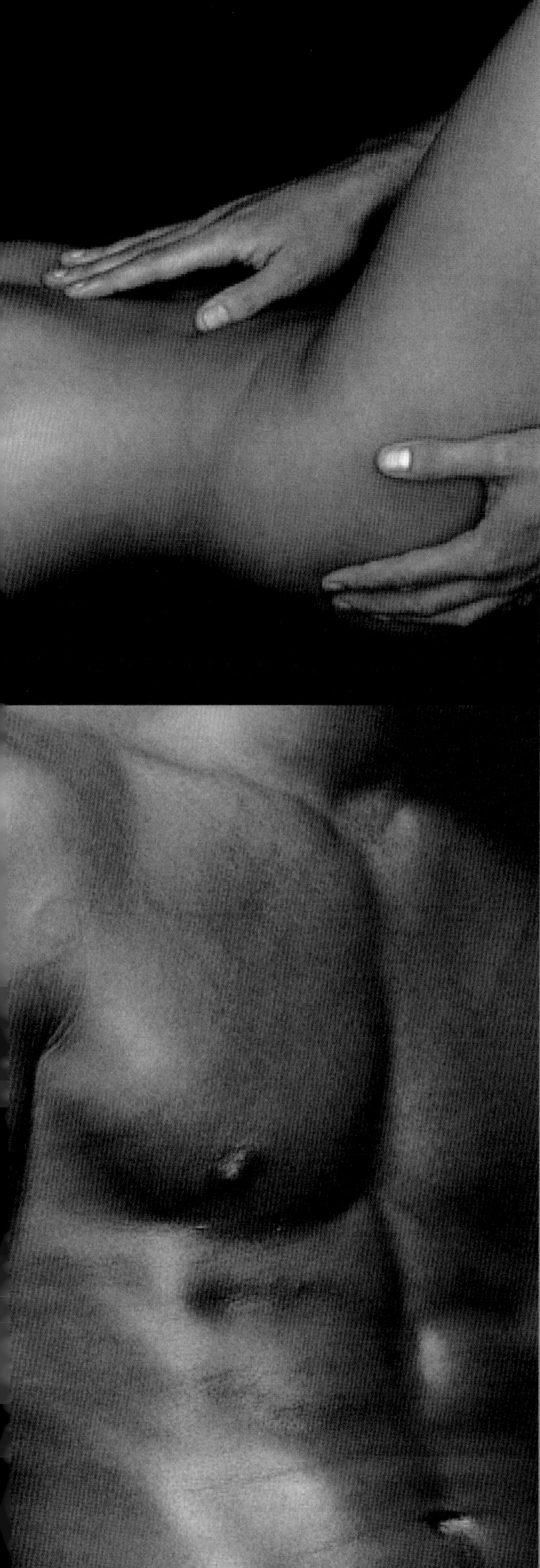

"Keep clitoral stimulation light, wet, rhythmic, and indirect."

neck There's something ever so sexy about being licked and nibbled in such a vulnerable spot. Start gently, then change the pressure from feathery to firm, and add in a few experimental "nips." If that gets a moan, she might well want you to bite!

breasts Stroke underneath her nipples, using your tongue, fingers, lips, and the tip of your erect penis as tools to tantalize. Try swirling your fingers over her breast without touching the nipples at all. Combine breast-stroking with rubbing her clitoris to zap her to a place she's never been before.

stomach Rub her lower abdomen, just above the pubic bone, as she's about to climax and see her face register an orgasm that shoots right off the raunch-Richter scale. Plant your hands on her lower abdomen and slide them slowly backward and forward, moving in opposite directions.

clitoris Most of you know we have one, but plenty of men still aren't quite sure what to do with it. As a general rule, keep all clitoral stimulation light, wet, rhythmic, and indirect (better to circle slowly around it than press it like an elevator button).

vagina The whole front wall of the vagina (the side nearest her tummy) is wondrously sensitive. See if you can find an area that feels like the outer skin of a kiwi fruit—that's the G-spot. Insert a finger and crook it to make a beckoning motion. Initial G-spot stimulation might feel weird to her—as if she's about to go to the bathroom. Get her to grit her teeth and wait 10 seconds—the payoff is worth it.

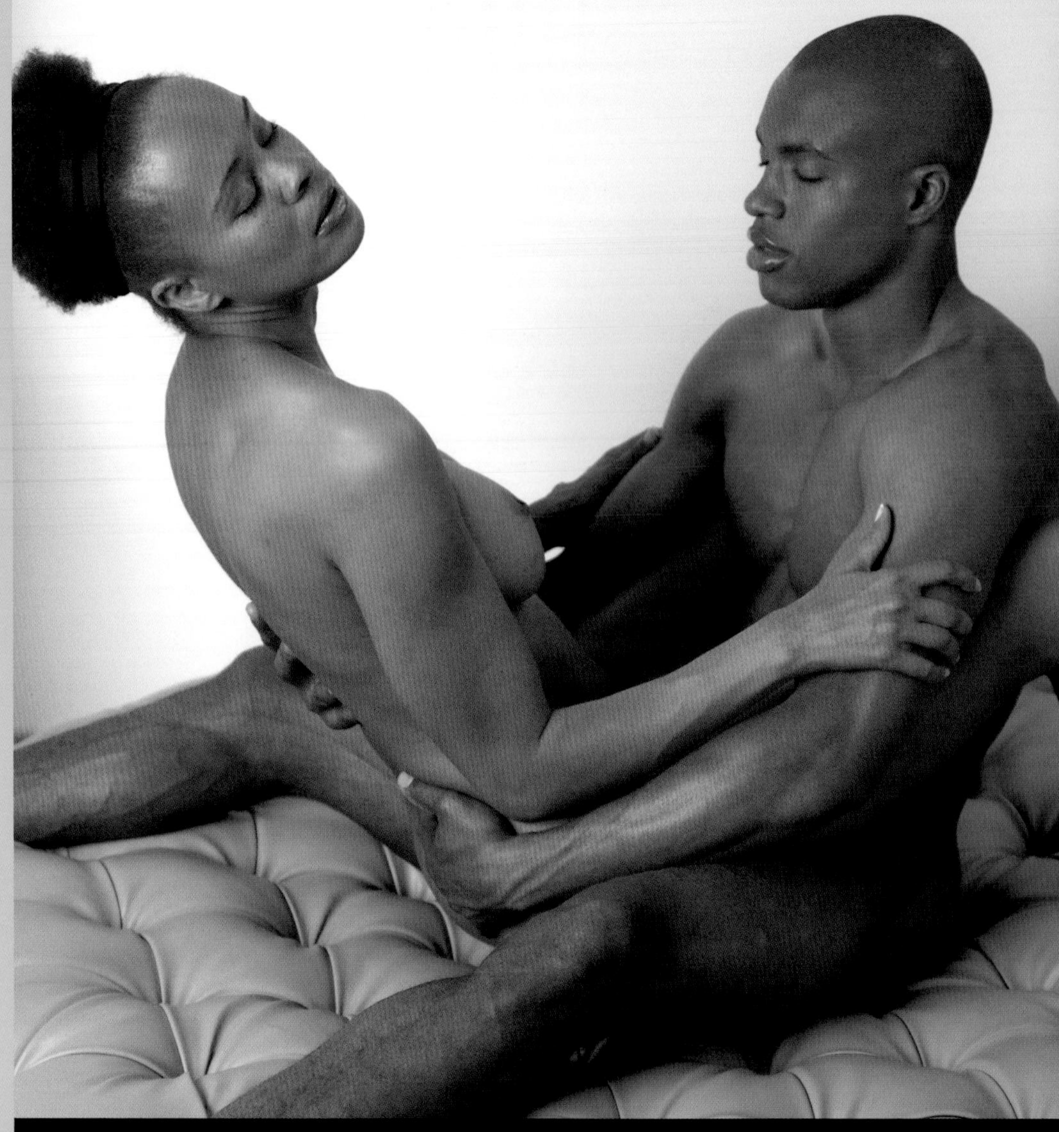

9

sexy seesaw

He sits with his legs extended and apart. She lowers herself on top, allowing him to penetrate, before sitting on his lap. She clasps his upper arms; he supports her back. This pose isn't actually intended to provide an orgasm for each of you, but instead offer a relaxing way to simply enjoy being sexually linked. It's all about appreciating each sexual feeling for its own value, rather than thinking that all roads lead to intercourse. (Bet you can't do it without wiggling!)

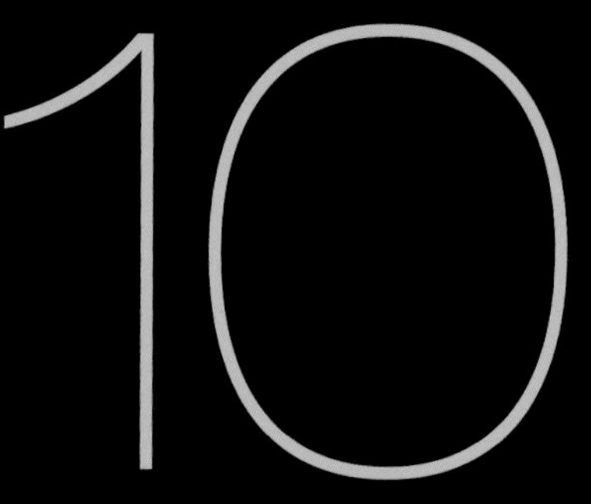

lazy days

Erotic but laid-back, with lots of sensual snuggling, positions like this suit days when you're aroused and interested but not frothing at the mouth for sex. There's lots of skin-to-skin contact and your hands are free to roam. This is a good one for grinding against each other without using the traditional in-and-out thrust. The theory behind trying a variety of positions—even if there are only extremely subtle differences—is to allow you to try a different thrusting style.

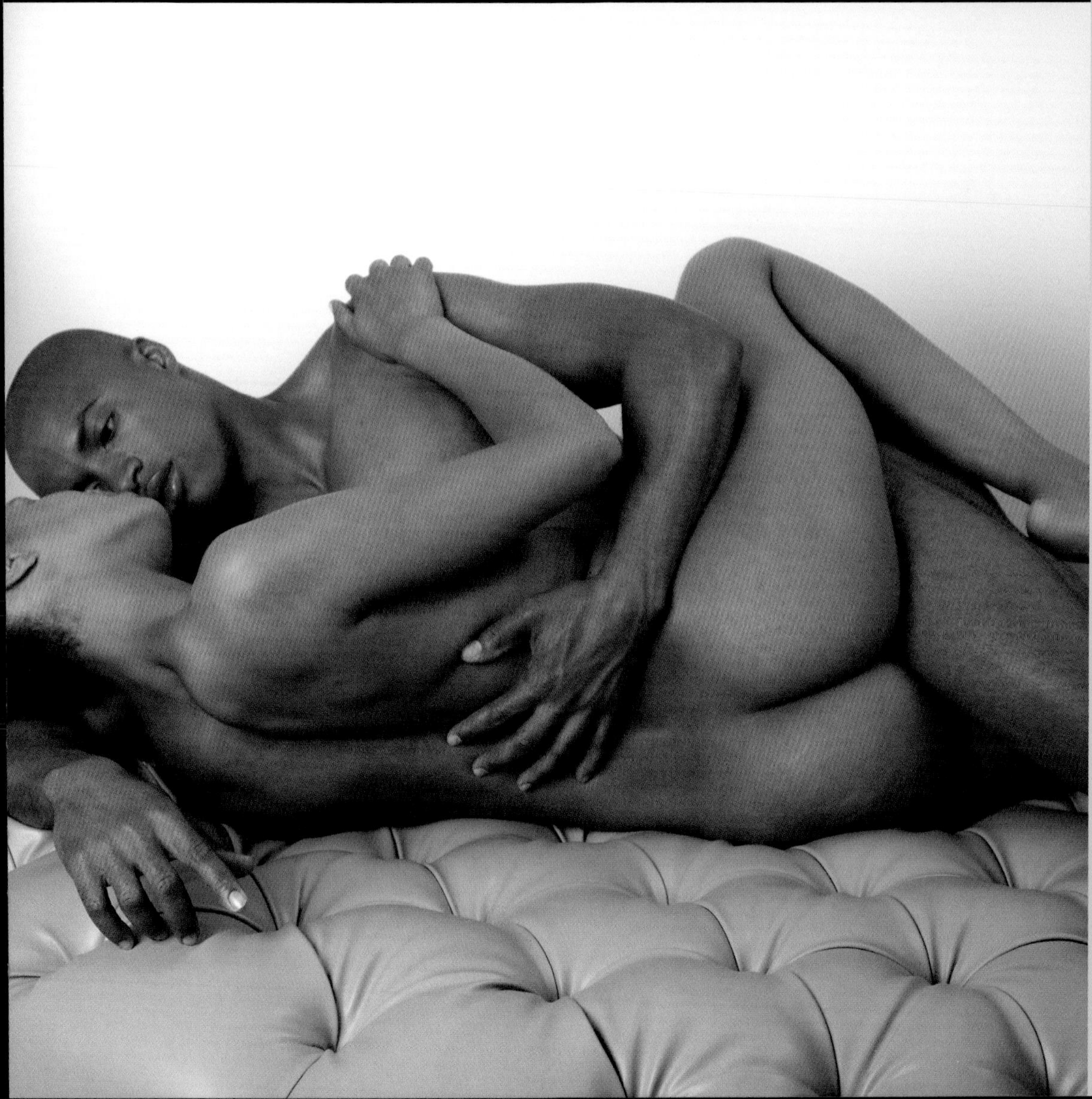

11 the ankle cross

This is a good one if his penis is on the small side: any position where she keeps her thighs pressed together rather than spread keeps her tight and creates friction. Crossing her ankles keeps her thighs in place during thrusting. Penetration is shallow—which has benefits for both of you. The first third of the vagina has the most nerve endings and, since it's the narrowest part of the canal, it guarantees him the tightest fit.

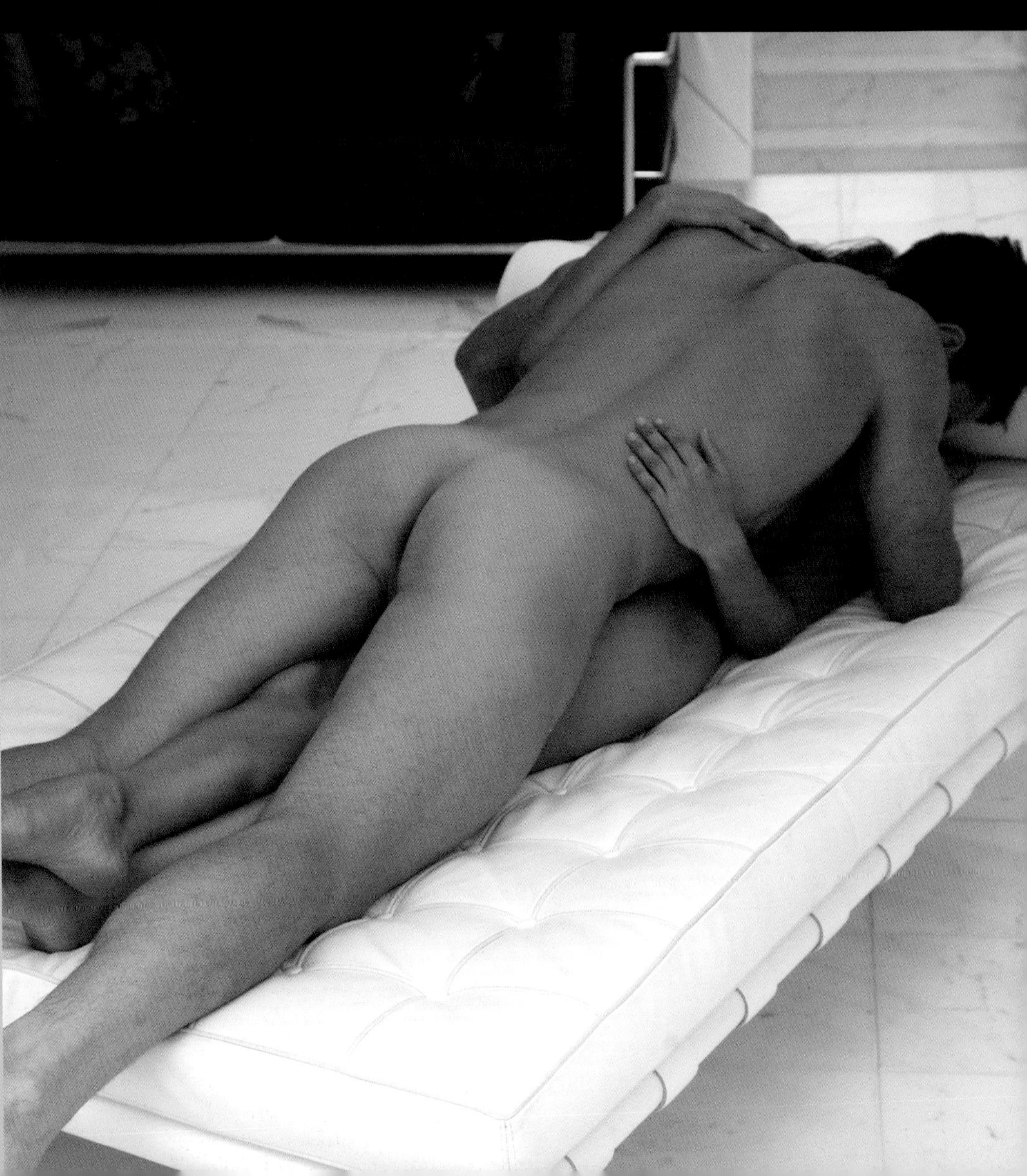

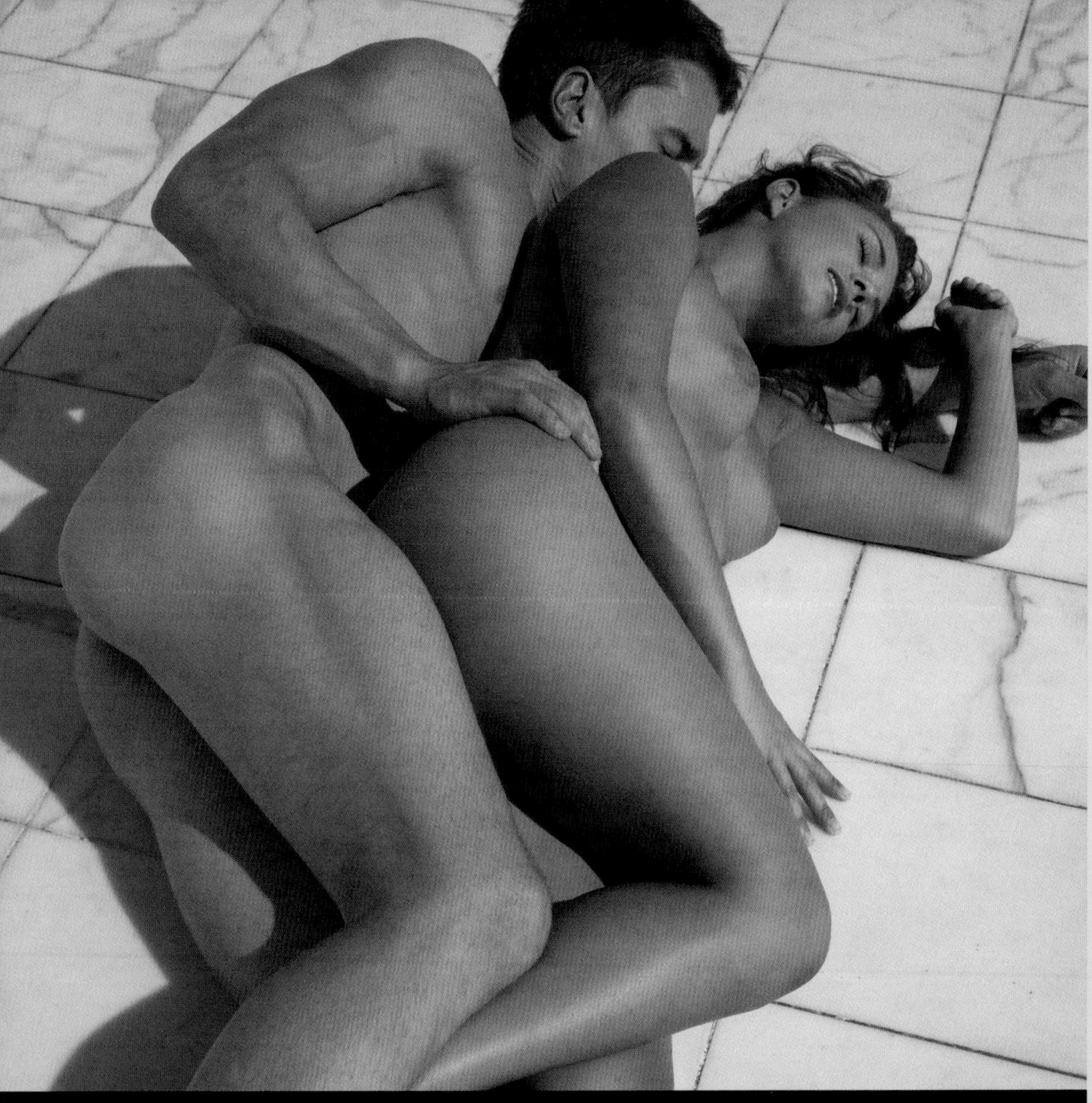

12 the weekender

Perfect for half-asleep-hungover Sunday morning sex, or post-boozy Sunday lunch sessions! This position is remarkably intimate, even though you're both facing in the same direction, because there's full body contact. He penetrates from behind, and she lifts her bottom and/or uses her hands to help him. He can kiss or bite her neck, easily reaching around to craftily play with her breasts or clitoris. It's a great position, too, if she's pregnant.

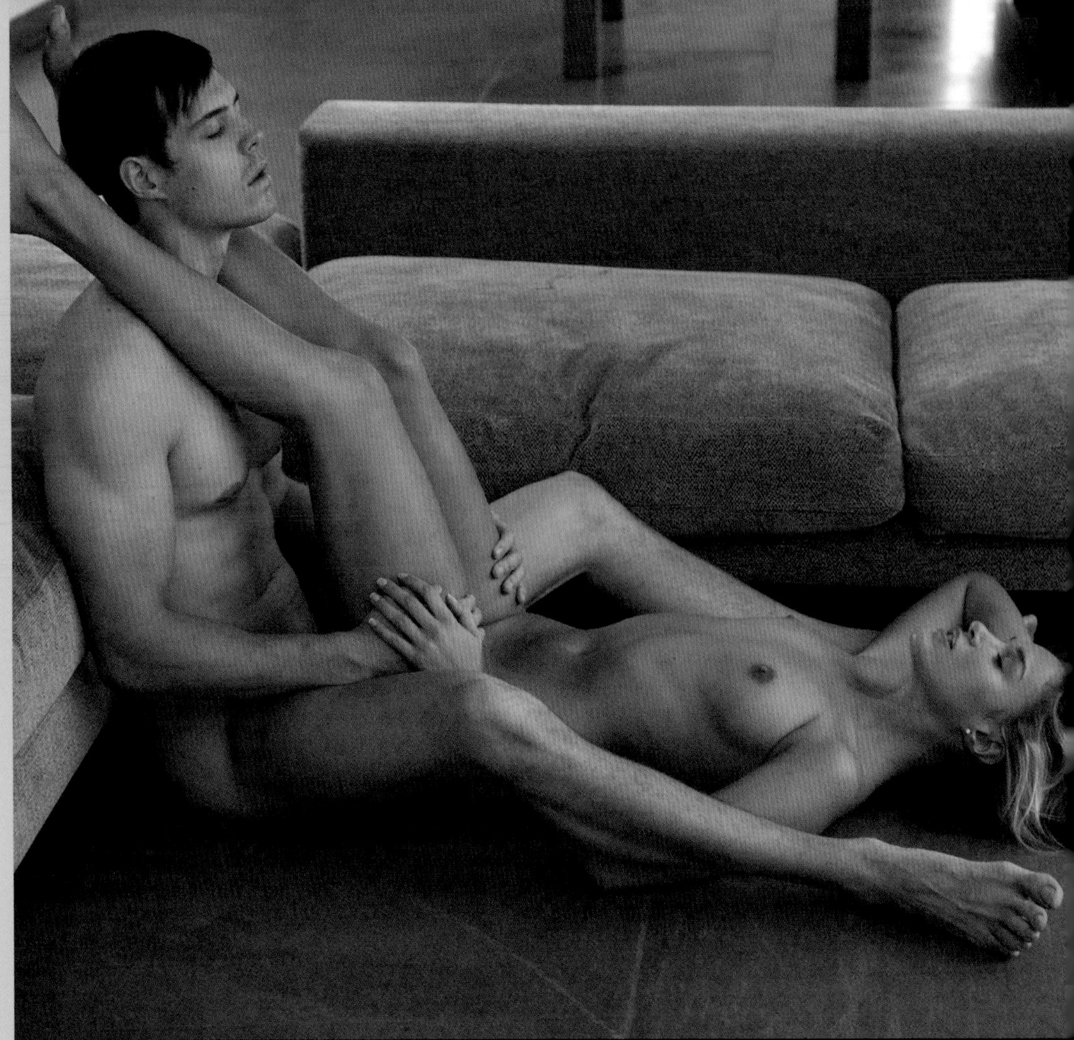

13

chill-out session

Too tired, too drunk, or too full up to have sex? Now you have no excuses! This position is invented just for those occasions. He leans back against some sturdy but comfy furniture, she lies in front of him, lifting her legs to rest on his shoulders and he then penetrates her. It's sexy because you both have a great view of each other's bods and penetration is deep and intensely satisfying. He holds her hips and moves them in time with his own. If he really, really wants to get her attention, he can reach down and play with her clitoris or anus as well.

14

wanton wiggle

This works on a (very stable) chair (minus arms) or on a step—all you need is for him to be able to sit down in the usual way, with her on his lap and both feet flat on the floor. She then lifts herself up and down to rock on his penis. There are obvious advantages to this: first, it can naturally morph from what began as an affectionate moment. Second, it's ridiculously easy for her or him to reach down or around to stimulate her clitoris. Meanwhile, she makes like a lapdancer, adding in as many wanton wiggles as she pleases.

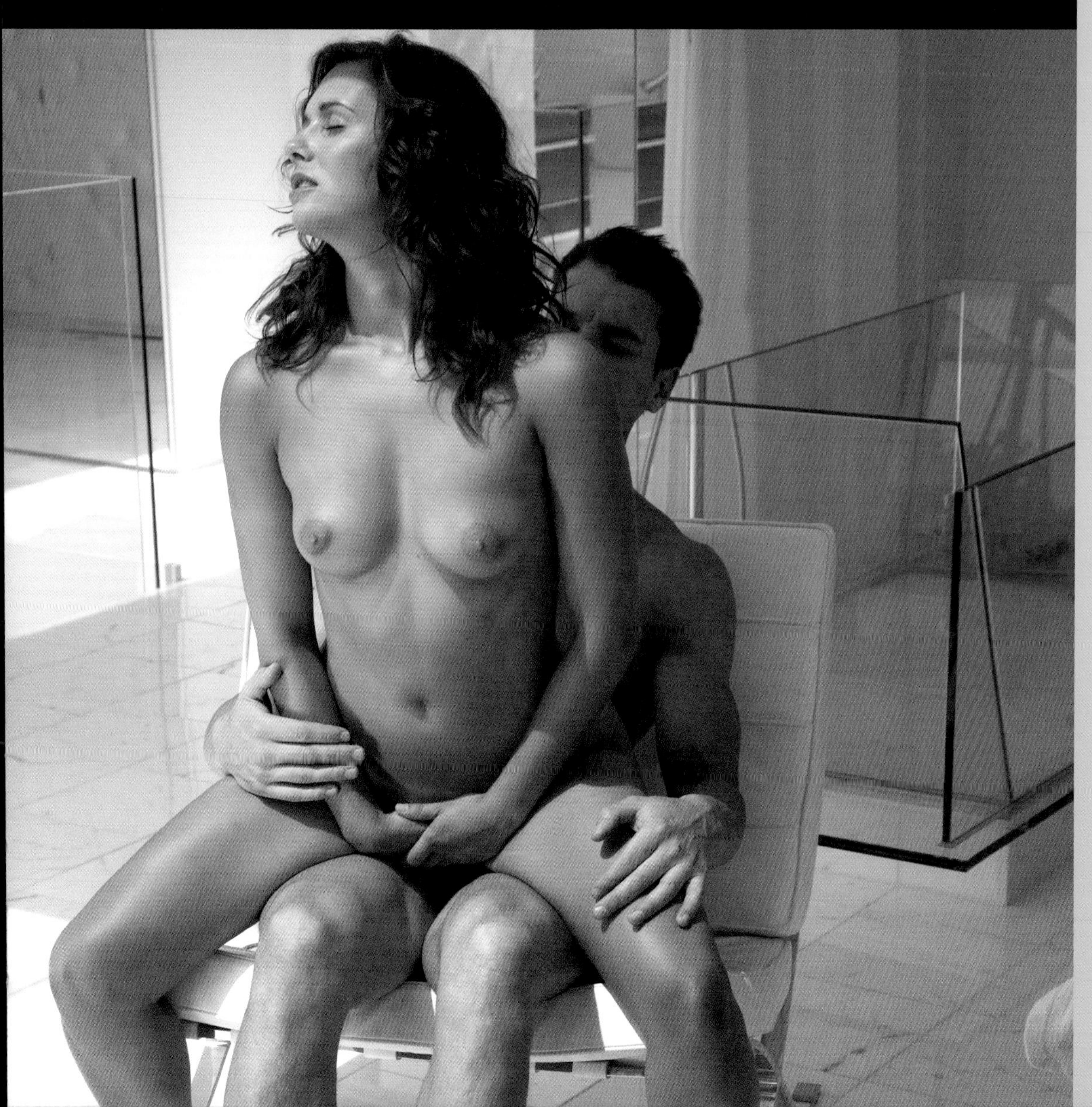

15

soul to soul

He might be on top, but winding a leg around his thigh puts her in command of the action for a soul-to-soul sexual smooch.

This small, but spiritually significant variation on the standard face-to-face position makes a big difference. She places one leg across his thigh to draw him as close as possible—and puts herself in the power position because she can now use pressure to guide the depth, rhythm, and pace of penetration. Up the difficulty level by doing this position standing up, where it magically transforms into The Vine (see page 53).

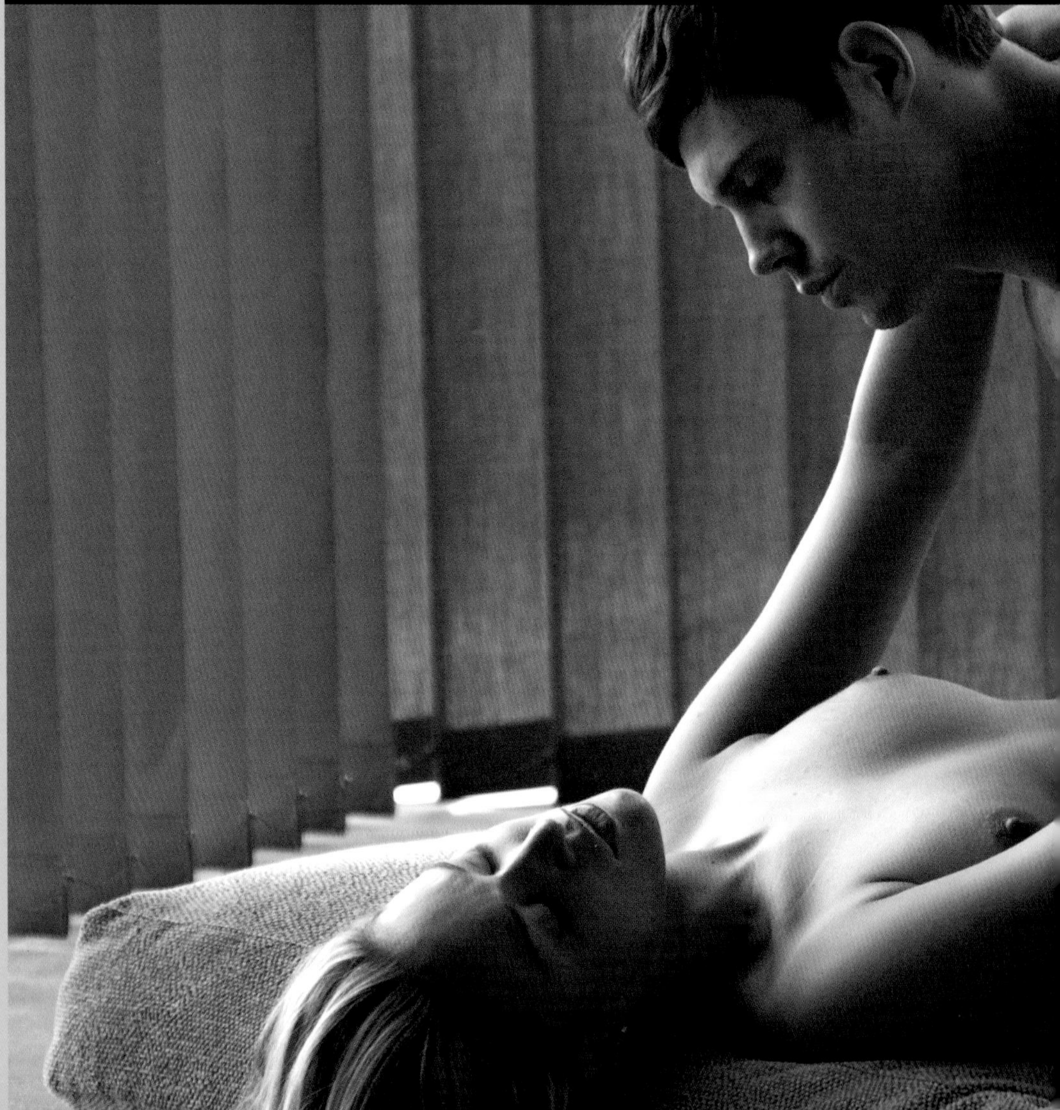

To alter the depth of penetration, she can move her leg higher or lower or turn on her side for an even tighter fit. For added pleasure, lean forward to allow your nipples to rub against each other, or try scratching his back. If she gently drags her nails across his skin, it's not just the hairs on his back that stand to attention.

Letting the female take control is nearly always a good idea, because she'll tend to slow down the thrusting pace. Make it last even longer by ditching traditional in-and-out thrusts for sexy circular grinding, Elvis-style.

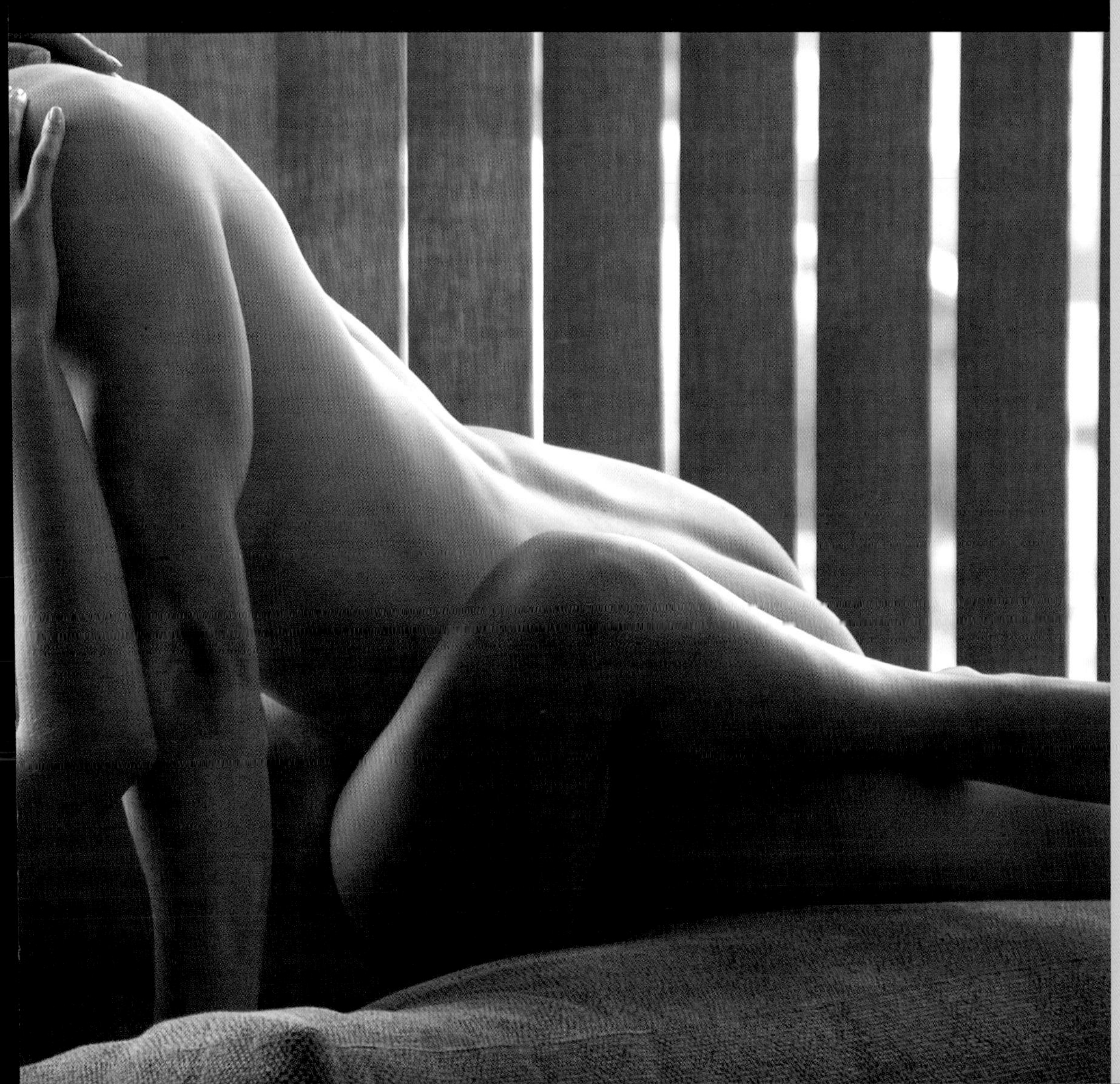

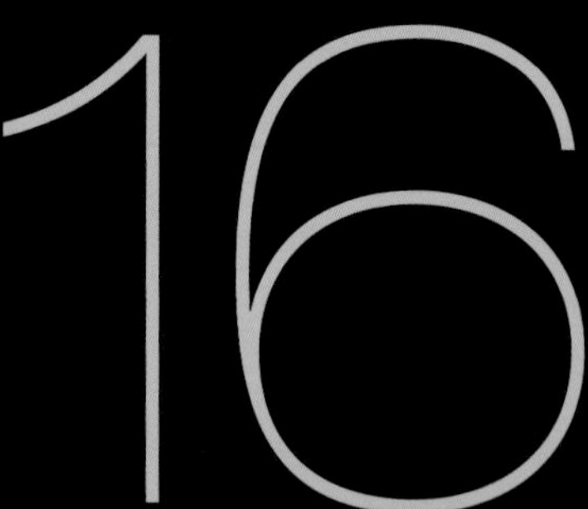

the plunge

Him on top nearly always makes a couple's top three positions because it's so versatile. Him kneeling instead of lying offers more range of movement, but it's the position of her legs that's vital for how this feels.

For deep penetration, she should put her legs on his shoulders—the higher and farther back, the deeper his penis plunges. Spread her legs wide and make sure he's fully pressed against her pubic bone and lower abdomen for a magic tugging sensation on the clitoris. Keep her legs straight and together with his outside hers, for a tighter fit for him, while he grinds satisfyingly against her mons and clitoris.

Most him-on-top positions are improved by putting a pillow under her hips or bottom, and he's better off using a rocking/grinding motion, unless, of course, he's been a very, very good boy and it's his turn to let loose in a good old-fashioned, go-for-it pounding!

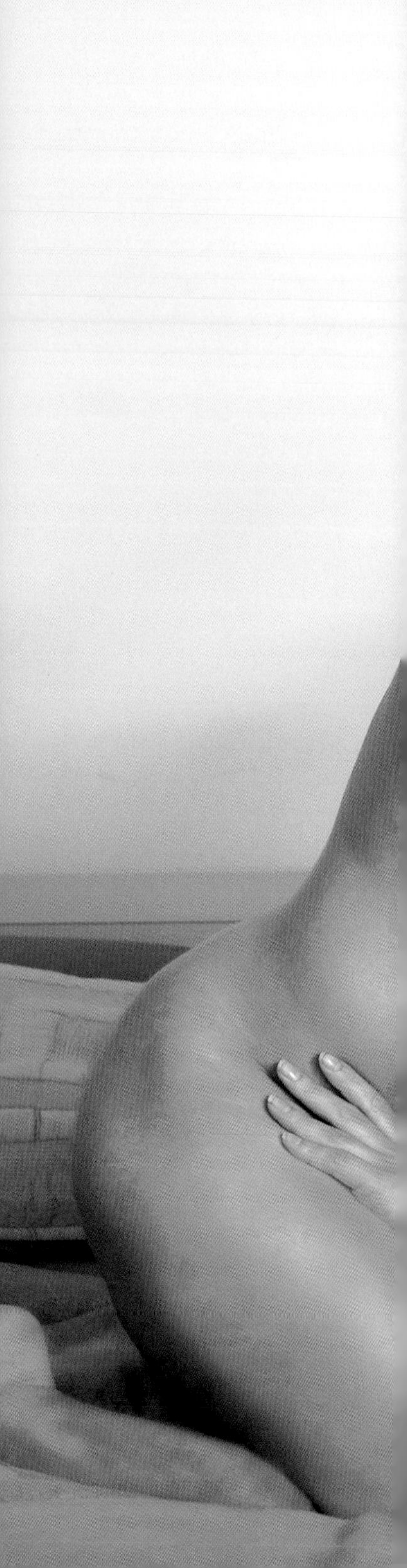

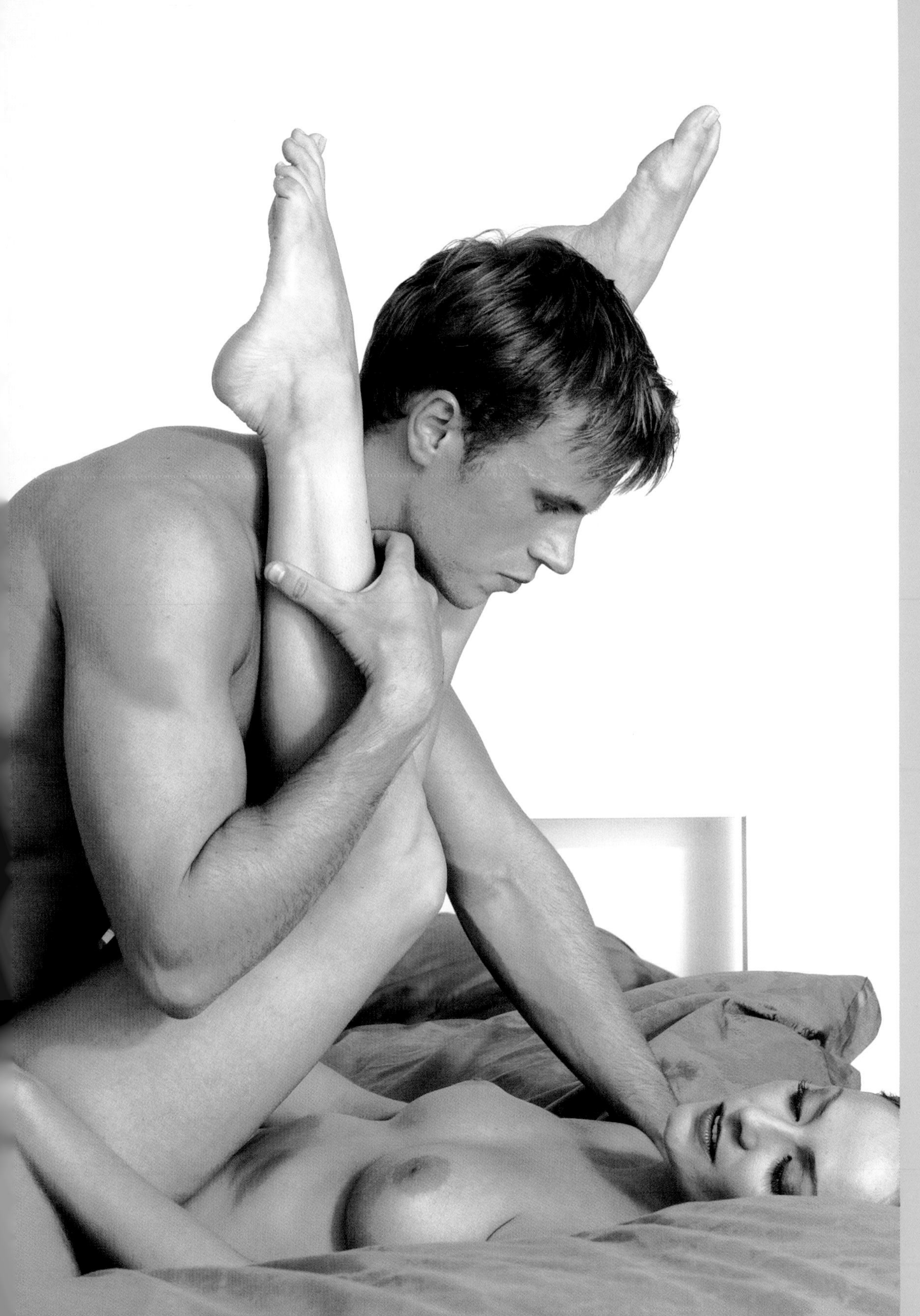

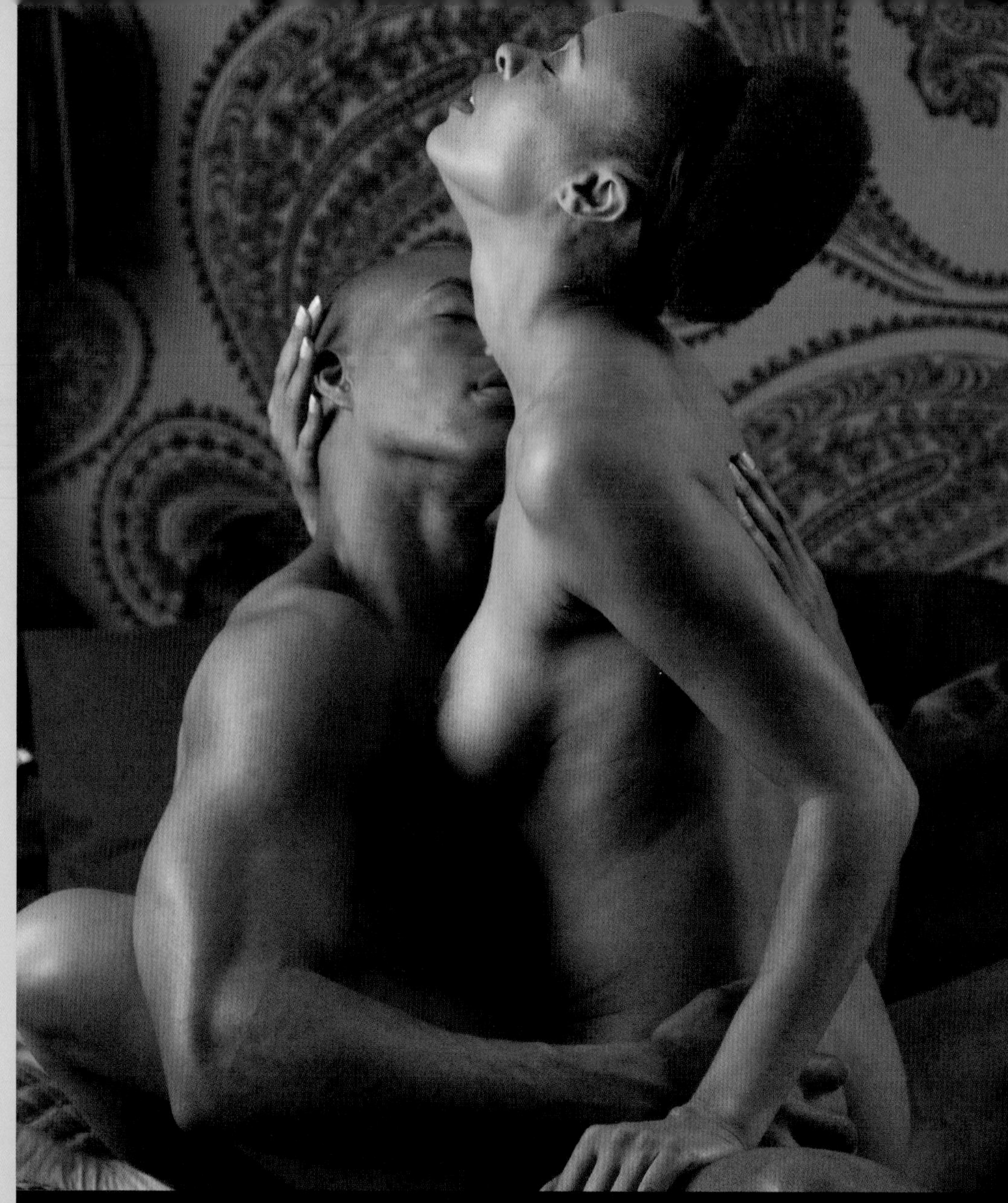

17 fleshfest

There's so much on offer to nuzzle and nibble in this pose, it's easy to see why it's often a favorite. Penetration is deep and straightforward. All he has to do is push her bottom toward him. If you can drag yourselves away from devouring each other's flesh, lock eyes.

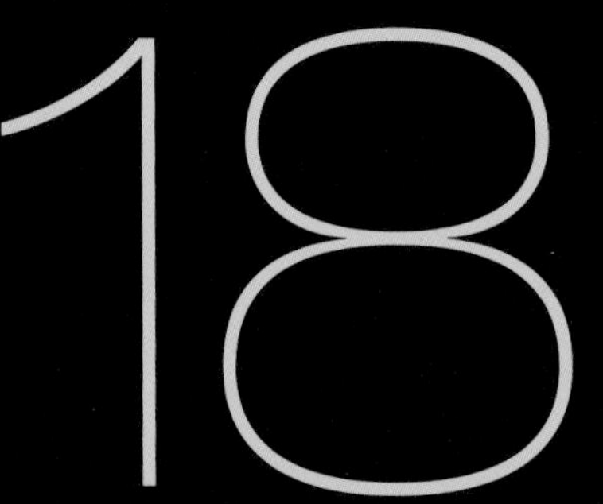

pace yourself

This is the laid-back version of the position opposite, where he's fully penetrated. Get there by letting him insert just the head of his penis before she wiggles and repetitively squeezes her vaginal muscles to draw him fully inside. To bring him to orgasm, she swings her hips from side to side. The thrusting roles are reversed, with her doing most of the work.

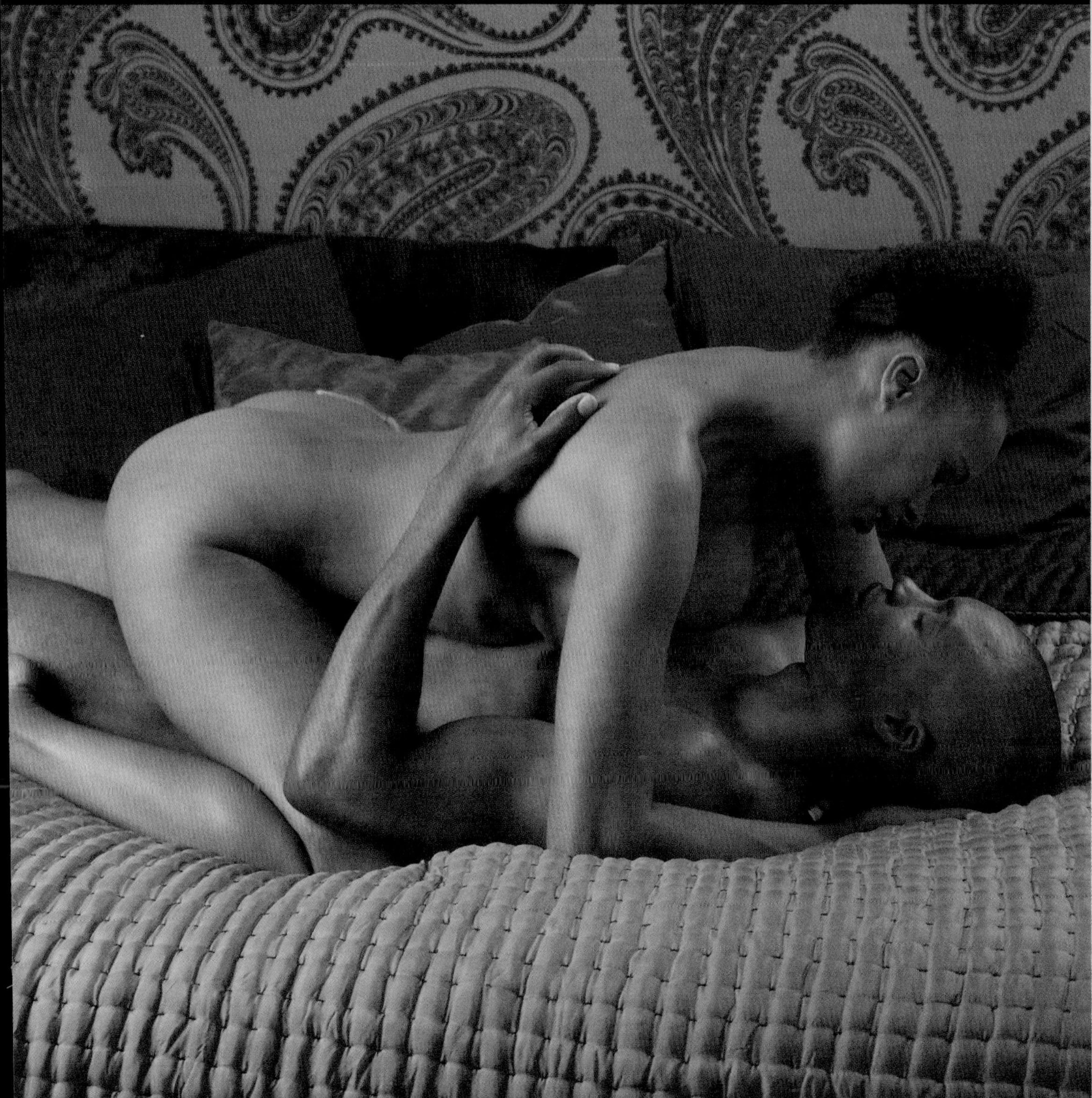

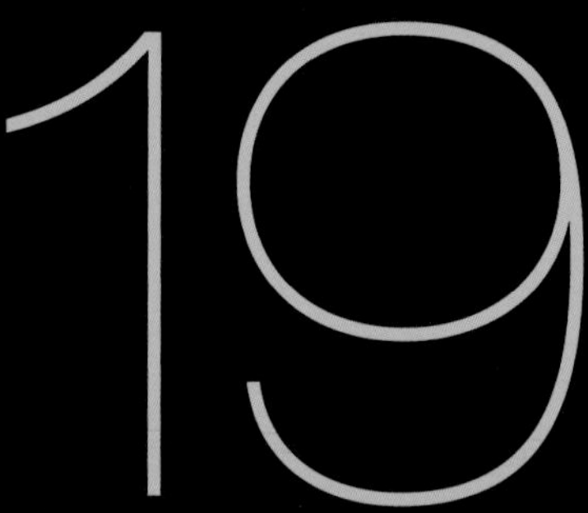

singing monkey

This is one of the 26 positions in a famous Taoist pillow book by Li T'ung Hsuan, nearly all of which are variants on four basic postures: Intimate Union (him on top), Unicorn's Horn (her on top), Close Attachment (side by side or face to face), and the Fish Sunning Itself (rear entry, and yes, really!). The position names are all intriguingly mysterious, some incomprehensible, but hey, the book has been around for centuries and we're all still going on about it, so go with the flow…

Think close and sensual rather than a lusty romp on this one. She climbs on top, getting him to penetrate in the usual fashion, then keeps her balance by wrapping one arm around his neck and placing the other on his leg. He leans forward, tensing his abs to stay physically connected to her. There's not a huge amount of freedom of movement, but she can move back and forth on his penis by tensing and relaxing her bottom and upper thigh muscles. If you want to stay true to the original Tao text, he should place his hand directly under her bottom and pull slightly to create some (rather delicious-feeling) friction on her genitals, perineum, and anus.

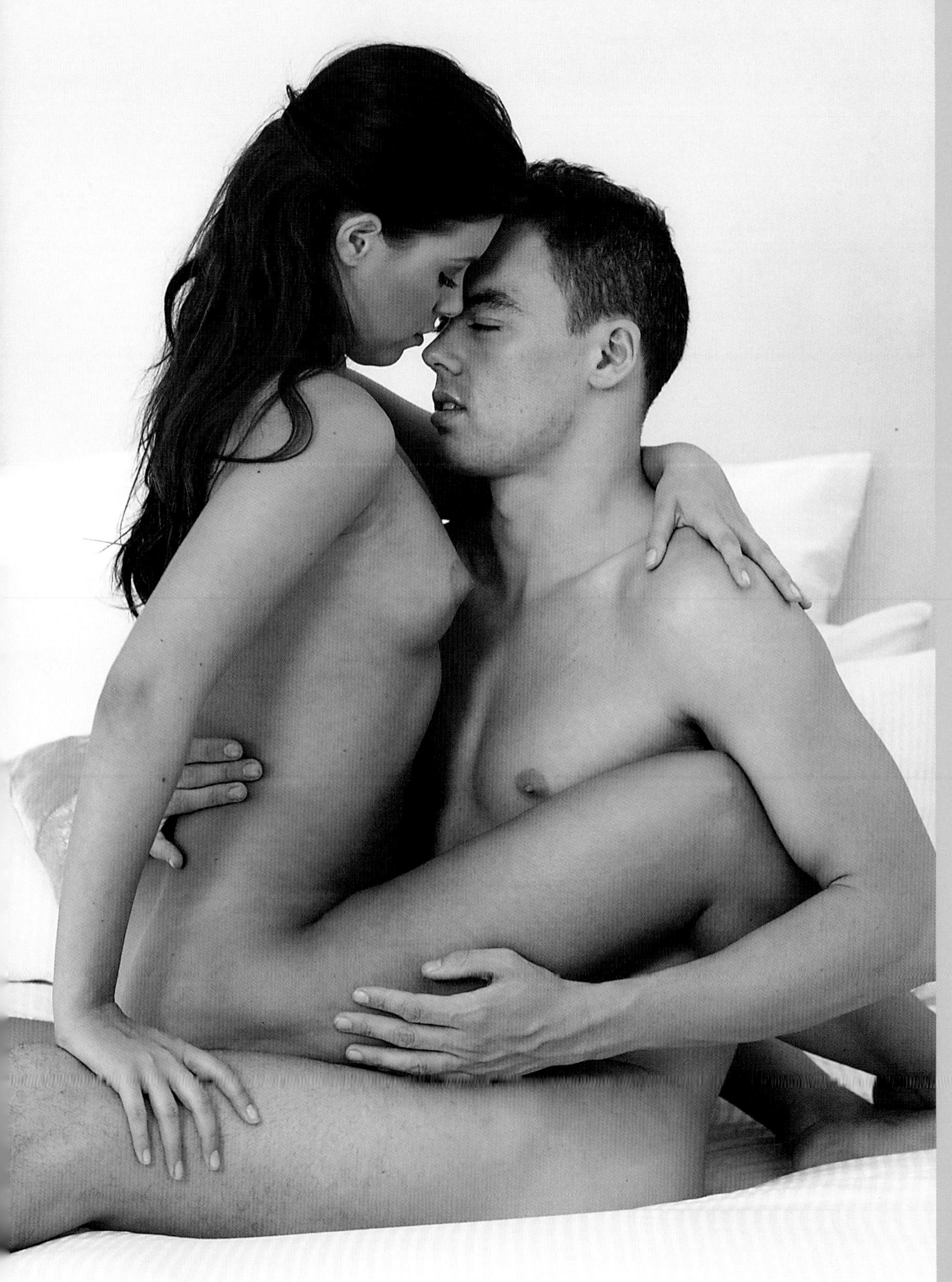

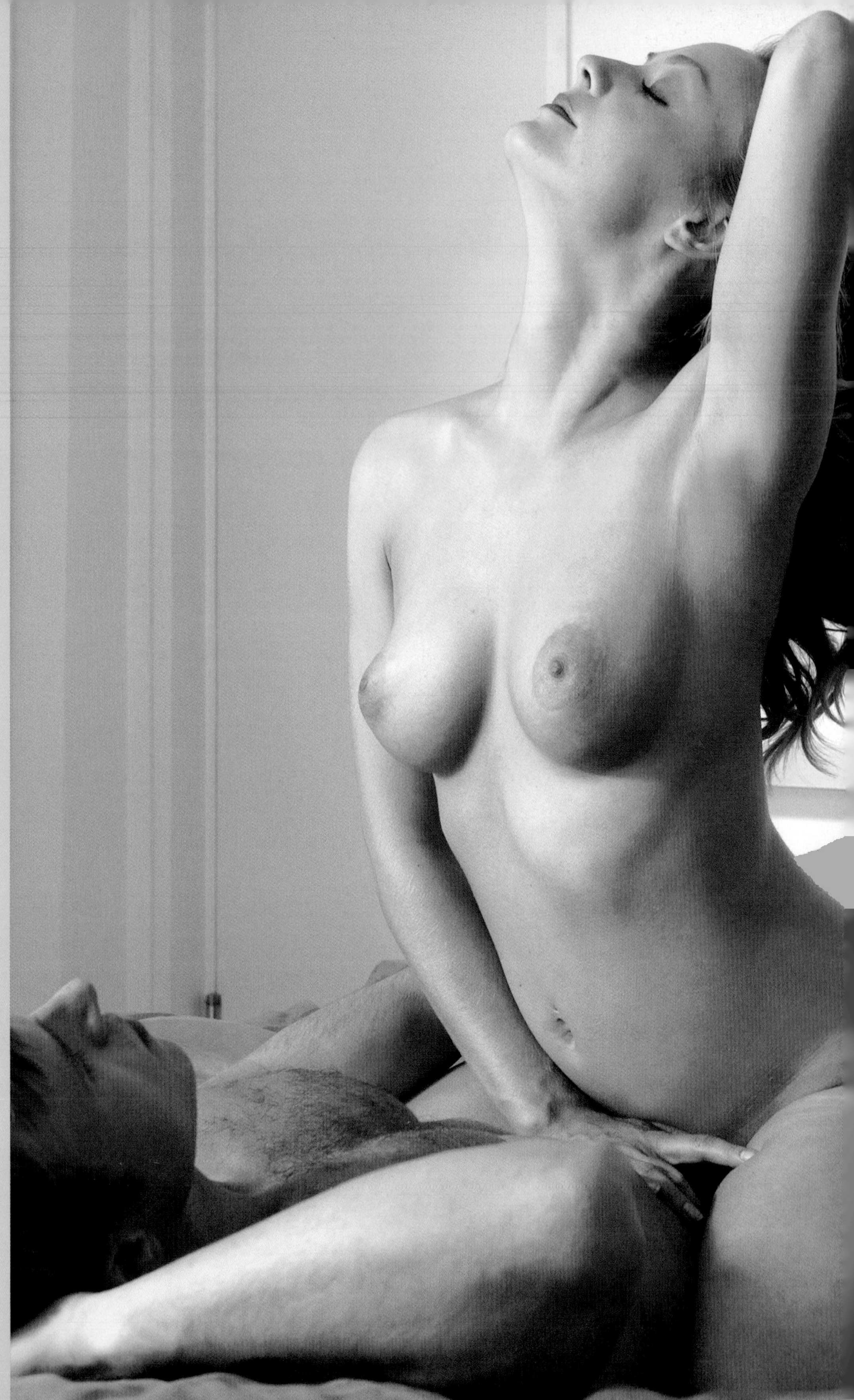

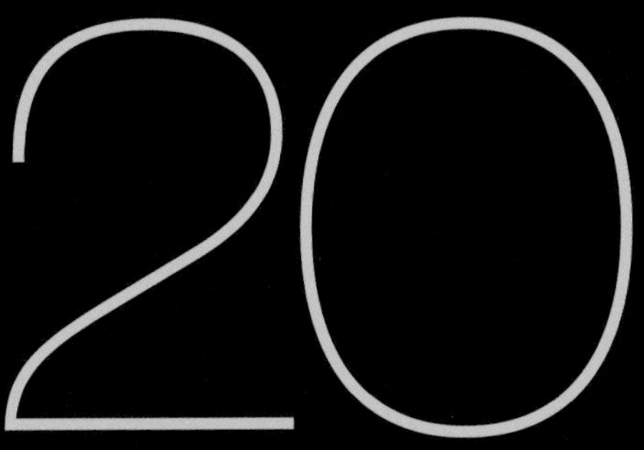

in her hands

You'd be hard pressed to find a reputable sex expert who won't advise you to add clitoral stimulation to any and all intercourse positions. But who does the best job—him or her? She usually wins the prize, simply because most couples opt for stroking, which is hard for him to keep gentle and consistent while he's thrusting. His hand often gets knocked off target without him realizing—she can feel if it's all gone AWOL.

Try making a "V" shape with the first two fingers of one hand and place them around the vagina so the penis slides in between. This stimulates the clitoris, inner labia, and urethra—as well as adding intensity for him.

help! I can't find her clitoris!

It's definitely the star of the show—but on some women the "little man in the boat" seems to be hiding in a hidden harbor. It is—it's under the clitoral hood. Here's how to coax it out:

works every time

* Be patient. If you're having trouble finding it, she might not be ready for you yet! The clitoris will swell and become obvious once she's aroused. If it's still not obvious then, say, "Show me where it feels good to you?" and you won't feel like you're the dunce of Sex School. Remember, you're looking at the top end of her vagina (nearest her belly, not her bottom) for a teensy-weensy marble that is tucked inside a hood of skin.
* When it's aroused, the clitoris usually comes out to meet you, but if it doesn't, try gently licking the hood itself to see if that works. Or put the tip of your tongue on the hood and move it in circles. If it still doesn't emerge, but she's pulling you closer, place the heel of the palm of your hand on her pubic mound (the fleshy part), fingers pointed to her belly, then push up toward her tummy. This stretches her and exposes her clitoris.

ta-da!

* Now that it's made an entrance, don't go berserk. Gently lick around the sides, make circles around it, or lap at the bottom. Don't lick directly on it and remember: wide tongue, wet, gentle, slow, slow, slow. (And did I mention—slow?)

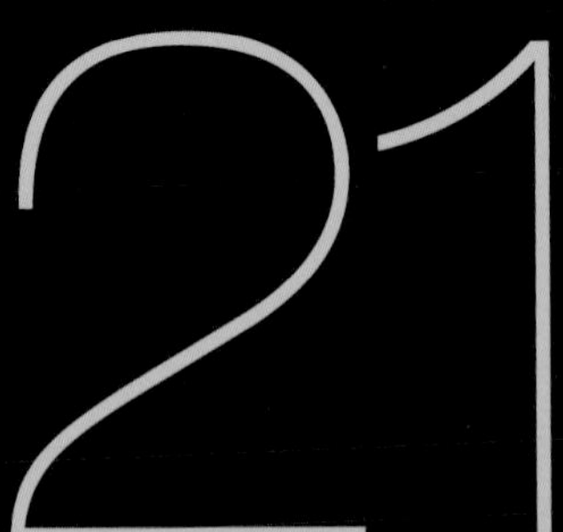

the twist

This position looks awkward because she's twisted, but it's actually surprisingly relaxing. Start by both lying on your sides and penetrate as you usually would in a side-by-side position. At this point, you're both facing in the same direction. She then lifts her top leg, winding it backward over his waist and thigh. You can hold hands, and if she puts her other hand up to hold his face, this can be super-romantic as well as sexy. Go with the mood. Don't be scared to turn what's supposed to be a lusty position into a loving one, or vice versa.

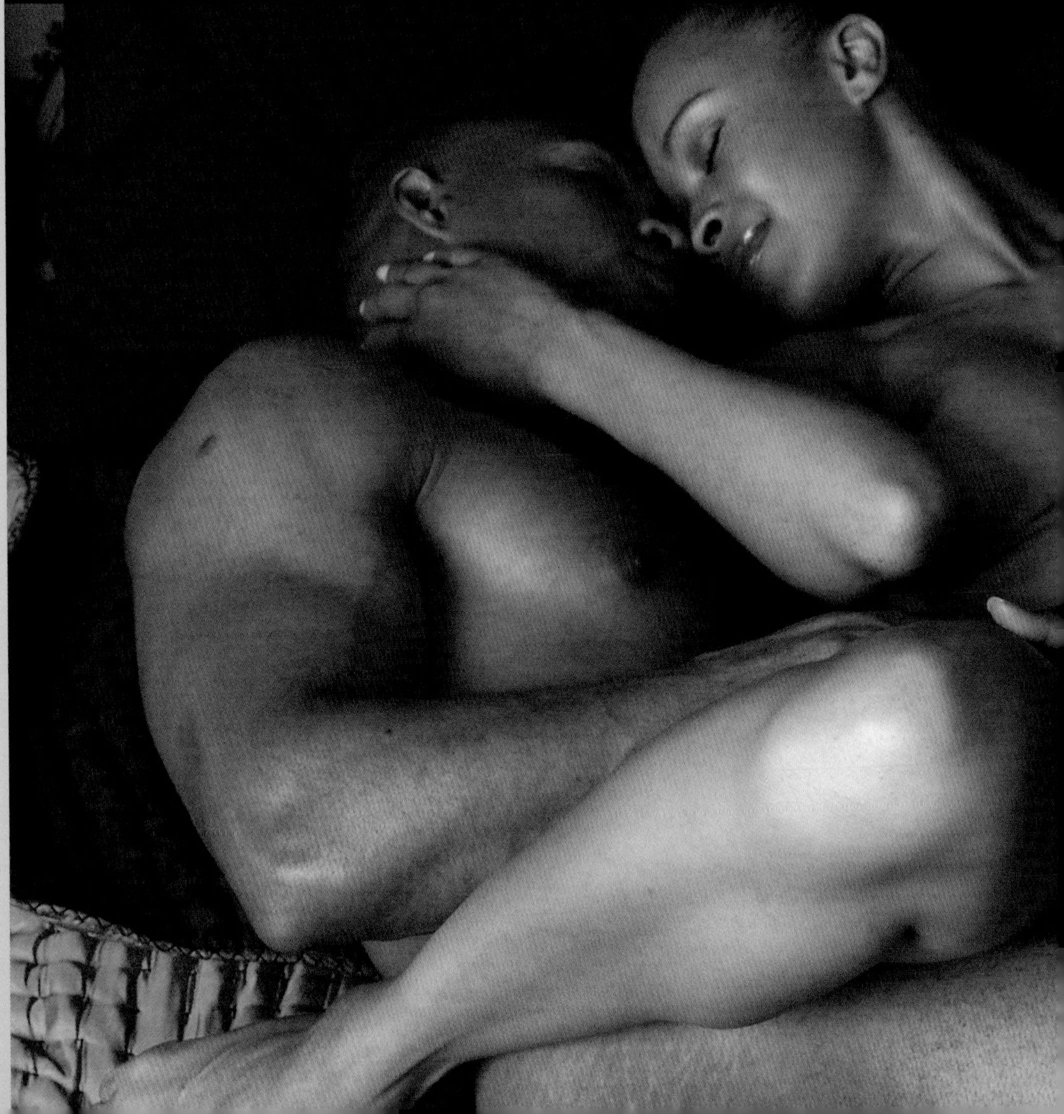

While we're on the topic of changing positions, I'm all for mixing it up a little in one session—moving easily from one position to another when they flow naturally—but radically changing position purely for the sake of it (read showing off) isn't so hot. Men are particularly fond of working through a routine that makes our morning yoga session seem like a rest period, thinking it's hugely impressive. It isn't. In fact, nothing's guaranteed to turn us off more than being thrown around like a rag doll. A lusty but loving pose like this one, however, might just win us over.

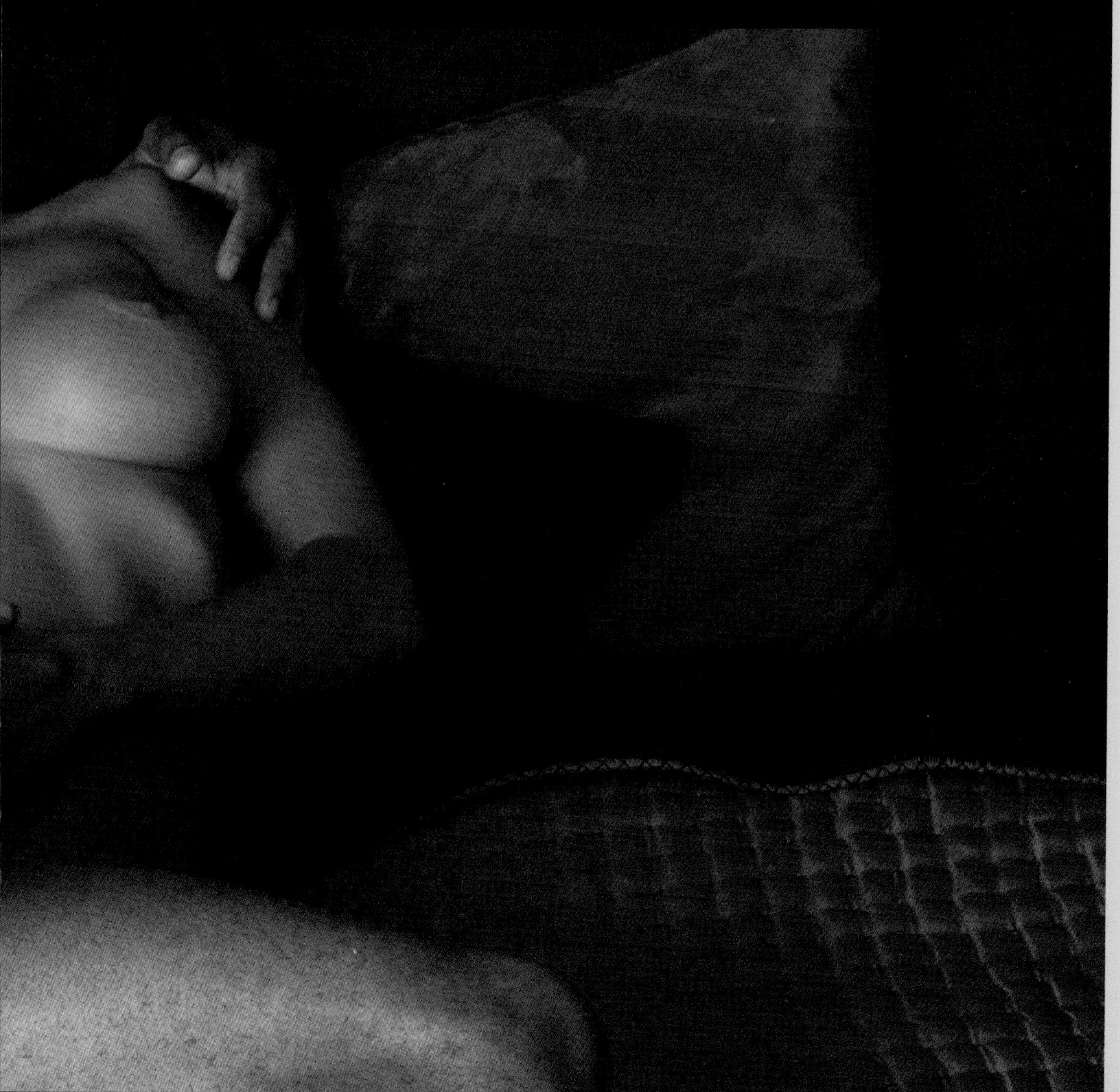

quick sex: the rules

Fast, frenzied sex will do many nice things for your relationship: it reminds you both how much you are attracted to each other on a purely physical basis; it's unplanned, impulsive sex that keeps the "Aren't we naughty?" buzz alive; and there is no argument against the fact that quick sex, rather than no sex, keeps you connected as a couple.

use a lubricant Most men can get an erection in the time it takes her to say "How about it?" Women's arousal systems are, sadly, somewhat slower. During relaxed lovemaking, there's time for the vagina to lubricate and expand: during quick sex you both need to be ready for immediate action.

Adding lubricant speeds up the female arousal process by instantly providing what her body usually takes a little while to provide naturally. With gentle but slippery hands, you can dive straight for her va-jay-jay , guaranteeing pleasure, not pain. Lubricant also artificially prepares her for quick penetration. Combine this with immediate, expert stimulation and you can shock her sexual system from "Whoa" to "Go" in under a minute. Leave tubes of lubricant in secret hiding places (behind a couch cushion, in the bathroom, in the glove compartment of the car, in the office). You can also buy little sachets of travel-size lubricant to carry with you, for whenever and wherever.

mix it up A good sex life is balanced and you need a variety of sex sessions to nurture all parts of your emotional and sexual selves. Lusty and loving. Long and short. It's totally acceptable to have quickish sex the majority of times you make love. But when

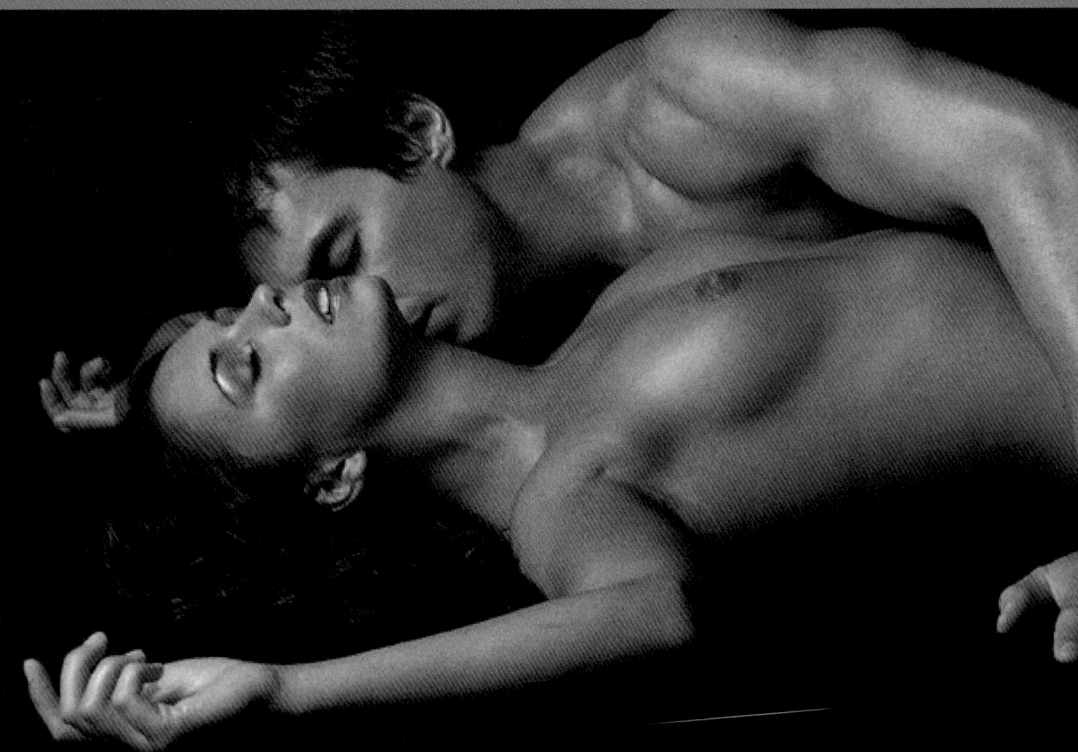

"Shock her sexual system from 'Whoa' to 'Go' in under a minute."

you do have time, make the effort. A sensible two-week mix for busy couples is to include four to six low-effort, minutes-long turn-ons, at least four quickies (anywhere from five minutes to 15), and at least one session that lasts up to an hour (or more). In total, that's around an hour and a half every two weeks. Considering most of us spend around two hours per night parked in front of the TV, that's a pretty effective use of time.

Vary where you do it: having sex in unusual places adds to the danger and urgency, and doing it outside of the bed forces you to try new positions and means of stimulation you wouldn't normally try.

change your attitude Rethink what you mean by "sex." A quickie means quick sex of any kind, not necessarily intercourse. Think of "sex" as anything that makes you feel sexy—teased as well as totally sated. Two minutes of oral sex is just long enough to get everything standing to attention... and wanting more, more, more when that mouth is taken away. Teasing each other physically—arousing your sexual systems, then leaving them to simmer—whets the appetite and encourages anticipatory sex. Spontaneity, often lost long term, gets replaced by something far more delicious: knowing what's coming and exactly how they're going to do it. A sexy, long, kiss with some neck kissing, a hot text from your lover that makes you instantly wet—all these things count as "sex" sessions.

Learn to enjoy parts of sex and parts of your bodies, rather than always devouring the whole thing. Impose rules to introduce limitations designed to get you both begging for more: hands-only sessions, tongues only, penetration only, breasts only, genitals only, she's only allowed to touch, he's only allowed to touch. Then stop—part company for a while if you have to—and enjoy the hot rush of desire you feel by *not* having it all.

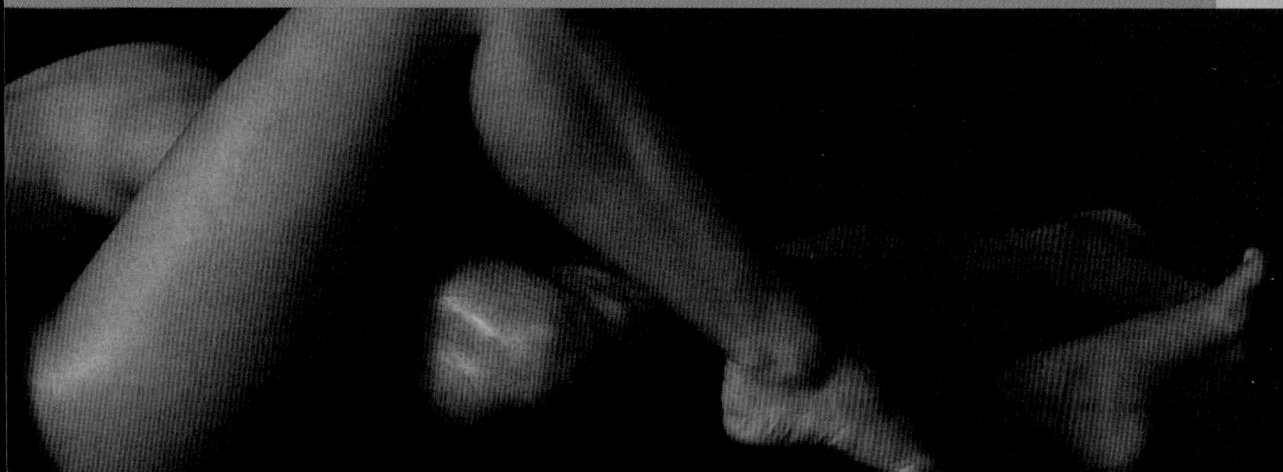

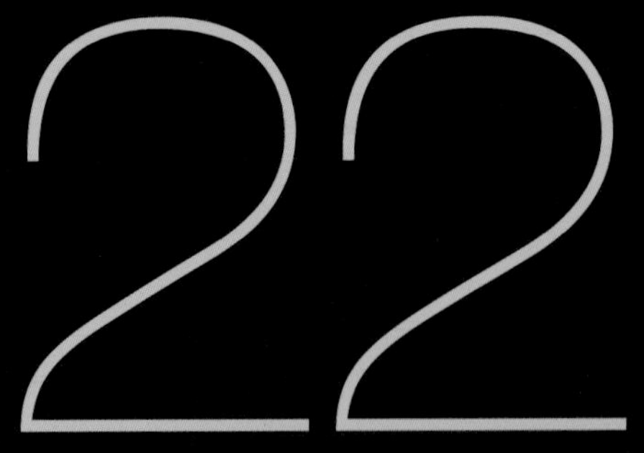

the leg lift

Being able to make intense eye contact adds intimacy to passion in this position, and her thighs being spread wide ups the eroticism.

She raises her legs in the air, making a wide “V” shape by holding her thighs open with her hands. He penetrates in the usual man-on-top position. Penetration is already pretty intense, but if she’s feeling particularly raunchy and wants him even deeper, she should bend her knees and bring them up to her chest. Some interpretations of this pose include her putting her feet in front of him, pressing against the top of his chest.

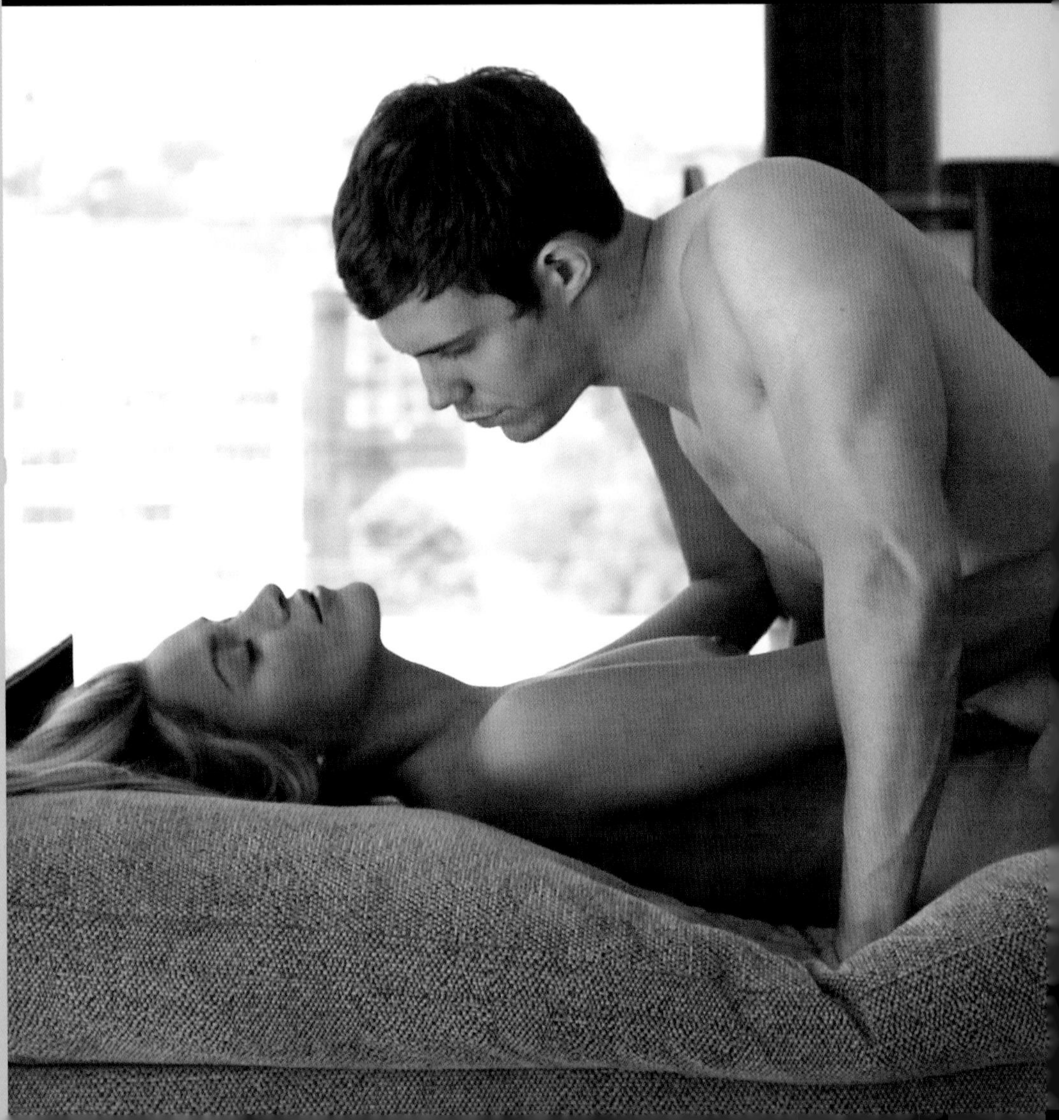

This position shortens the vagina, making her feel tighter so it's a good choice if she has a large vagina and he has a small penis. It's all in the angle of her legs—if he hits so deep it's more *owww* than *ahhh*, she should try legs together pressed on his chest and thighs squeezed, rather than parted.

It captures the essence of one of the pluses of "spiritual sex"—soul—and proves that missionary-inspired positions don't have to be boring. Sex and intimacy become bed fellows again, without the rose-petals-on-the-bed, yuk-inspiring sentimentality.

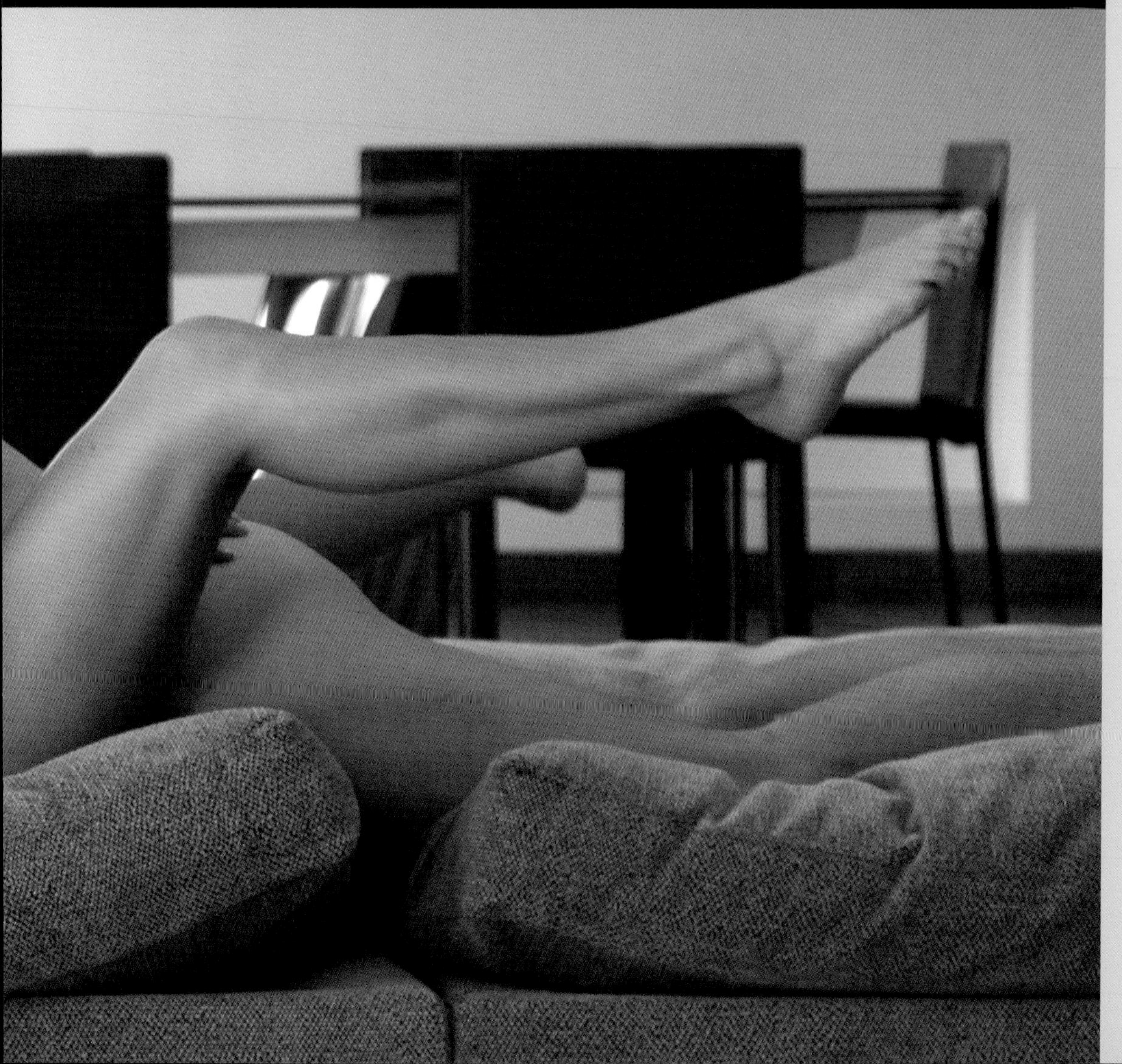

stand and deliver

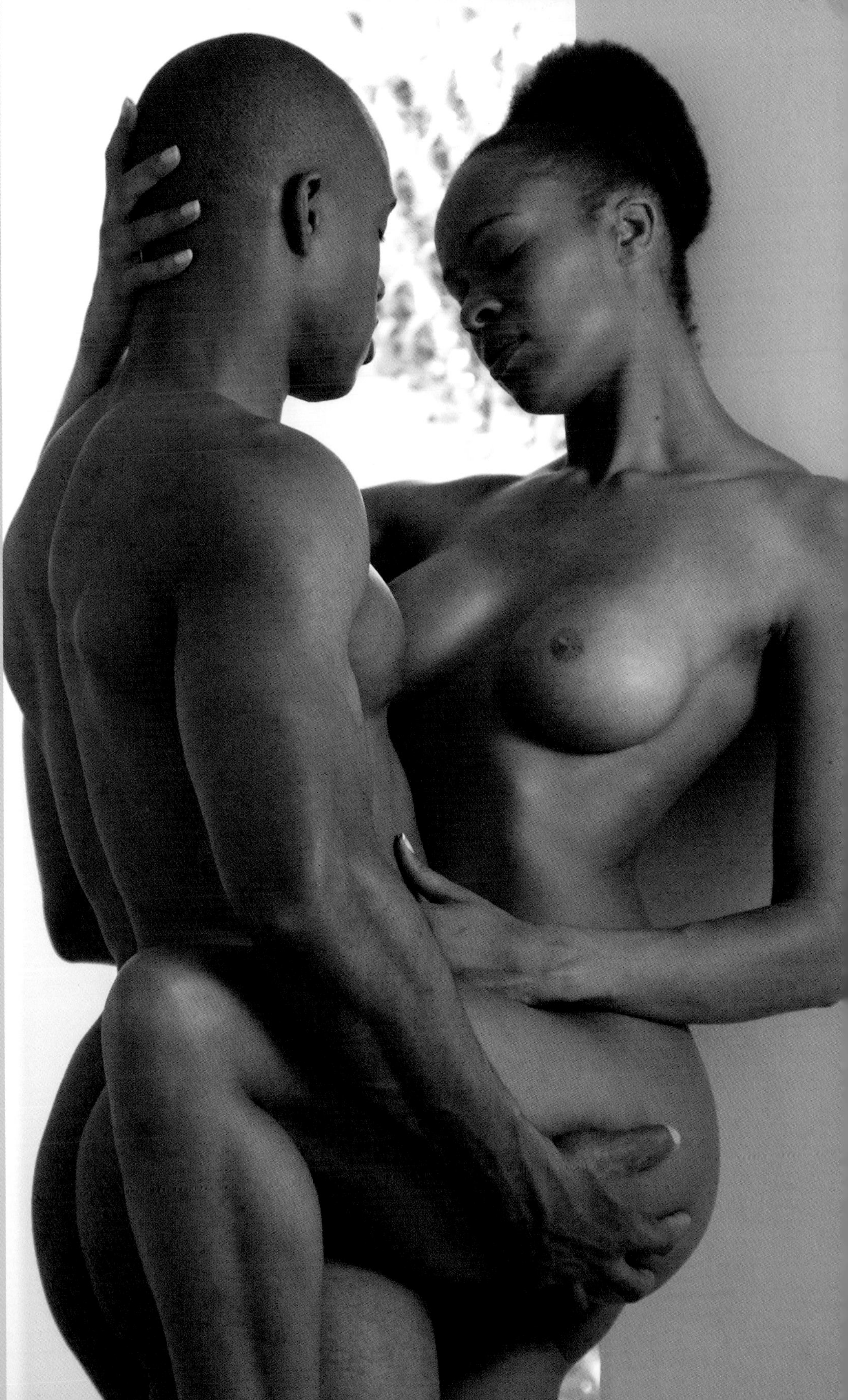

23

the vine

This one is a bit of a carnal challenge, but for fast, urgent, spontaneous sex you can't beat it. It's terribly manly: he feels strong and she feels outrageously ravaged. It's also perfect for a quickie: no need to remove clothes, just hurriedly and feverishly push them aside!

She leans against a wall, lifting one leg to help him penetrate and he stands between her thighs, holding her raised leg under her bottom and upper thigh. She leans into the wall for stability and to allow him to thrust away with abandon. The higher she lifts her leg on his thigh, the deeper the penetration.

This one's tricky if you're completely different heights. If you're having trouble getting into position, try penetrating while she's seated on the side of the bed and lifting her up from there.

I want an orgasm!

We've all been there. It starts off fantastically, he's thrusting away and you're both having a great time, but an hour later you're still at it, both pretending still to be having a great time but secretly praying like hell one or both of you will hurry up and finish! Here's how:

we're doing it…

✻ Missionary style: The traditional "jackhammer" style of thrusting is about as effective at getting her to orgasm as using a bread knife to shave. Instead, have her grind against his pelvis and move in circles, rather than up and down. Thrust short and shallow, rather than deep and fast.

✻ Standing up: If you're standing having sex at least one of you felt an urgent need. This lends itself nicely to talking dirty.

✻ Doggy style: She lifts her bottom high so he hits the super-sensitive front vaginal wall, he reaches forward to play with her clitoris, she reaches behind to play with his testicles.

✻ He's on top: Spread her vaginal lips once he's inside and make sure they're pressed against him to get maximum friction on the clitoris and the area surrounding the urethra. It's also packed with nerve endings.

✻ She's on top: The most likely position to result in orgasms-for-two, since she's in control. To come together, he should be alert to a tightening of her vagina. When she's around a level 8 on a 1–10 pleasure scale, her vagina will often grip his penis tighter.

chapter

2

steamy

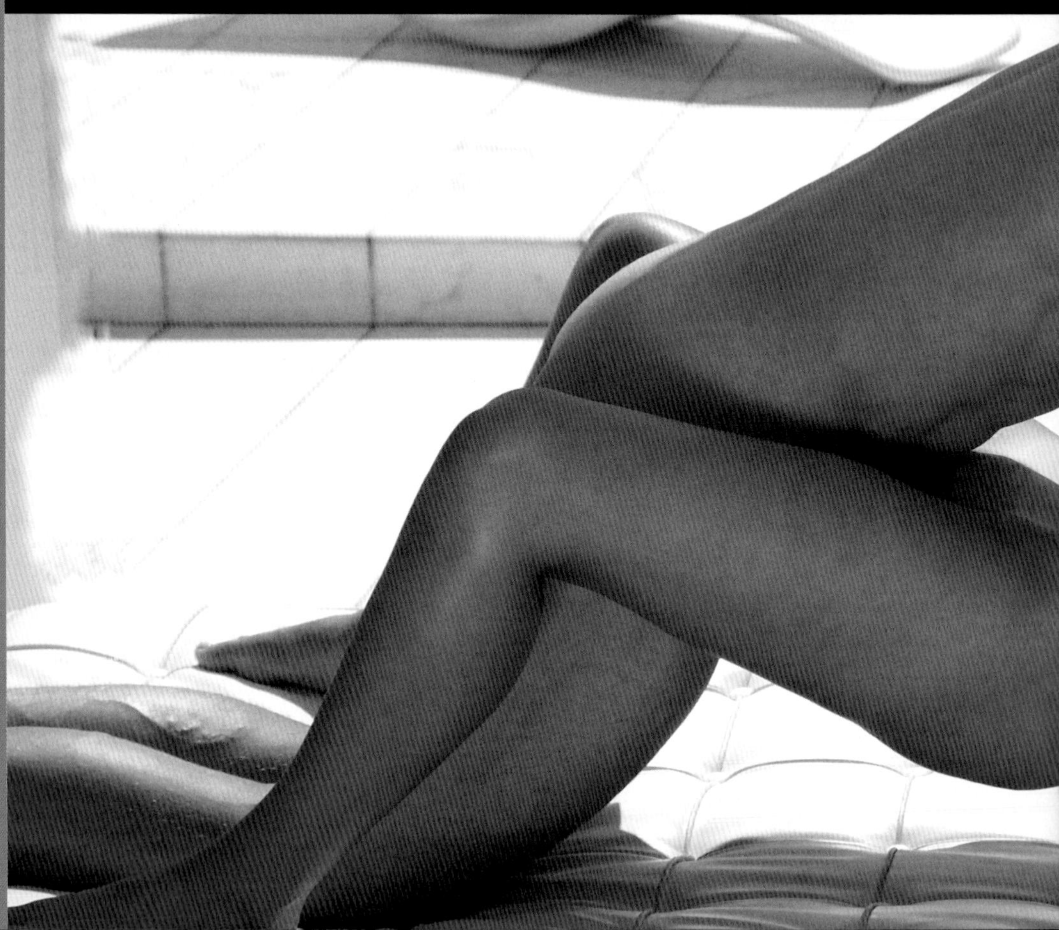

Turn it up a few (thousand) notches and get ready for some spirited sex that's deliciously raunchy.

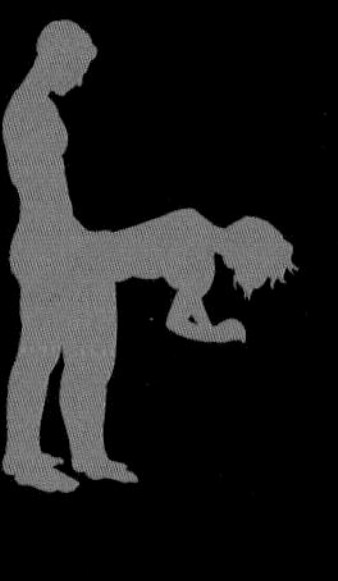

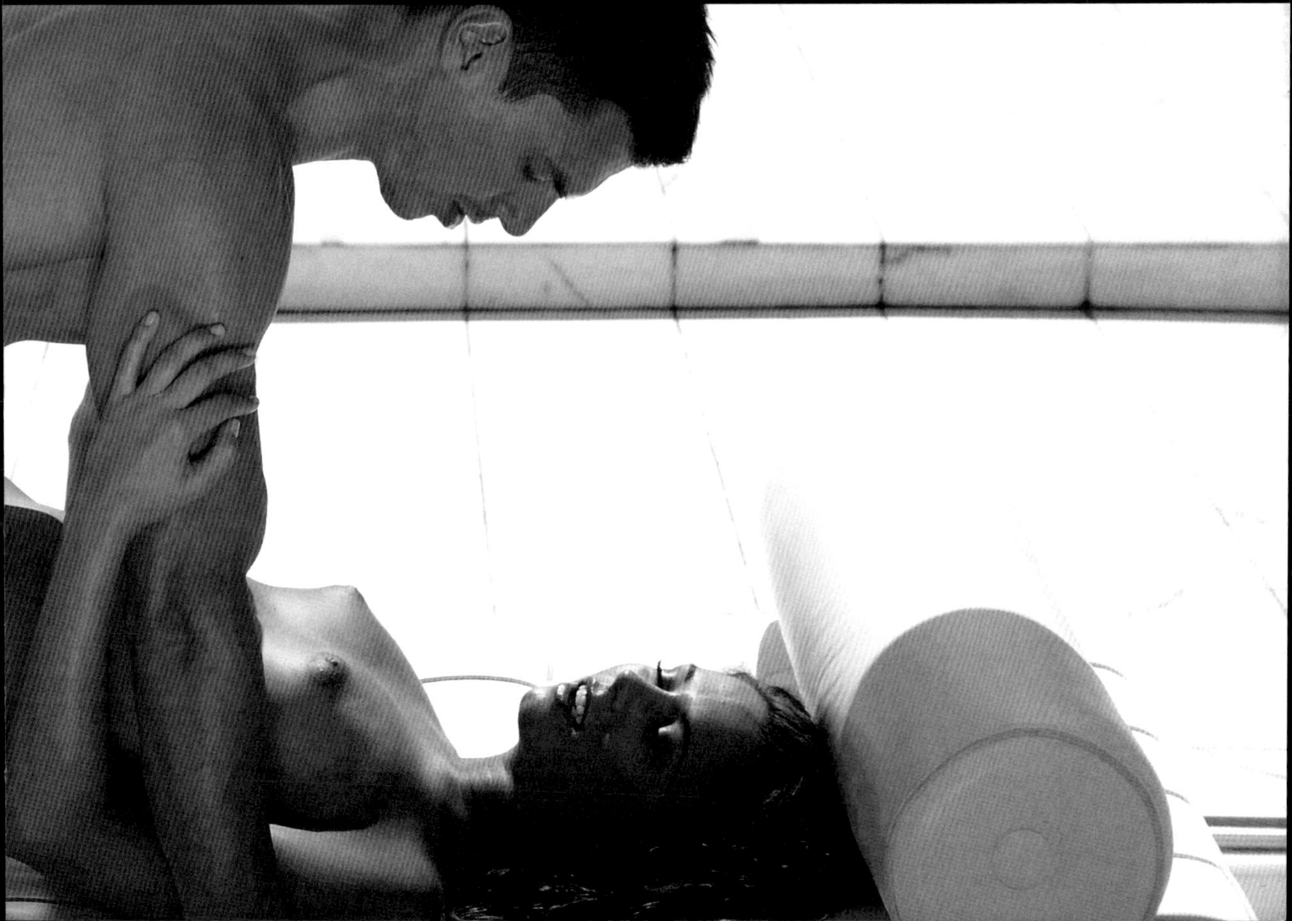

the flutterer

1 He kneels with his legs bent underneath him, she climbs on to his lap and the two of you embrace. He penetrates right from the start, but no thrusting just yet! Yes, you're sensing a theme here—the idea is to draw things out rather than rush straight into it. Savor the moment.

2 She starts to gently move up and down on his penis, but it's her pelvic-floor muscles that are doing the main work, rather than her thighs. By quickly and repetitively squeezing and releasing them, she's "fluttering," just as a butterfly flutters its wings. Awww!

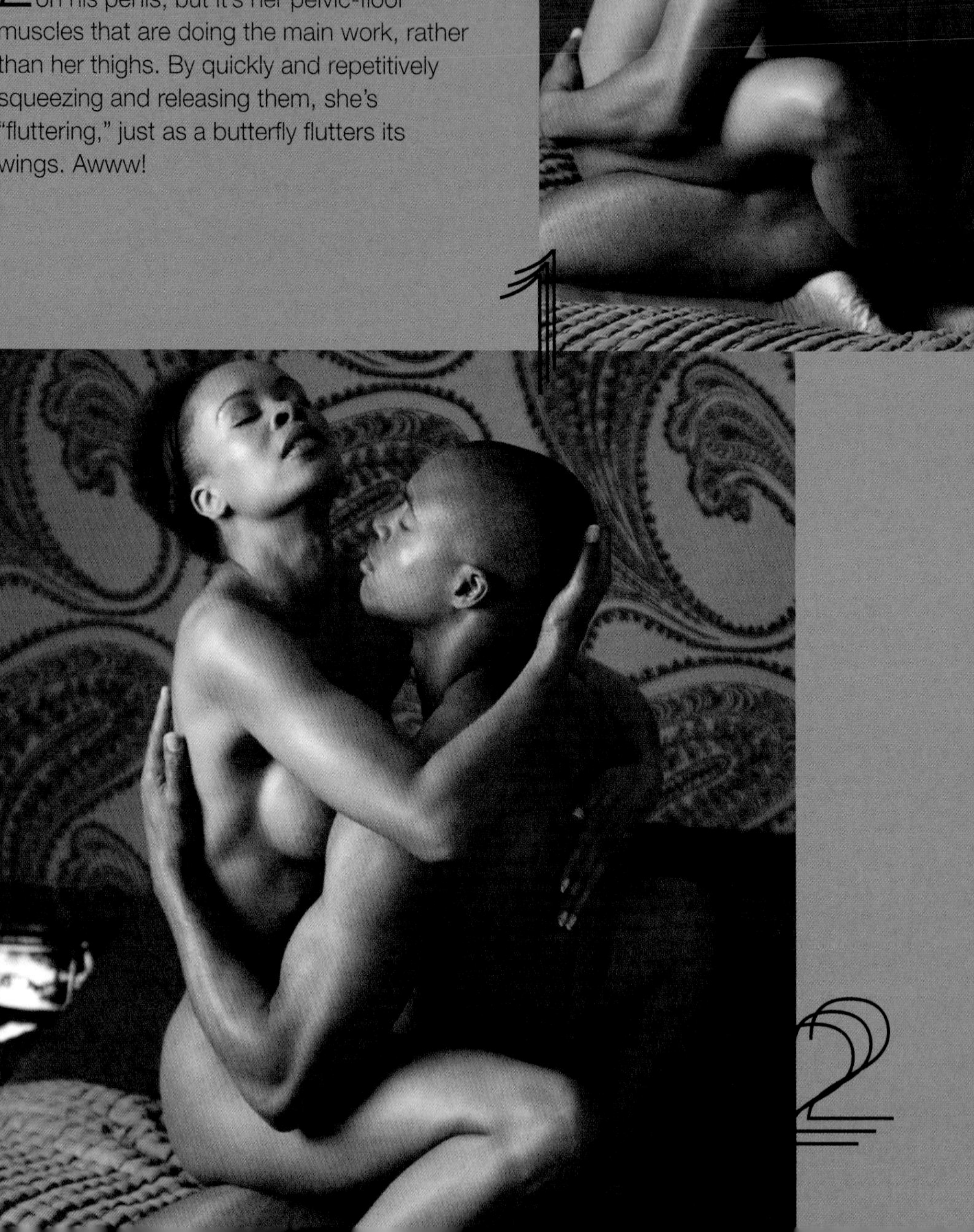

24

3 He lifts himself so he's "standing" on his knees, one foot flat on the bed. She stretches out her legs, just as a butterfly does its wings. Now, unless he spends more time pumping weights than pumping her, movement is limited, but closely clamped genitals and a unique penetrative angle more than make up for it. The farther she leans back, the greater the pressure. His knee keeps him grounded and she can move slightly until she finds a natural balance point.

3

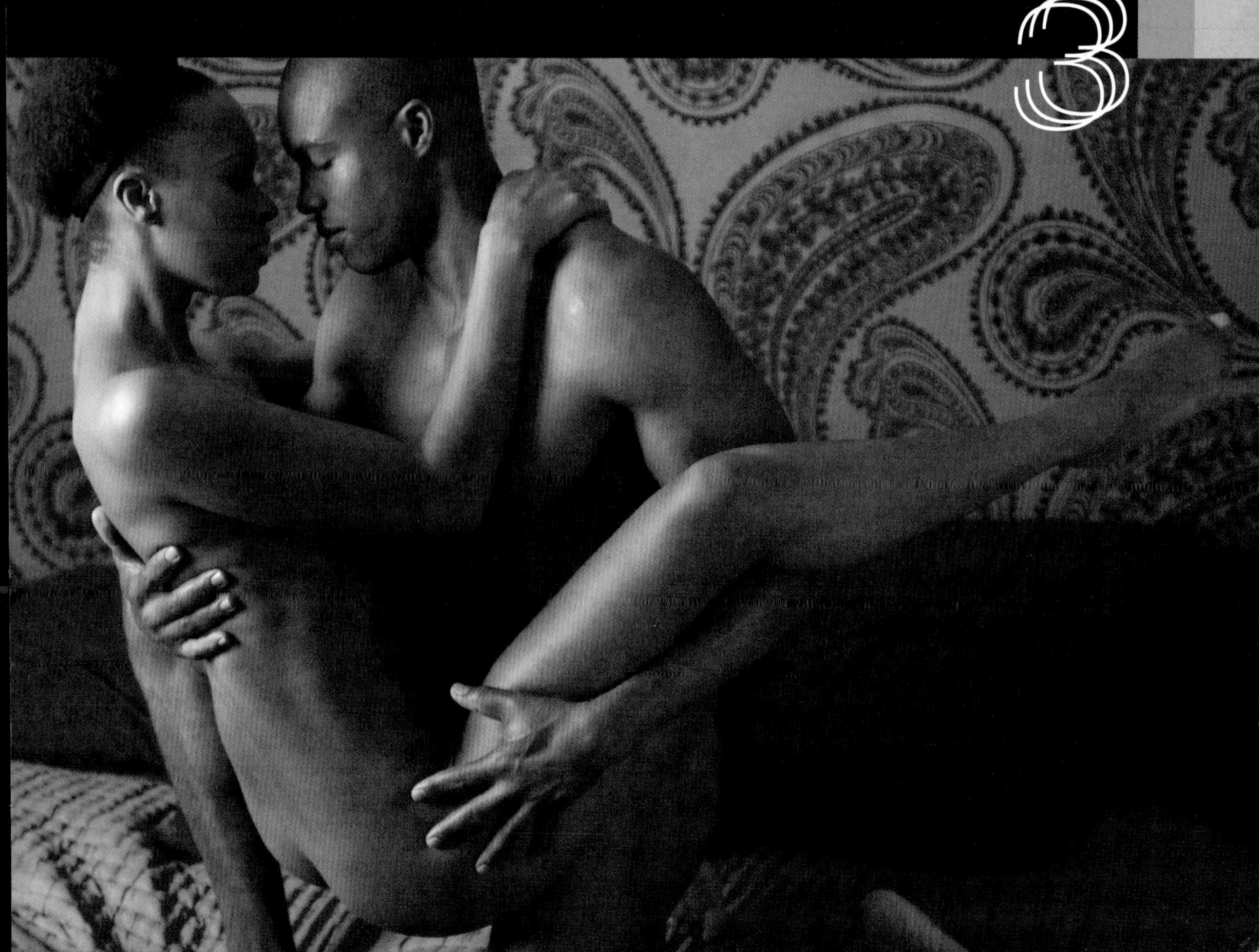

25

eyes wide open

A lift of her hips and a curve of her back means constant clitoral contact—and one very happy woman! Holding her hips high gives him the feeling that she desperately wants him inside her.

She arches her back and lifts her bottom, legs opened wide. He props himself up on his hands for support. Like all face-to-face positions, this one's derived from the missionary, except that instead of having their bottoms planted on the bed, they're lifted high in the air. Not only is this a great workout for her thighs and bottom (bonus!), but it also

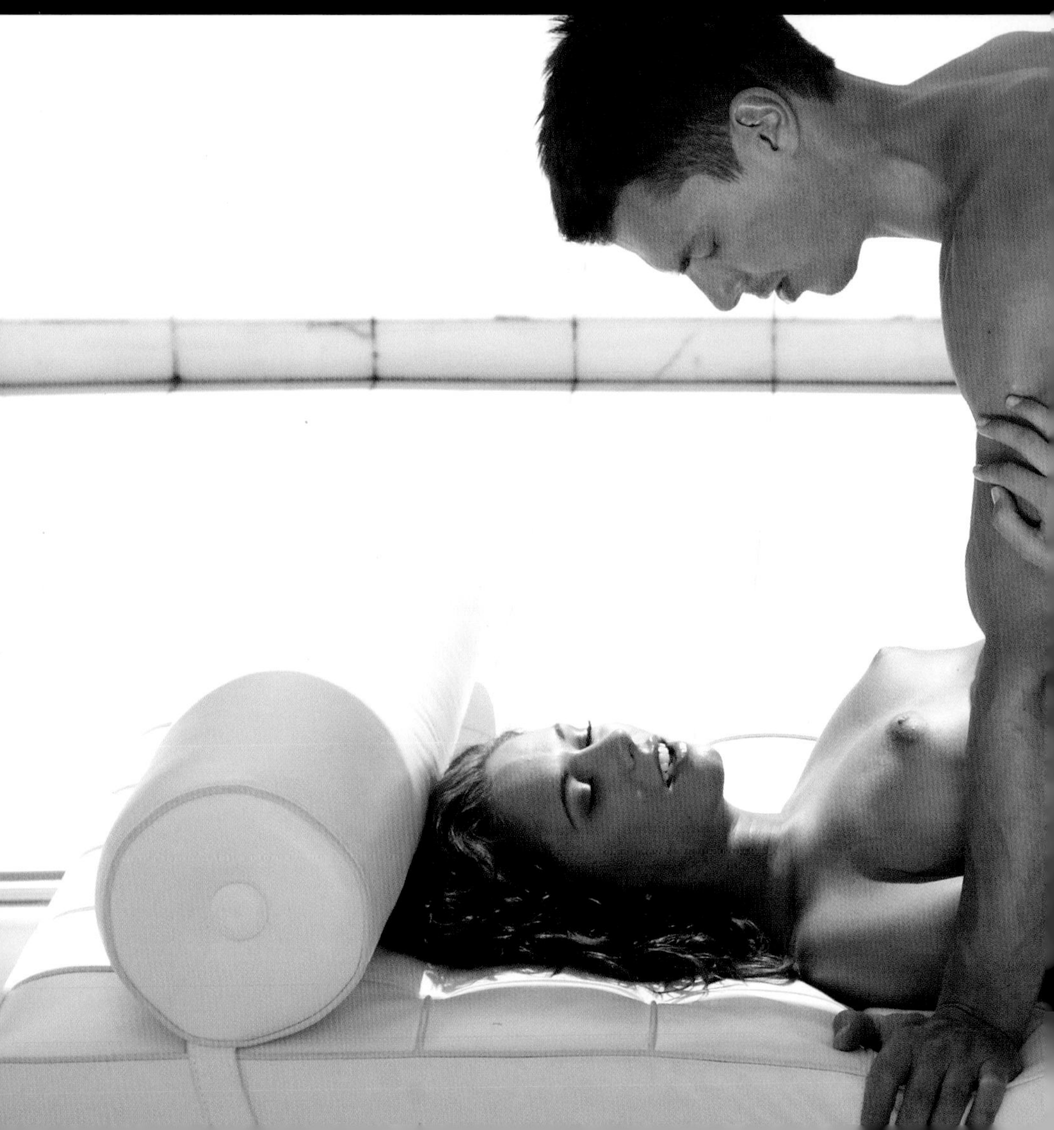

pushes the clitoris against the base of his penis, providing friction during thrusting. If her thighs or bottom start to ache, put some firm pillows under her (rather grateful) bottom.

This is a great position for eye contact and for watching each other orgasm. Research shows that 70 percent of couples have sex with their eyes closed and only 15 percent open them during orgasm. So you're tuning each other out when you should be intimately connected. Silly, right? This position is a perfect opportunity to try it out. So eyes wide open, please, fixed and focused from start to finish.

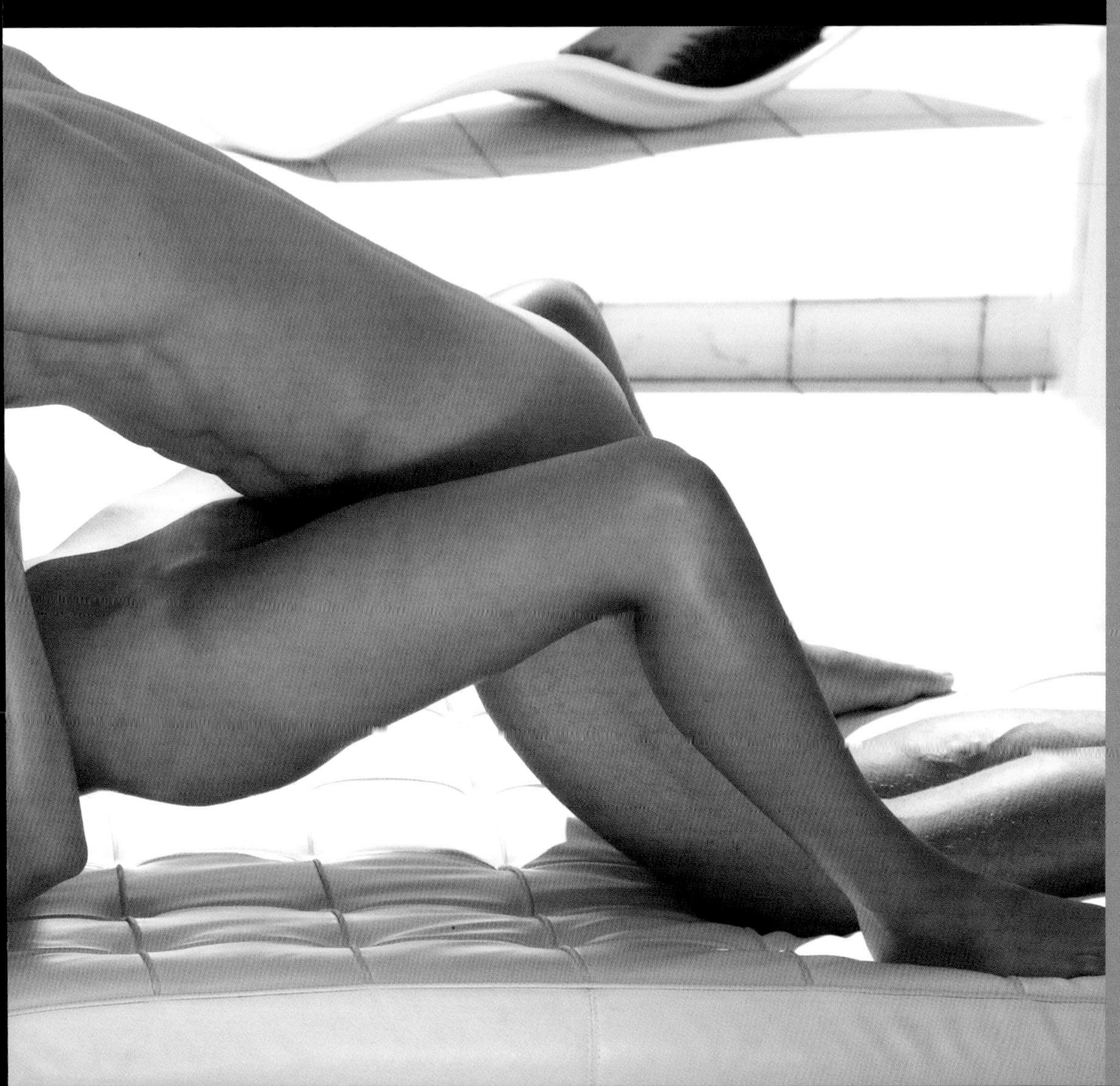

graceful straddle

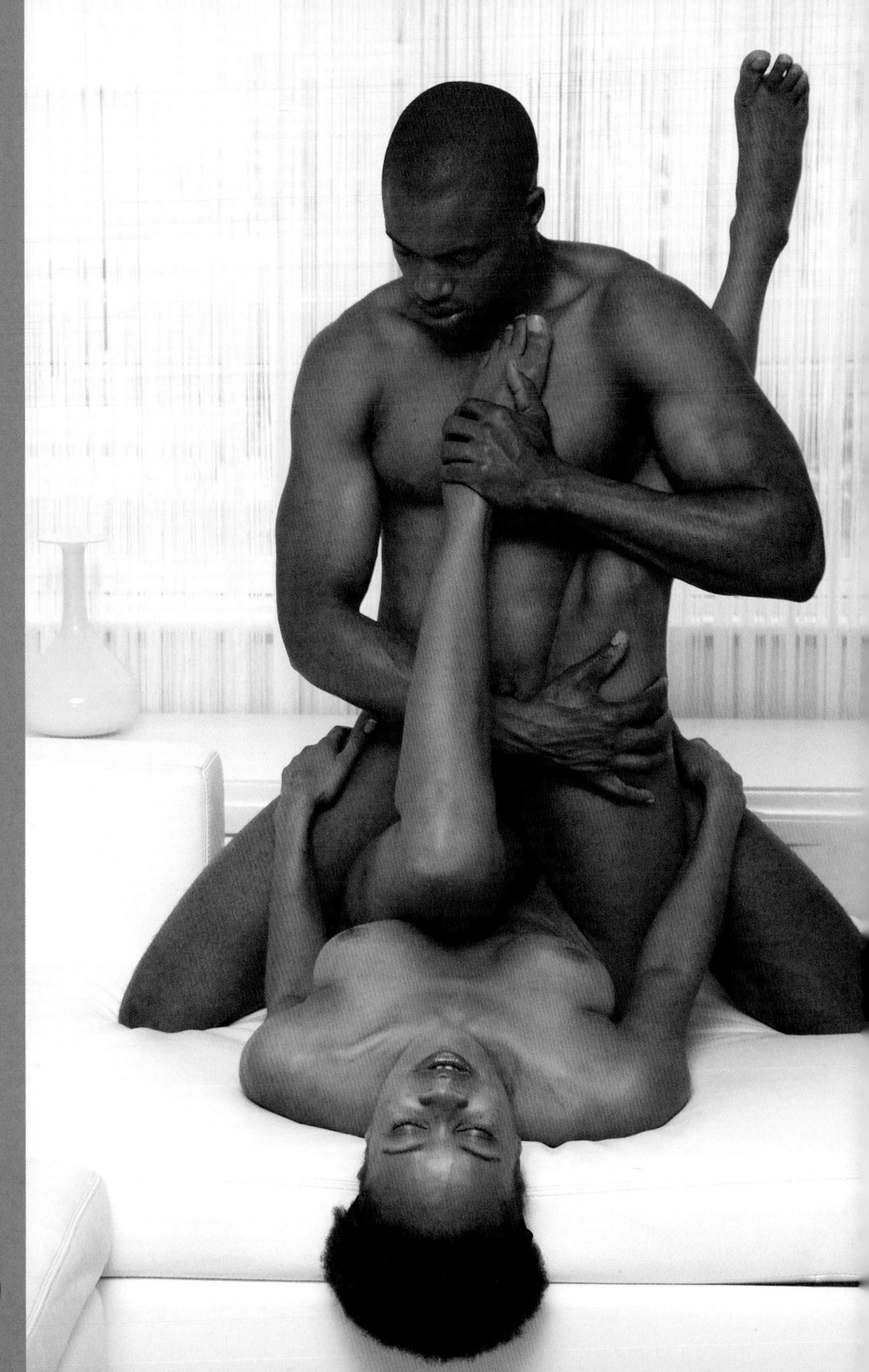

26

target practice

Elegant and balletic, this position looks splendidly choreographed but it is actually quite easy. She lies on her back and he kneels in front. Hanging on to his thighs for balance, she bends one knee, placing the sole of her foot on his chest, and stretches the other leg out as far as she can. He thrusts carefully (the angle is unusual, so experiment with shallow thrusting first).

Her clitoris is in direct contact with his lower stomach. By rolling her pelvis, clitoral stimulation is pretty much guaranteed—and we all know clitoral orgasms are the easiest to come by (so to speak), so that's no small advantage! Her unsupported leg may start to ache, but think about how toned it'll be! Or, alternatively, position yourselves so she can rest her leg against a wall.

the lowdown on lube

Want to improve your sex life dramatically—and instantly? Use lube. Don't just drag it out for intercourse, use it for handjobs, anal play, with sex toys—for everything!

which is best?

✱ Saliva—yours or theirs—is natural and good for everything. Add some to reactivate lube and give it another lease of life.
✱ Hand cream, Vaseline, baby or massage oil, and olive oil work well in movies but aren't so fab in real life. Some eat condoms; others upset the pH balance of vaginal secretions and cause infections. Others are messy and smelly and nearly impossible to get out in the wash.
✱ Water-based lubes feel and look natural and are great all-arounders. They're safe to use with condoms and toys and come in flavored varieties, so you're not gagging if you end up giving oral after applying them. They're nonirritating and don't stain sheets.
✱ Silicone lube is more expensive, but it lasts much longer than water-based lube, which means it's the only choice for anal. Silicone is really slippery and it works in water. Silicone lube sounds like a match made in heaven for silicone sex toys, but, instead, it just damages them. Stick to the water-based variety.

and another thing

✱ Lube makes safe sex safer: a drop inside a condom makes it less likely to tear.
✱ It's crucial to use the right amount. Use too much and you reduce all friction. So add a little, then add a bit more later, if necessary.

sure-thing sex positions

This is for the 70-odd percent of women who can't orgasm without oral sex or masturbation. (If you're one of those lucky women who *can* orgasm purely from penetration, then I'm very pleased for you. OK, and maybe a bit jealous.) As much as orgasms are delicious any way you can get them, it would be nice to have one during intercourse, when he's having one, too.

get real The point of all these sexual positions is to shamelessly up your orgasm quota by using a combination of techniques to hit both internal and external hot spots. Never one to leave much to chance, I'd suggest we hedge our bets by mounting this campaign on two fronts: with words and action. Like, how about we debunk the myth and let him in on the secret, huh? You know, the one about the penis being the almighty satisfier. Because it's... well, just not the case. Be honest. If you can only climax during intercourse when he's stroking your clitoris as well, tell him! Explain that it's not his fault, but that lots of women are built this way and it's just a matter of biology—it has nothing to do with his sexual technique. If he's got a problem, tell him to take it up with God, or failing that, Mother Nature.

educate him Does he know exactly where your clitoris is? Has he had a good look at it in broad daylight? Don't get all shy on me, please! It's dark down there and it's easy for him to lose his bearings as you change positions. I'm not suggesting that you should lie down spread-eagle on the kitchen table just as your neighbor drops by for coffee, but it is a good idea to have the lights on when he's giving you oral sex. Get him onside and clued up, then try your luck with these...

lie down Zap life into the laziest lying position by going head to toe. This one's simple as can be. He lies on his back. Facing his feet, straddle his hips and lower yourself onto his erect penis. Then extend your legs backward and lower your torso down until your feet are next to his head and you're lying on top of him. You're facing one way; he's facing the other. His feet are near your head; your feet are near his. Try slow thrusting, so you can feel every inch of his penis as it slides slowly back and forth.

For a different type of clitoral stimulation, slide off him for a second, look him straight in the... feet (i.e., feel free to fantasize like crazy!), and use your hand to slide the head of his penis up and down to stroke your clitoris. Use your hand (or his) to continue to stimulate your clitoris manually while his penis is inside you—but stop just short of orgasm to let his thrusting trigger off the orgasm itself—and you've done what's officially called the "bridge maneuver." What this does is form a "bridge" between clitoral stimulation (how most women orgasm) and a penetrative orgasm (how men would like them to). Smart girl!

get on top Women who can orgasm through penetration alone generally do it when they're on top. Ask him to sit up, his legs extended out in front of him. Climb on top, cowgirl style, and let him penetrate. Now fall back as far as you can until the top of your head is just resting on the bed. Reach backward until you can grasp his feet. Not only does your tummy look amazingly flat in this position, it's also

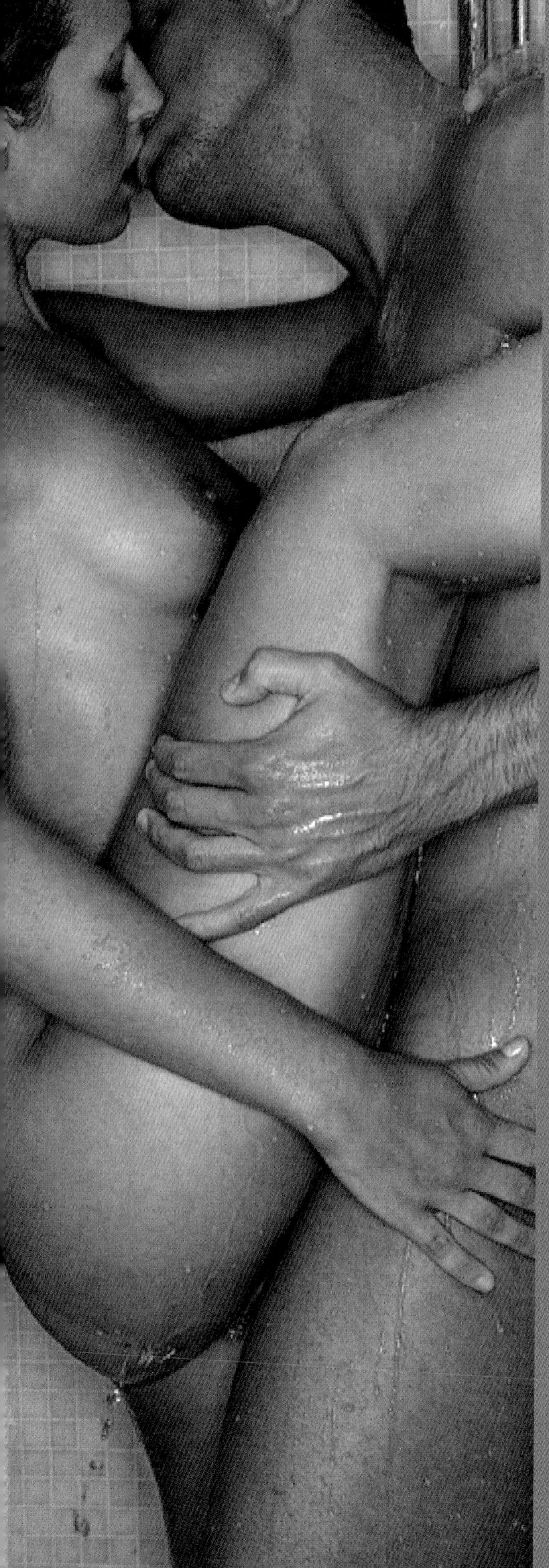

> "This position is bouncy, sexy sex—perfect for teasing."

incredibly easy to turn it into a killer workout if it reminds you that you should be at the gym, rather than lying around having sex.

Instead of straddling him and resting on your knees, squat so your feet are on the bed. Stay leaning forward, then you do all the work—as in thrusting—and the only way to do this is to lift your heels and use those thigh muscles. Whatever, this position is bouncy, sexy sex—perfect for teasing him. Start with a fast up-and-down action before shifting gears and going for wide, circular motions. Will he like it? Excuse me? Your body is on full display so he gets to admire a full-frontal view because this position lays it all right out in front of him! He also gets to watch his penis go in and out, which is always up there on his Things I'd Like to Do Today list. (And the reason why he'll no doubt lose it within seconds.)

turn your back on him The front wall of the vagina is incredibly sensitive, which is why rear-entry feels great for women. Him-from-behind positions alter the angle of the vagina and give him a direct shot at your G-spot. Try to arch your back as far as you can, widening your legs so his penis has perfect access.

Give yourself a helping hand by reaching down to stimulate your clitoris and feel free to fantasize. There's no eye contact, so both of you can fantasize about anyone and anything you like (without feeling guilty when opening one eye to see your partner gazing lovingly at you). The rear-entry position is wonderfully primitive, perfect for those slightly pervy, don't-even-admit-to-your-best-friend type fantasies that suit dirty sex.

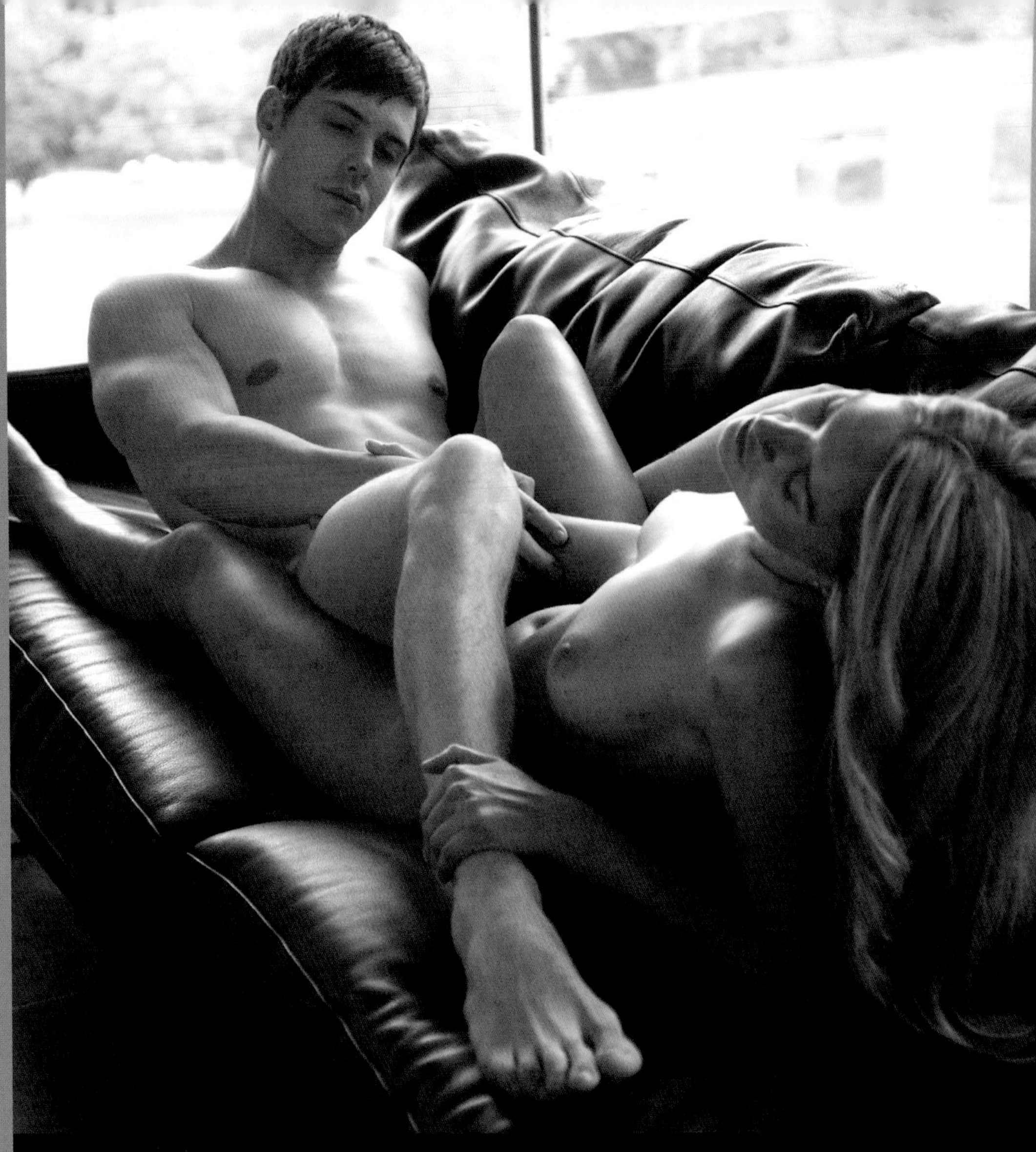

27 lazy crisscross

This position is unusual enough to catch your interest, but also appealing if you're both feeling tired. Lie with your heads at opposite ends, both open your thighs, and move into a scissor position before he penetrates. It's perfect for her to stimulate her clitoris and the scissoring of legs provides pressure on your perineums. The downside is you can't hug, but you need to weigh that up against the excellent, all-over view you get of each other.

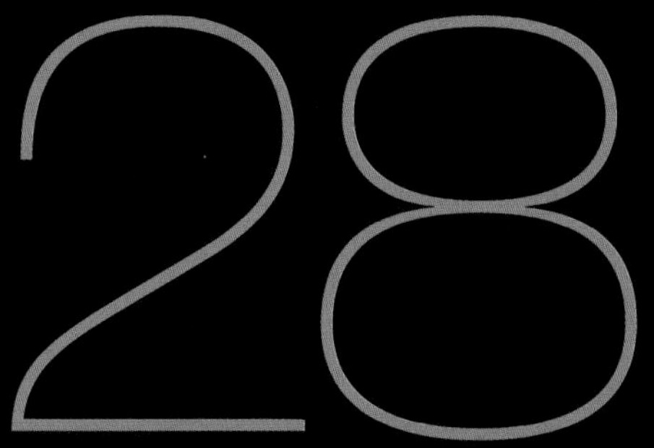

torrid tease

No, he doesn't have a gi-normous penis that is penetrating from that distance! She's provocatively poised in the just-about-to-let-him-penetrate position to ensure that he's at the if-you-don't-let-me-inside-you-I'll-die stage. Tease. Such an innocent word. Such a powerful tool sexually. The *Kama Sutra* is all about waiting until your partner is practically swooning with desire—frothing at the mouth, in fact!—before even thinking about going there. Good plan.

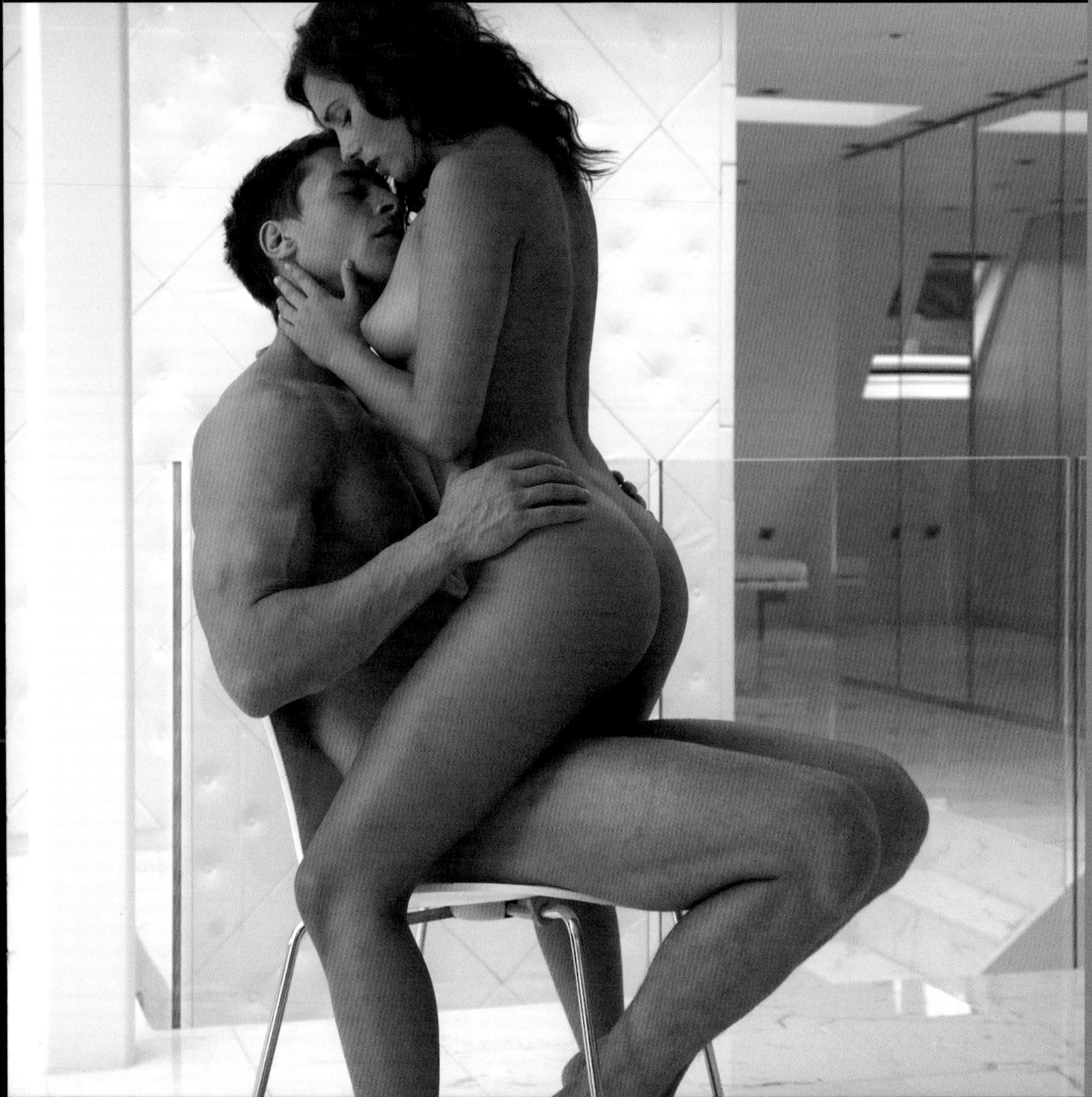

ride 'em cowgirl

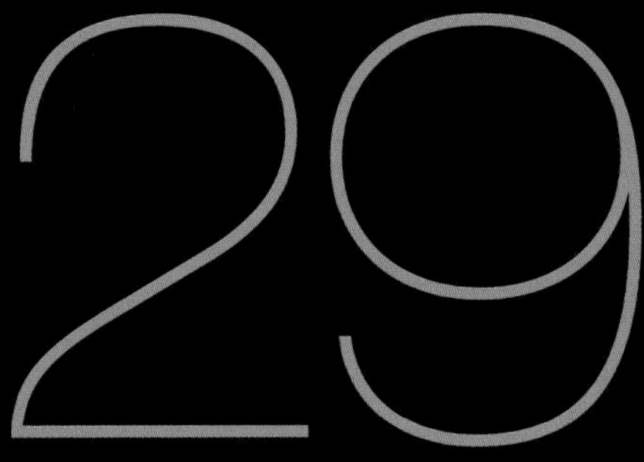

be a better buck

Jump on top and give him the ride of his life, literally milking each moment of this erotic roller coaster. The trick to this one is more about technique than position because it's what's happening on the inside that's more important. This is when all those pain-in-the-ass but oh-so-effective Kegel workouts (see right) come into their own (dreadful pun intended). Because this is when the clench-and-release pelvic-floor pull can pump his penis to orgasm.

Facing away from him, she places her bod in a fabulous fondling position. Start with a strong, girlpower grip and proceed to put on a frisky floorshow by touching your own breasts and clitoris—or get him to reach around and do it himself, if he'd prefer to play rather than watch.

muscle up

The fitter and more toned her pelvic-floor muscles, the greater the sensation for both of you. The vagina grips the penis tightly—better for him and intensifying her orgasms. These workouts increase arousal by improving blood flow to the pelvic area and upping lubrication.

the workout

- To develop a vicelike vagina, you need to train. The joy of female PC contractions (unlike male ones) is that you can feel if you're doing them correctly and/or improving by putting a finger you-know-where.
- Sit or lie down and insert two fingers into your vagina up to the second knuckle, then squeeze hard. Feel anything? A slight contraction means they're working, a good old squeeze means you're in good shape. (Don't panic if you feel nothing at all—you will after a week or two of exercising them.)
- Breathe in and relax the area around your vagina and anus. Breathe out and draw up the area until you feel a lifting sensation.
- Repeat 10–20 times, 3–4 times a day.

make it harder

- Repeat the above, but now hold each squeeze for 10 seconds.
- Alternate these slow sets with fast ones, by squeezing and releasing as fast as you can.
- During intercourse, squeeze and relax to "milk" the penis. But save some strength for when he's happy to orgasm, because that's when you squeeze hard.

countdown to a fab first time

You're about to get naked with someone new and trying to convince yourself it's no big deal. You've done "it" before—lots of times—so how come you feel so... well, utterly petrified! If, other than your ex, no one but the cat has seen you in your birthday suit in the last decade, keep reading...

on your mark... Thinking someone's awfully sweet/drop-dead gorgeous does not mean you won't wake up with an awfully painful not-so-gorgeous blister on your what-not, so think about contraception and safer sex.

Do it when you feel ready, not because of the silly "three date rule" thing or because your friends say you should. Take your time and get to know each other first. Then, once you're ready, set the scene—too much styling and it'll look contrived, but you can make sure there are clean, crisp sheets on the bed.

get set... Penetrative sex is often the most frightening part for both of you because: a) her "good girl" dilemmas rush to the fore; and b) he requires an erection to do it. The more time you spend easing into it, the better. It gives his penis time to get past the shyness stage, plus, if he's still calling after pretty intense petting/oral sessions, she'll be reassured he's not just in it for the sex.

Remember, sex isn't an exam. You're not going to be graded pass or fail (and if it feels like you are, you're with the wrong person). So stop stressing and thinking "This has got to be perfect." Sex is supposed to be fun! If it feels like you're about to take your driving test, talk about it. Say, "I've been waiting so long for this moment, but I so want it to be right." If you're with the right person, they'll instantly jump in with reassurances. Perfect sex only happens on the soaps; normal people muddle through the first time.

"Sex isn't an exam—you're not going to be graded pass or fail."

go... If you're self-conscious, dim the lights or take your clothes off under the sheets. Now show how much you want them because sincerity is sexy. Let them know that, even if their technique isn't perfect, you're being sent to heaven simply by the fact that it's their hand/penis/tongue touching you. Don't feel you have to perform like a show pony. Working your way through an entire repertoire—ice cubes, chocolate sauce, acrobatic positions—will only make you look like you're trying too hard. The slightly pervy/kinky/intense stuff can wait a little while. I'm not suggesting you both stick to the missionary position (although it does tend to be the most favored position for first-time sex). But, aside from not knowing the other person well enough to define what they think is "kinky" and what will freak them out, what's the rush?

How you cope with a less-than-perfect performance can set the trend for your relationship. Even if the sex is disastrous, laugh it off, snuggle up, and say "Oh well, we'll do better next time." And resist the urge to ask "How did I do?" Remind yourself that the really, really good sex invariably happens four to six sessions in. Try not to panic about it or the relationship (that's what next-day phone calls to friends are for).

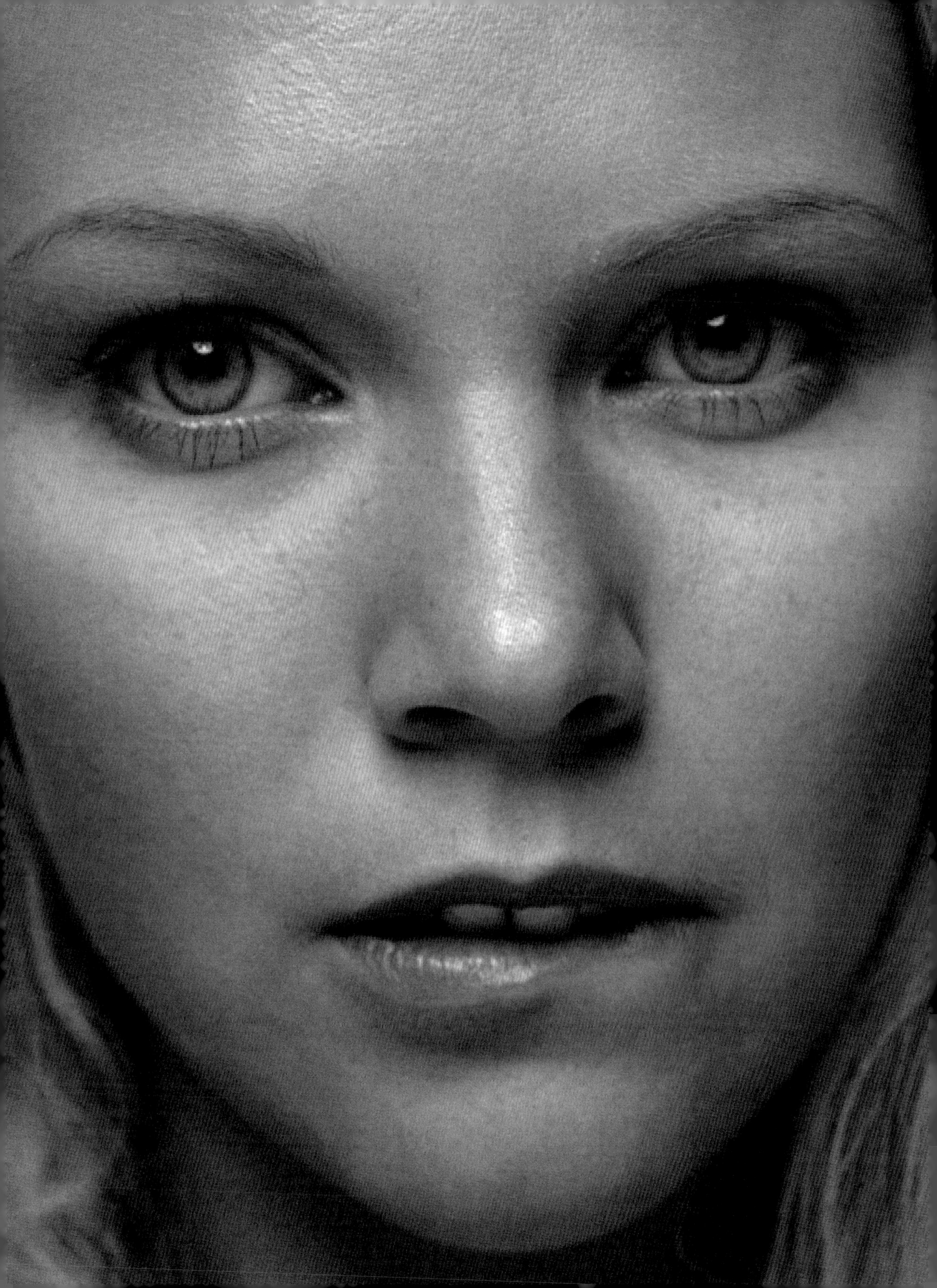

30

elephant

Animalistic, primitive, and positioned to hit supersensitive spots, this one puts him in charge of her pleasure. According to the *Kama Sutra*, if you're looking for new, exciting ways to make love, look no further than the animal kingdom.

This position is inspired by the mating of elephants (except you won't have to laboriously mount with a penis of that size!). She lies on her front on the bed, pressing her thighs together, rather than apart. She can lift her upper torso off the bed to get closer to him or lie flat. He penetrates from behind, supporting his weight on his arms, straddling the outside of her thighs. There's no clitoral stimulation for her, but he'll hit the sensitive front vaginal wall, so there's a greater chance of a vaginal/G-spot orgasm. The higher she tilts her bottom, the more directly he'll hit the front vaginal wall.

This and all rear-entry positions score high on most people's "must-do" list because they're fantastic for indulging dirty fantasies—that don't necessarily include your partner. You're free to pretend that your partner is whoever you want him or her to be!

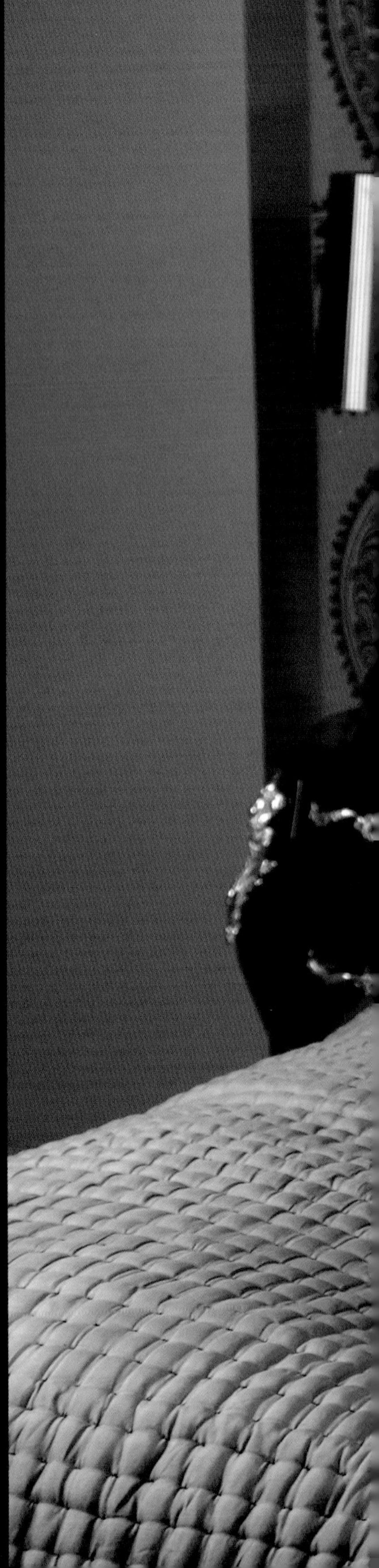

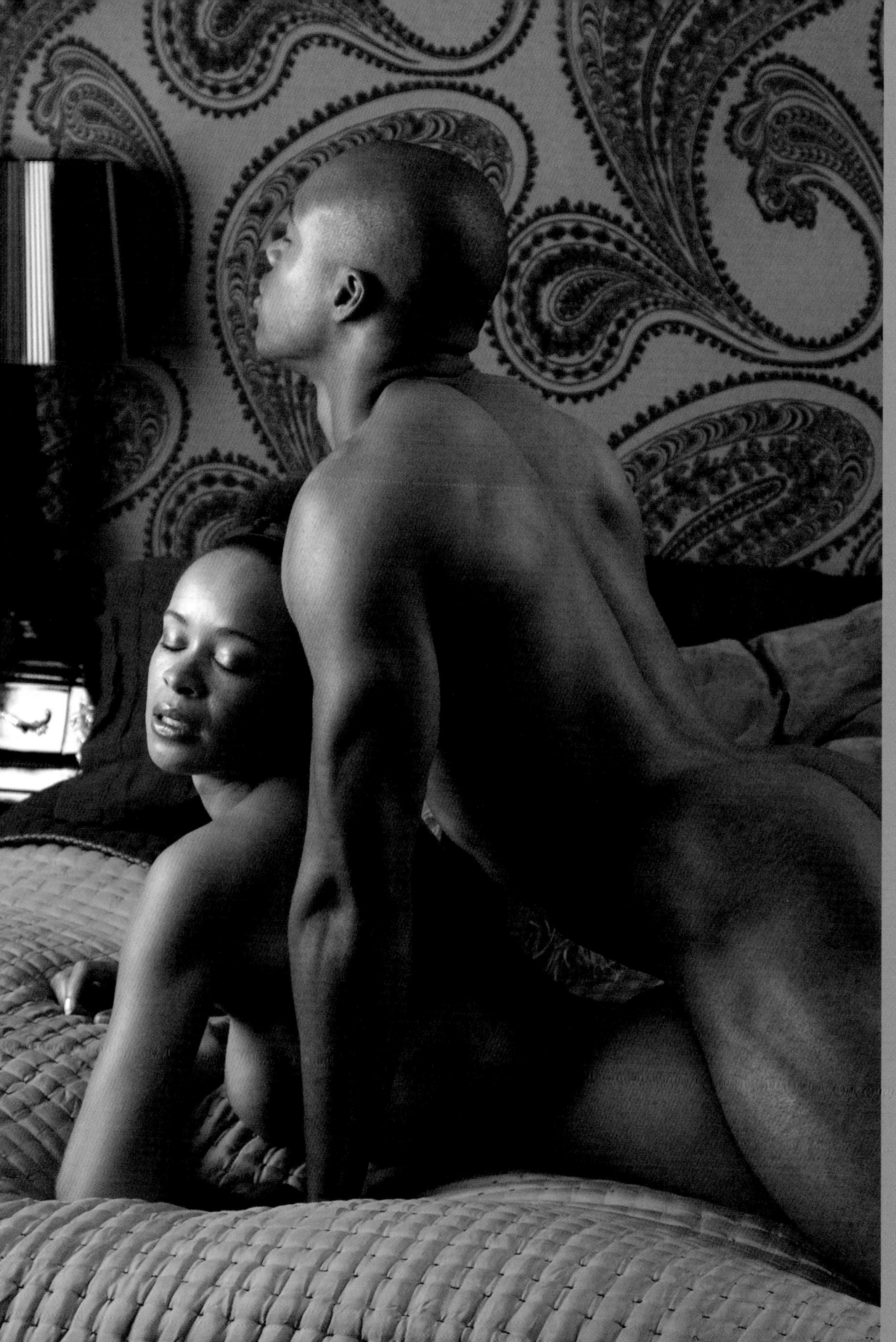

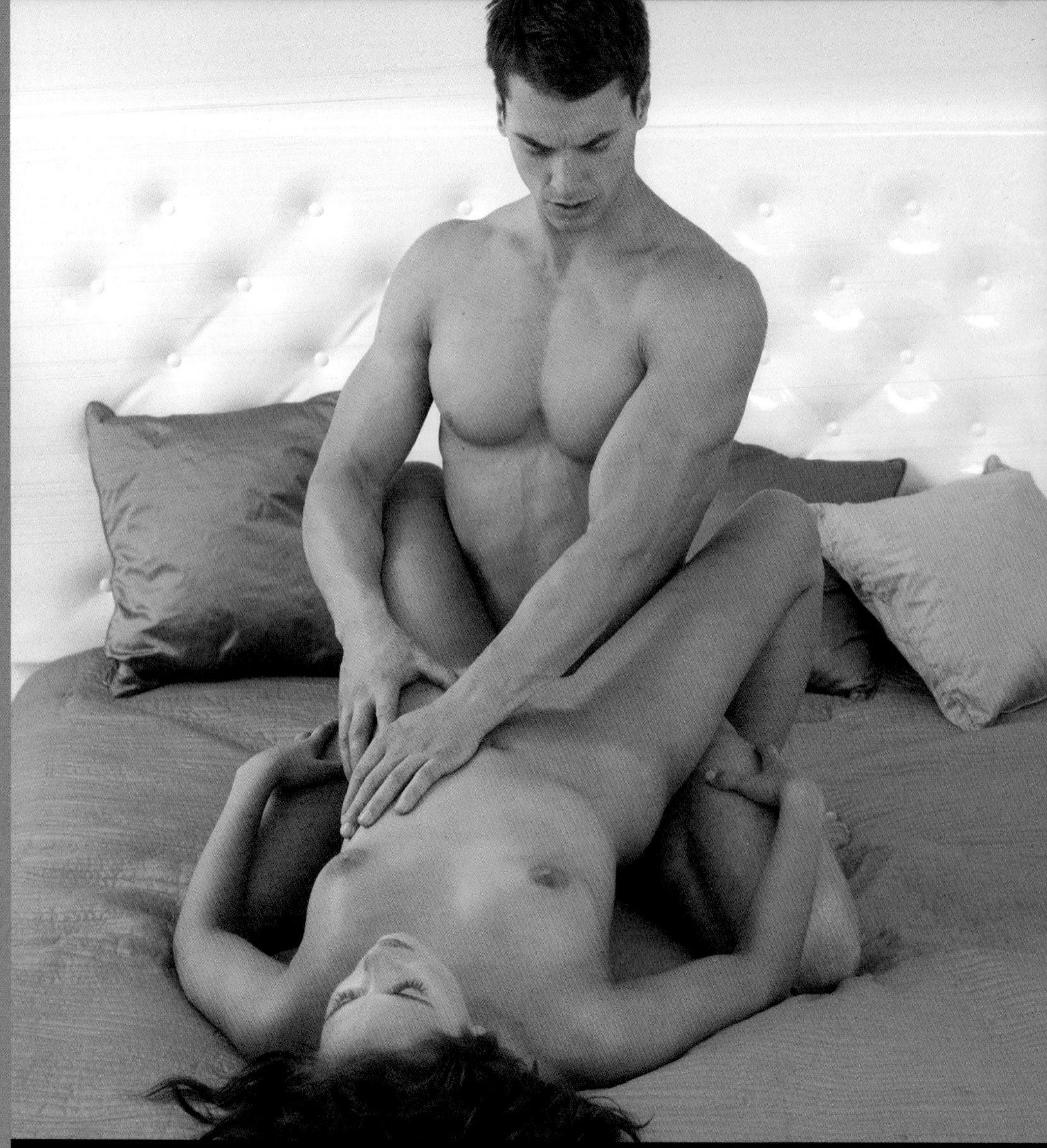

31 mission possible

This is a twist on the standard missionary position that makes it way more comfortable for him because he doesn't have to support his own weight on his elbows. Another bonus: he gets a fabulous view of her bod and complete control over his thrusting. She can vary the sensation on her end by opening her legs wide or wrapping them around his waist. For deep penetration, she can pull her knees up to her chin and put her feet on his shoulders.

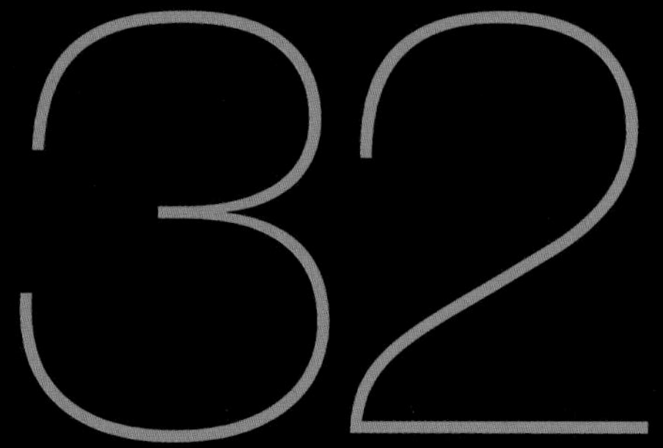

best for big boys

She lies on her back and he kneels in front between her legs. She then lifts her bottom, allowing him to enter. He pulls her toward him, she reaches down to hold her ankles as he supports her by holding her hips. If she's flexible enough to take a firm hold, she can hold her legs open far wider. This is a good position if he has a big penis and she has a small vagina (both a bit smug, are we?). She's opened wide and by raising her hips, he's pushed deep inside.

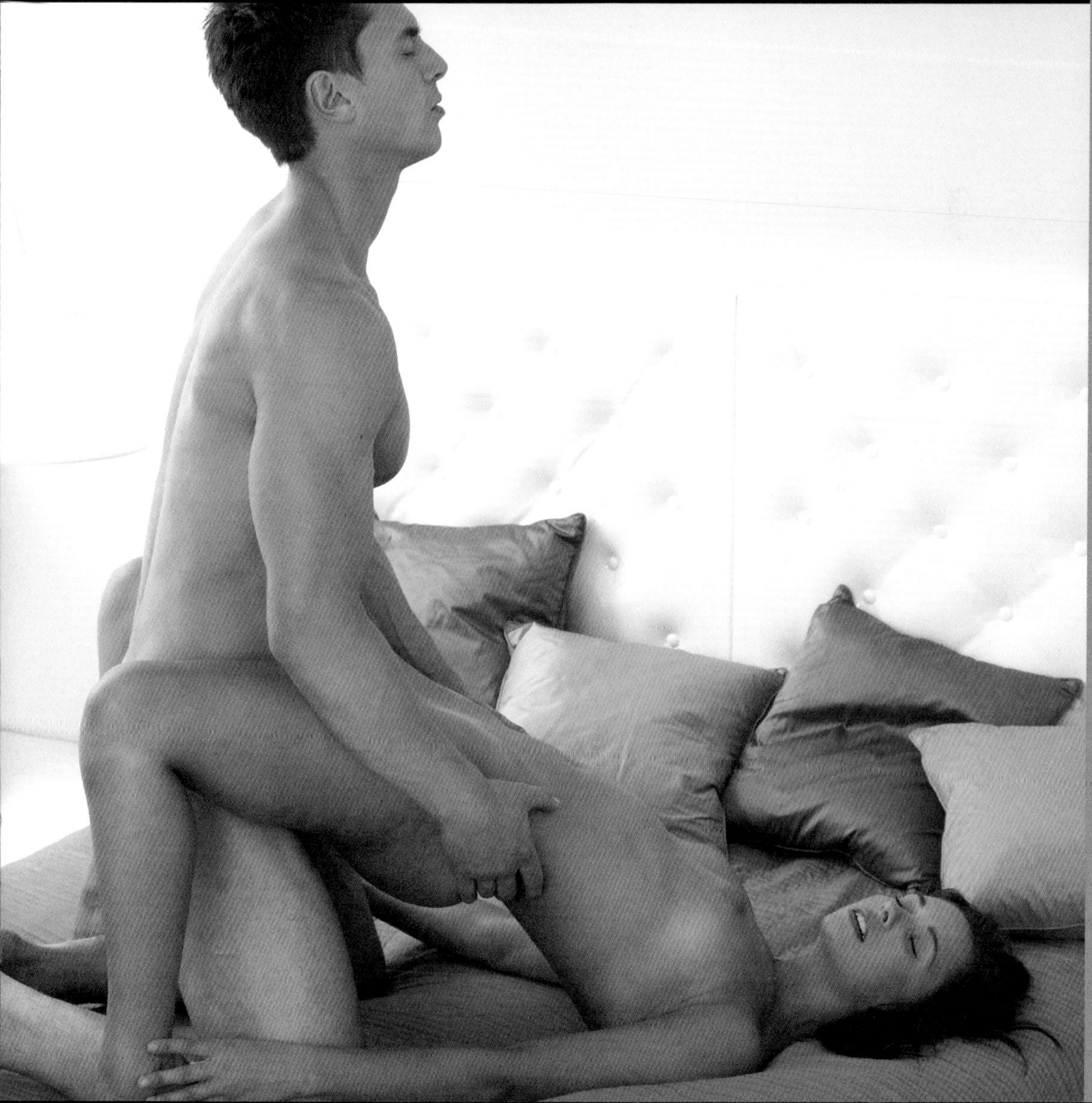

female superior

1 She sits opposite him, with her legs over his thighs. Embrace but don't start any funny stuff just yet—you're simply settling into some slow, sweet necking as you both arouse each other fully in preparation for some good old-fashioned rutting.

2 He lifts his legs up until they rest on her shoulders and now penetrates. She lays her hands on the top of his lower legs and waits… pushing herself forward into this wonderfully dominant role.

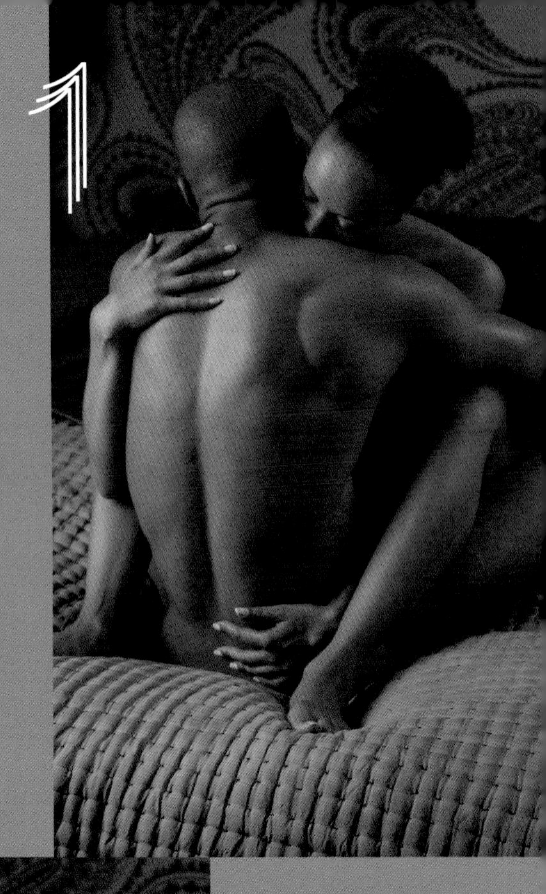

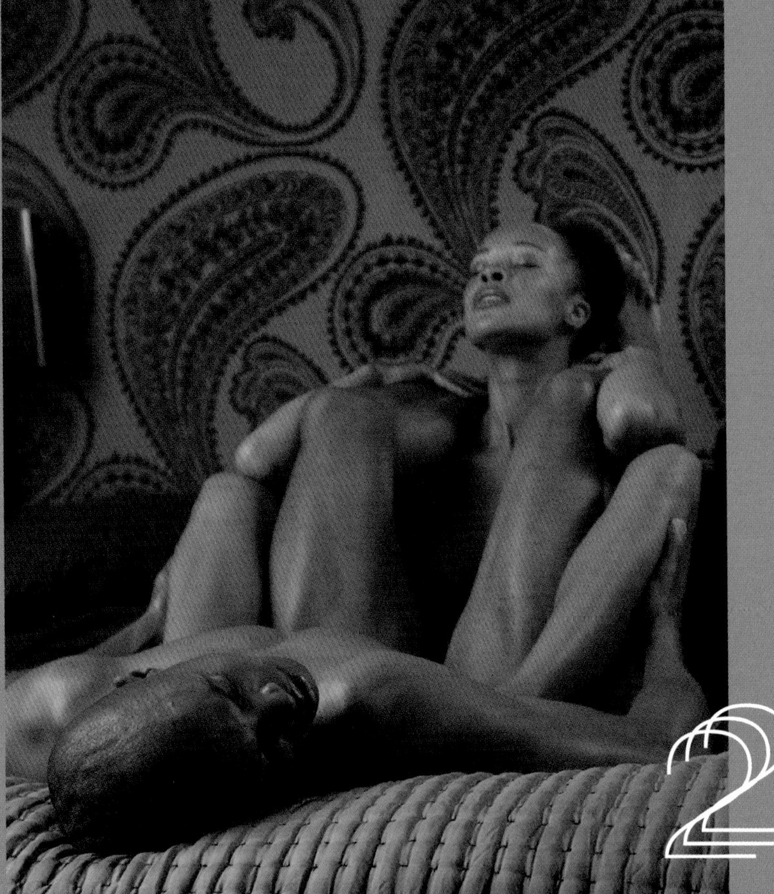

33

3 She's now in the "male" position, while he gives in to her wickedly wanton ways and becomes vulnerable. Still struggling to figure out how penetration happens? Well, I struggled with this one (or my boyfriend did, anyway). My (boastful) best friend, however, managed it no problem with hers (you can guess what that means!). But penetration isn't always the object with spiritualists, who're more concerned with where the mind and imagination are traveling, rather than with your you know whats.

3

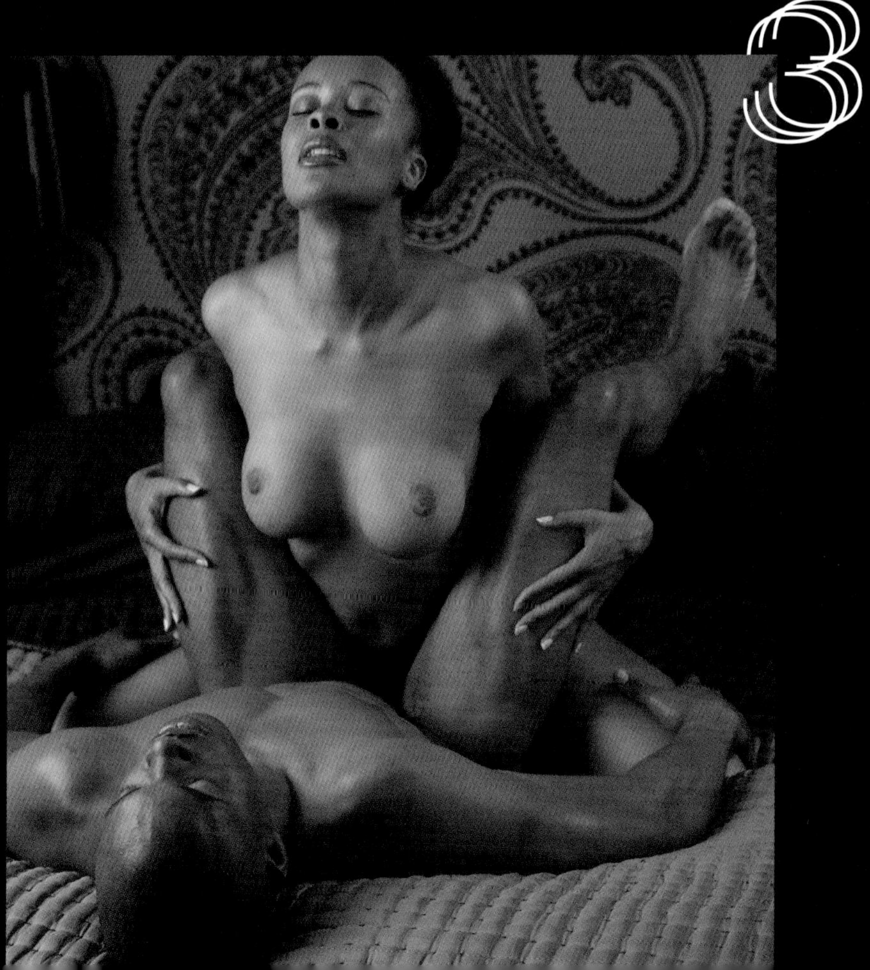

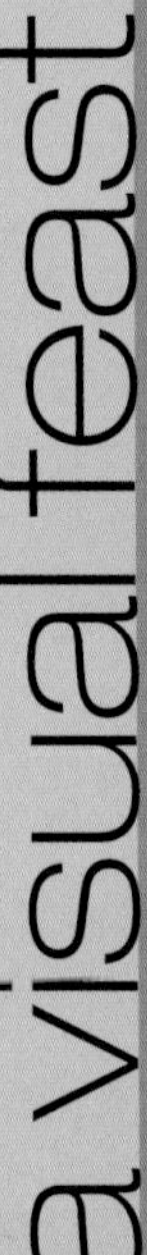
a visual feast

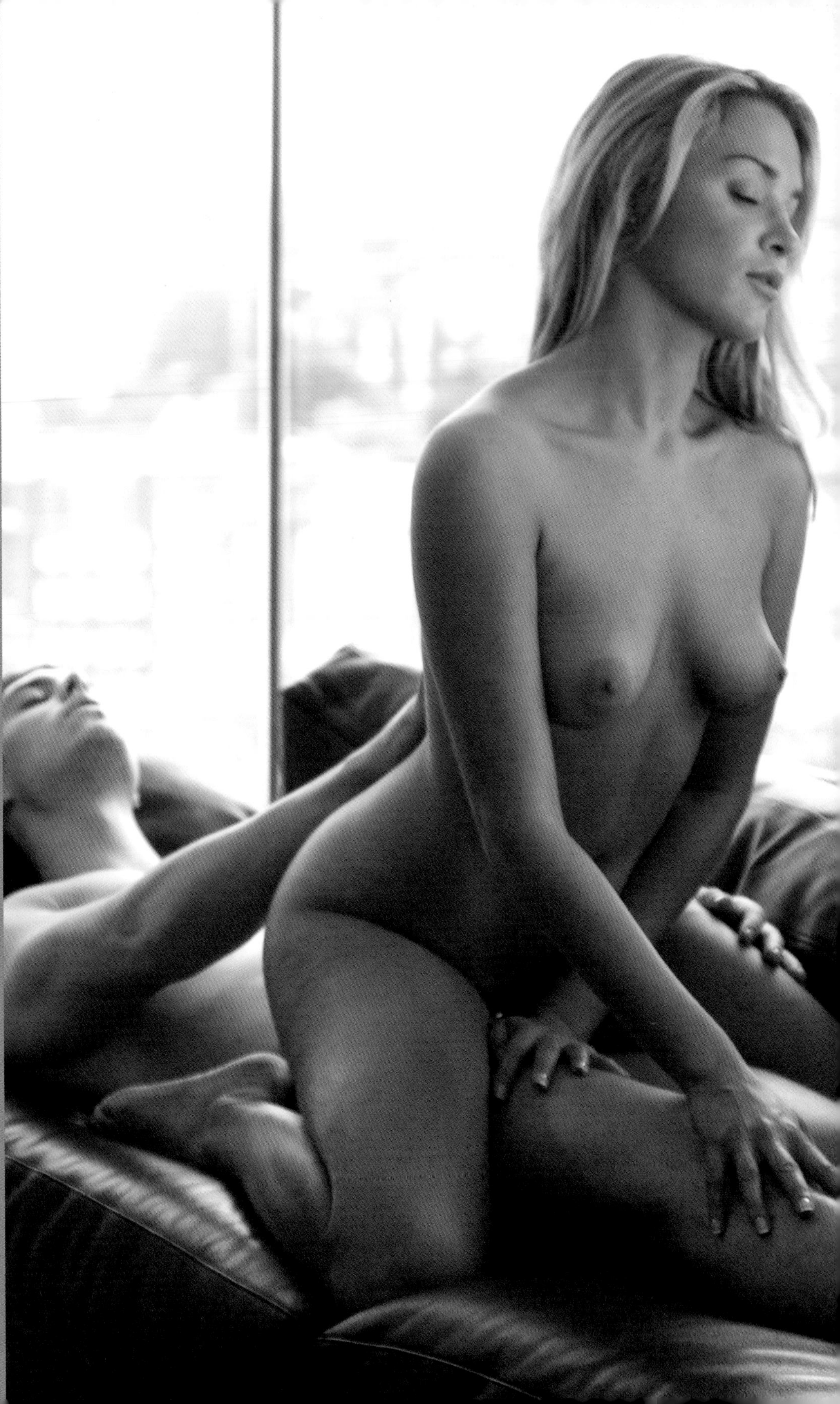

34

rock-a-bye baby

He lies back, she faces his feet and lowers herself onto his penis, with knees bent and calves folded back toward him. She leans onto his thighs for support—he lies back and relishes the steamy sight of her bottom lifting up and down and swinging from side to side before him. This one's more for him than her, because there's a visual feast for him, but little in the way of clitoral stimulation. On the other hand, turning him on so much is a huge turn-on for her!

Now, face-to-face contact means you can feel but not see your partner, adding an erotic "anonymous" edge. She can either sit up or—if she's feeling a bit pervy—lean forward, resting her weight on her hands to expose both her vulva and anus. But be careful: leaning forward too enthusiastically will leave both of you feeling oddly empty. That'll be because his penis has popped out!

given up on your G-spot?

A lot of the positions in this book deliberately aim his penis for a direct hit to the front vaginal wall, supposed home of the "G-spot." If you've tried but failed to find anything up there that feels even vaguely good, you might want to give a specially designed G-spot vibrator a try. Use it to pinpoint your hot zone and it'll be easier to angle him to hit the right spot during intercourse.

the cheat's way

* The curved tip of the G-spot vibe points toward your top wall. Don't move it in and out of your vagina like you might a normal penetrative vibe; instead, make a rocking motion so it starts to feel like a firm massage.
* If your vibe has a ball at each end, hold it by one of them, insert it, then use your grip on that ball to roll the other ball (the one inside you) from side to side. If you like the sensation, try using your G-spot vibe while he's licking you. Don't be surprised if you need clitoral stimulation as well as G-spot stimulus to orgasm—it's not unusual.

a helping hand

* Further intensify your orgasm by getting him to press down lightly on your lower abdomen while the G-vibe's in there. This provides extra pressure on the "back side" of the G-spot (this also works during intercourse or when his fingers are inside you as well).

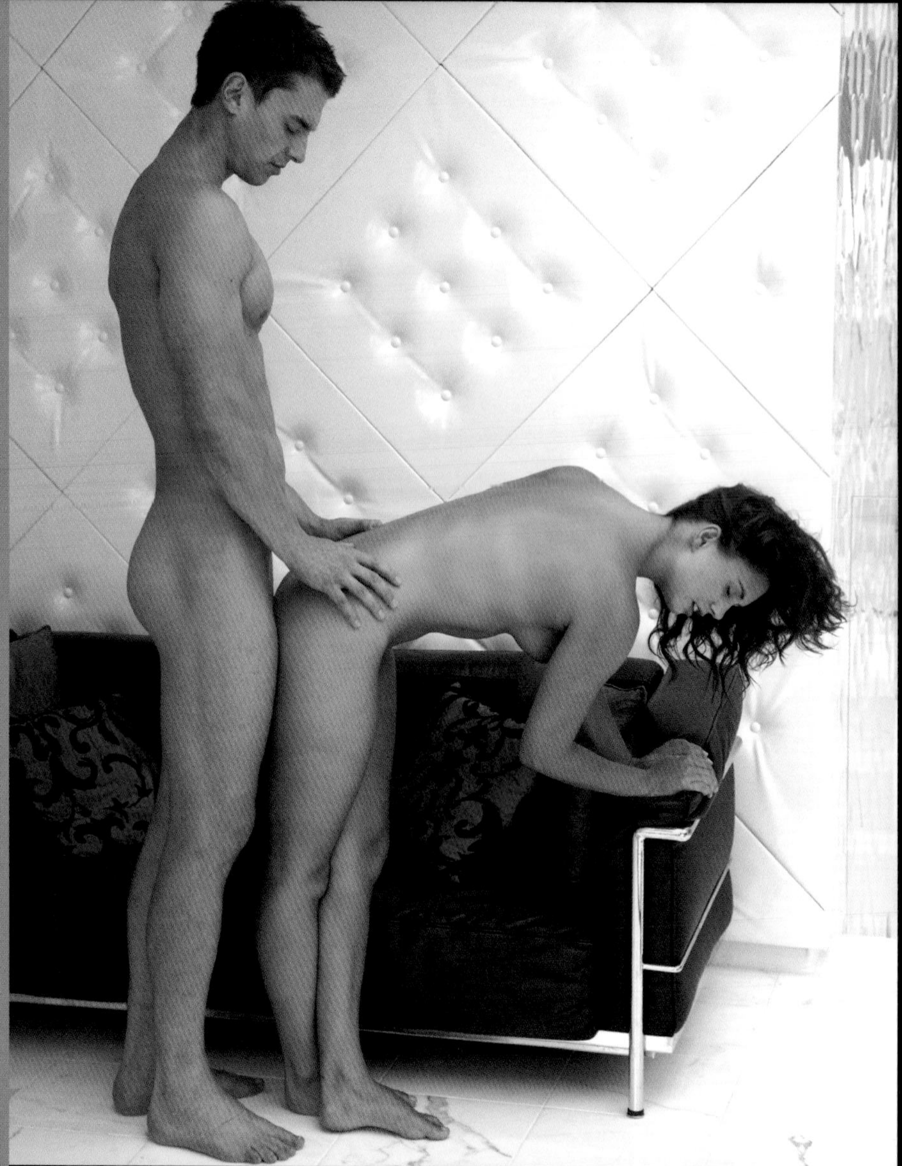

35 the bendover

It's an elegant version of rear entry that feels fabulous for both of you. He penetrates from behind, she leans forward, holding onto a piece of furniture for support. Crossing her ankles keeps things tantalizingly tight and by squeezing her vaginal and buttock muscles around his penis, she can up the sensation even further. It's versatile, too, since you don't really need props, other than something for her to hold onto.

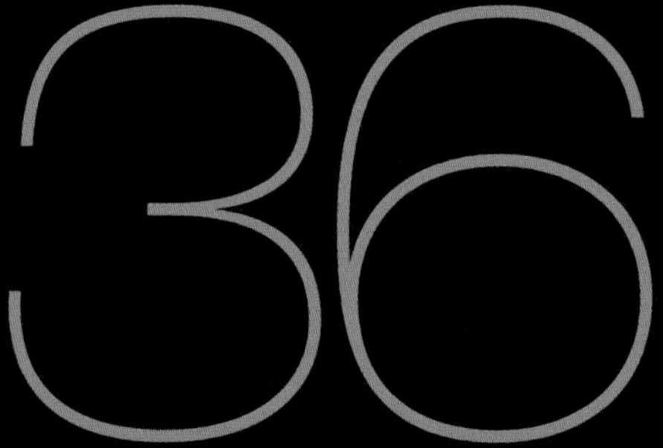

side saddle

She's still on top but sitting side-saddle, which alters the angle of the vagina, providing a fresh, new feeling for both of you. Granted, it's hard for her to move but he can, by pushing up his hips. Instead, she sits back and looks beautiful in this body-flattering pose. It's traditional name is "The Swan," because this position is graceful and reminiscent of a swan gliding elegantly across still waters.

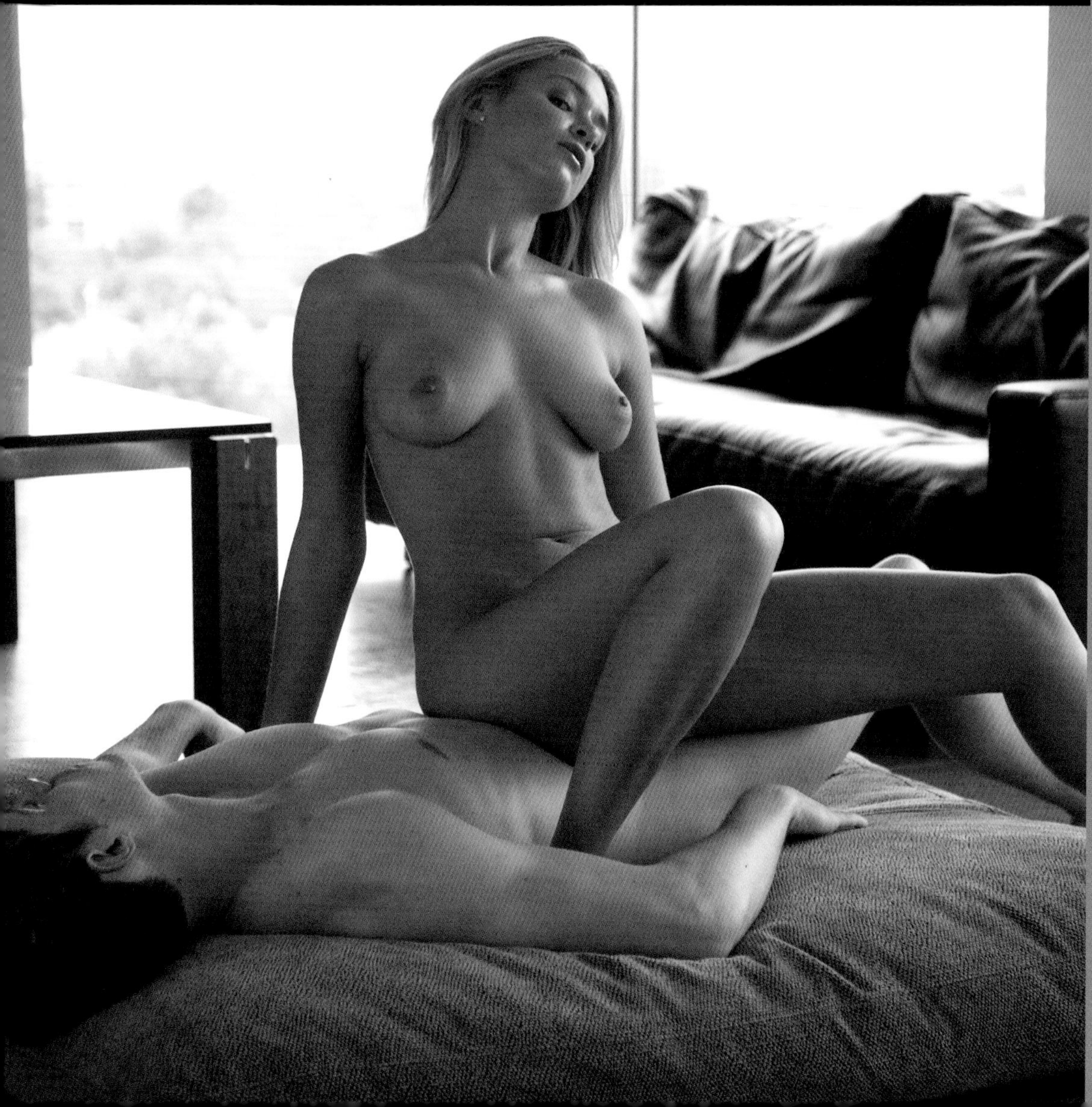

37 the rock 'n' roller

Switch to the CAT (Coital Alignment Technique) and you'll double her chances of climaxing—and slow him down by about the same rate. A winning combination! It's slightly harder work than the "pumping" style of thrusting and takes practice, but give it a try...

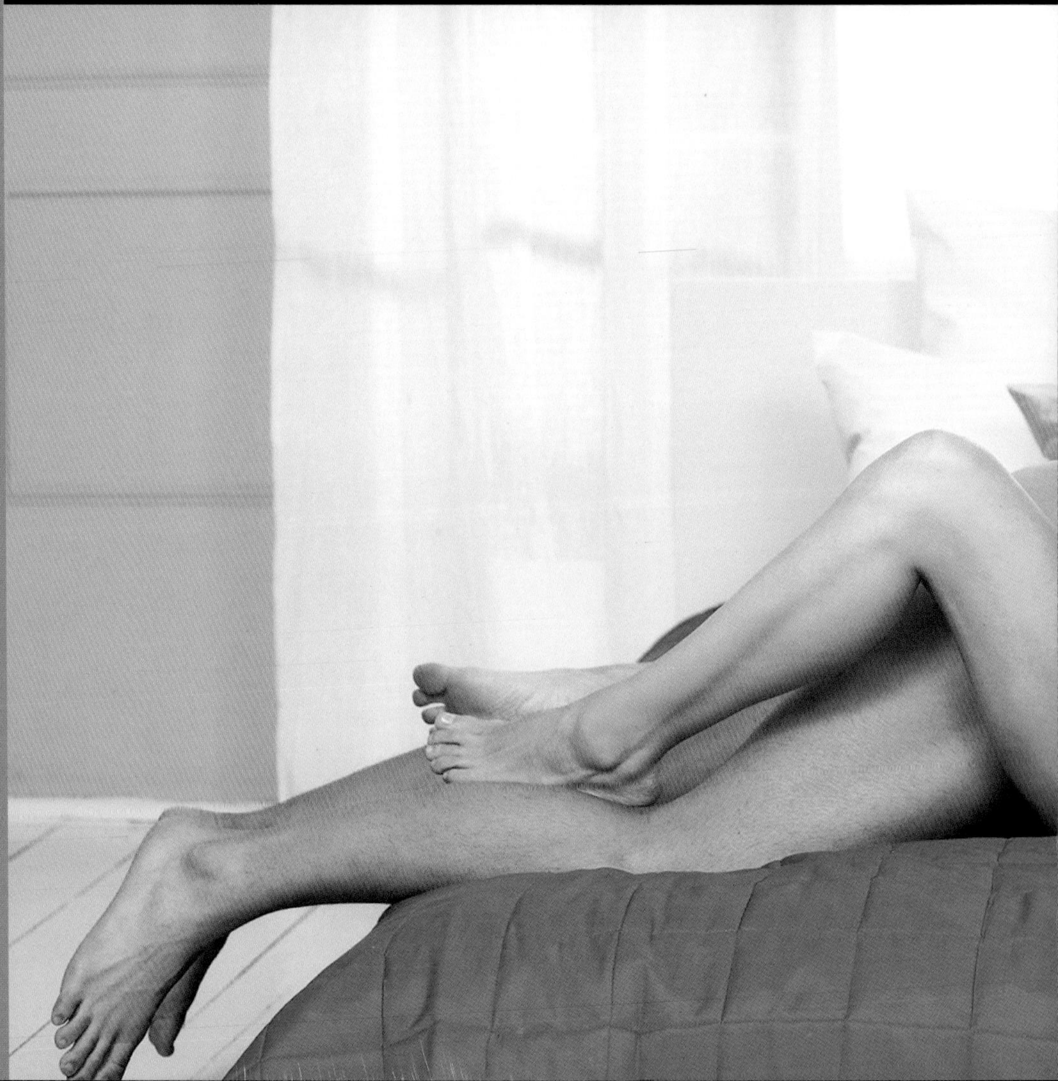

He's on top of her but riding high, his body moved up toward her head, and he's close rather than holding himself up on his arms. The pelvises are close, so the base of his penis rubs against her clitoris and stays there as they move together. Picture an even-paced rocking-chair movement: she

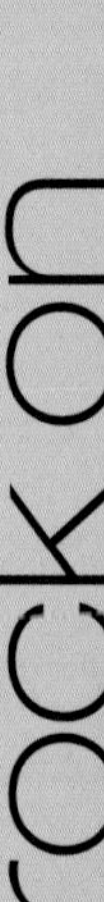

leads in the upward stroke, pushing up and forward to force his pelvis backward. He forces her pelvis backward and downward. It's pressure and counter-pressure, not thrusting, with deep, not shallow, penetration.

Yes, it's complicated. You have to think very much "outside the box" to stop from doing something that's become second nature after years, so while some devotees don't have intercourse any other way after mastering it, most couples (sensibly, I think) only use it when they're feeling particularly energized and motivated.

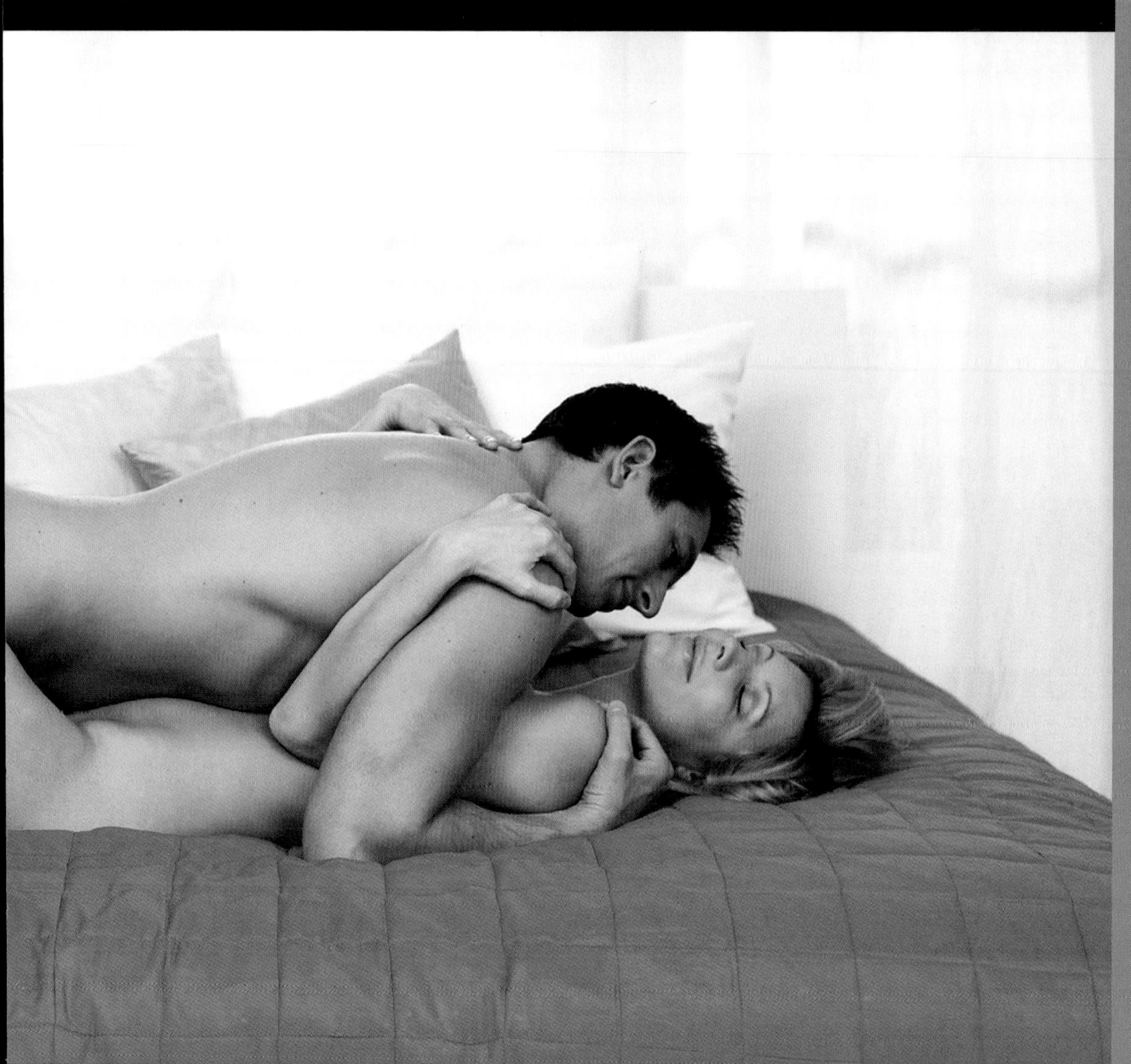

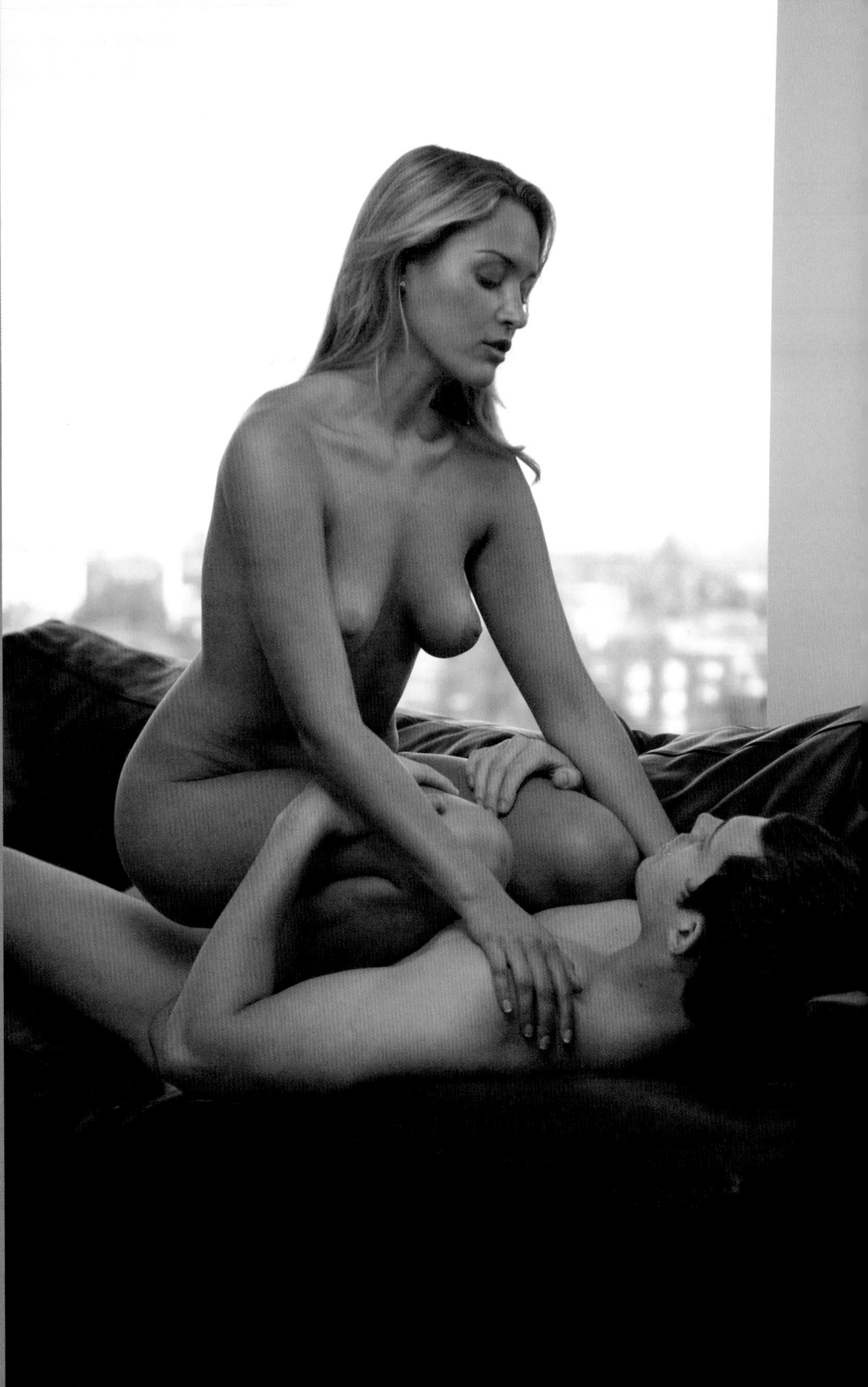

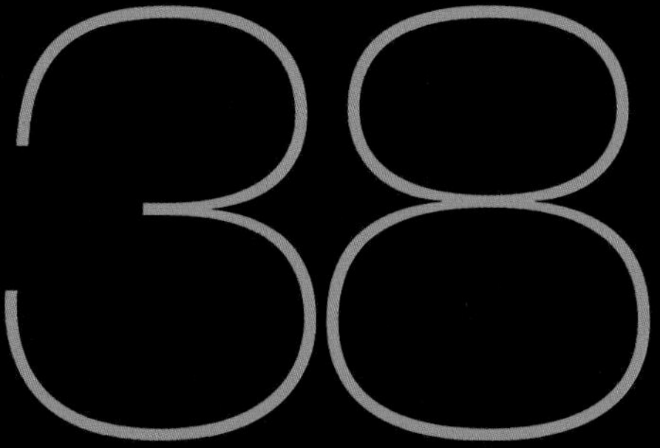

she comes first

A twist on the usual her on top, here she sits astride him with her knees and calves supported and squats rather than kneels. Not as comfortable—but it's far easier to move. Which means she's in charge of satisfying herself.

This sounds like effort, but so isn't, and it's a strong theme of all my books. The reason why sex works best if she's in charge is that it's easy for her to rub herself against him, back and forth, providing much-needed friction on the clitoris. Assuming her thighs can take the pace, she's in control of how deep he goes, the angle he penetrates, and how fast and hard he pumps.

intercourse orgasms

So all girls climax through penetration, huh? And pigs can fly. In fact, only 30 percent of women can reach orgasm without additional stimulation. But you've got a much better chance if you're highly aroused before he penetrates.

to tip you over...

* Get him to penetrate immediately after an orgasm that he's given you with his hands or mouth. This can sometimes set off another wave of contractions and some women orgasm more easily the second time around.
* Get him to use his fingers on your clitoris (use lots of lube) and bring you almost to the point of orgasm. He then quickly penetrates and continues using his fingers on you after he has, with only a few seconds' break.
* After he penetrates, move immediately into a girl-friendly thrusting style (rock or roll with full contact of the pelvis) or grind pelvises. If you're intent on sticking with traditional "pump-style" thrusting, get him to aim for your G-spot and cross your fingers.

if all else fails...

* Get out her vibrator. Either hold a small finger vibe or classic vibe on your clitoris while he's penetrated, get him to wear a vibrating penis ring, or consider a wearable vibe like the butterfly or "We-Vibe" that stays on during intercourse (see page 98).

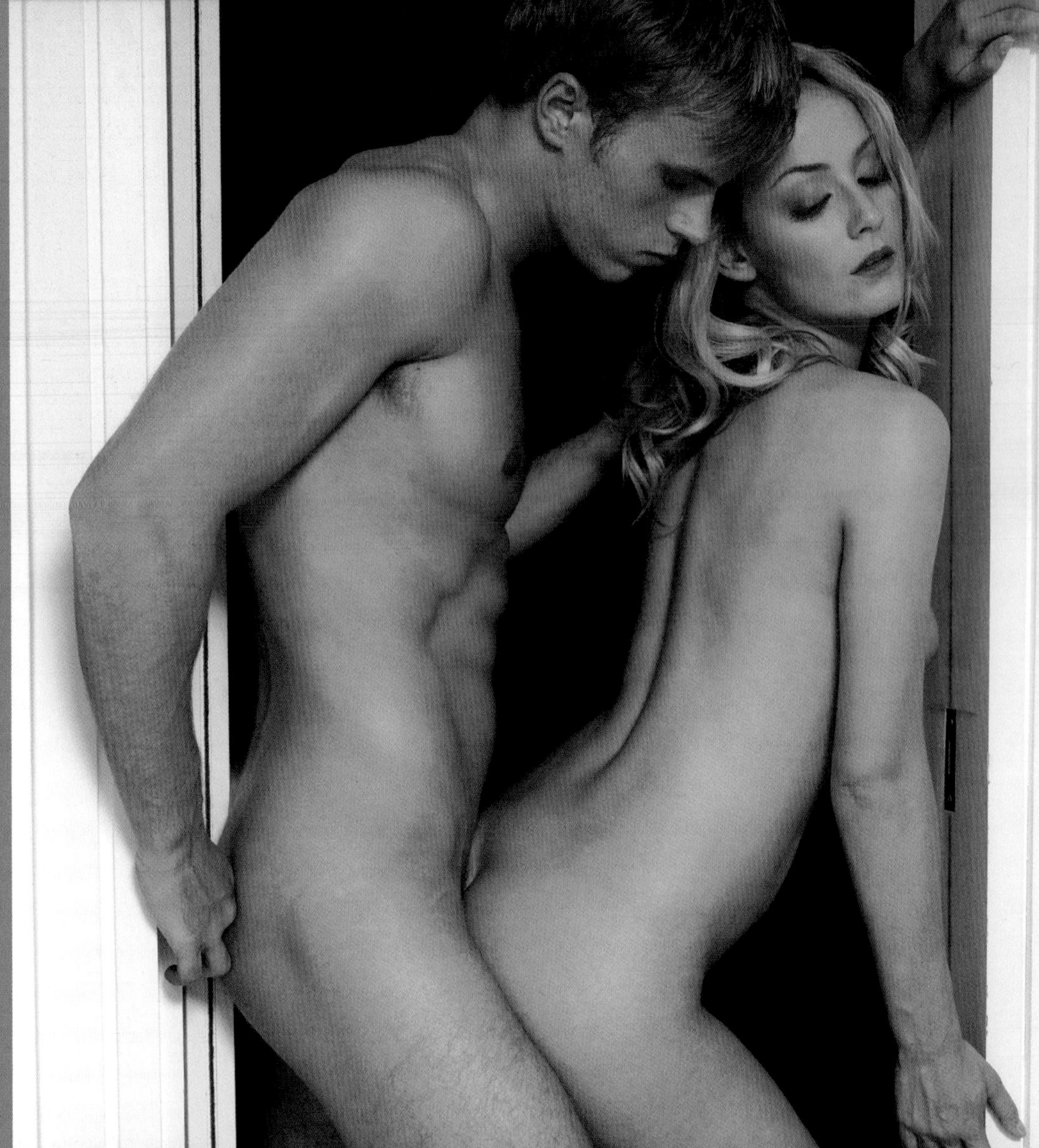

39

doorknobbing

Where you're having sex is almost as important as who you're having it with. Move the mundane missionary to the bathroom floor and suddenly it becomes more primitive than killing a beast with your bare hands. You've probably christened each room, but what about the doorways? He leans against the doorframe, she backs onto him, pushing her bottom high in the air. Look at every space, surface, and item of furniture in your house as a possible place to have sex improvise.

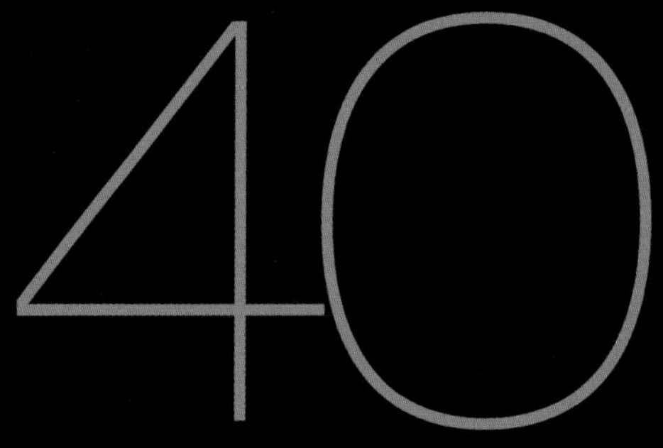

the cave

Not one for girls who find touching their toes a challenge—rubber, supple, s-t-r-e-t-c-h-e-d limbs are a necessity. Usual thrusting is impossible; instead, rock in a seesaw motion. With legs closed, the vaginal canal becomes invitingly narrow; she spreads her legs for wider access and deeper penetration. The Cave is great for men with short penises because it raises, tilts, and exposes the vulva, making it feel better for both of you.

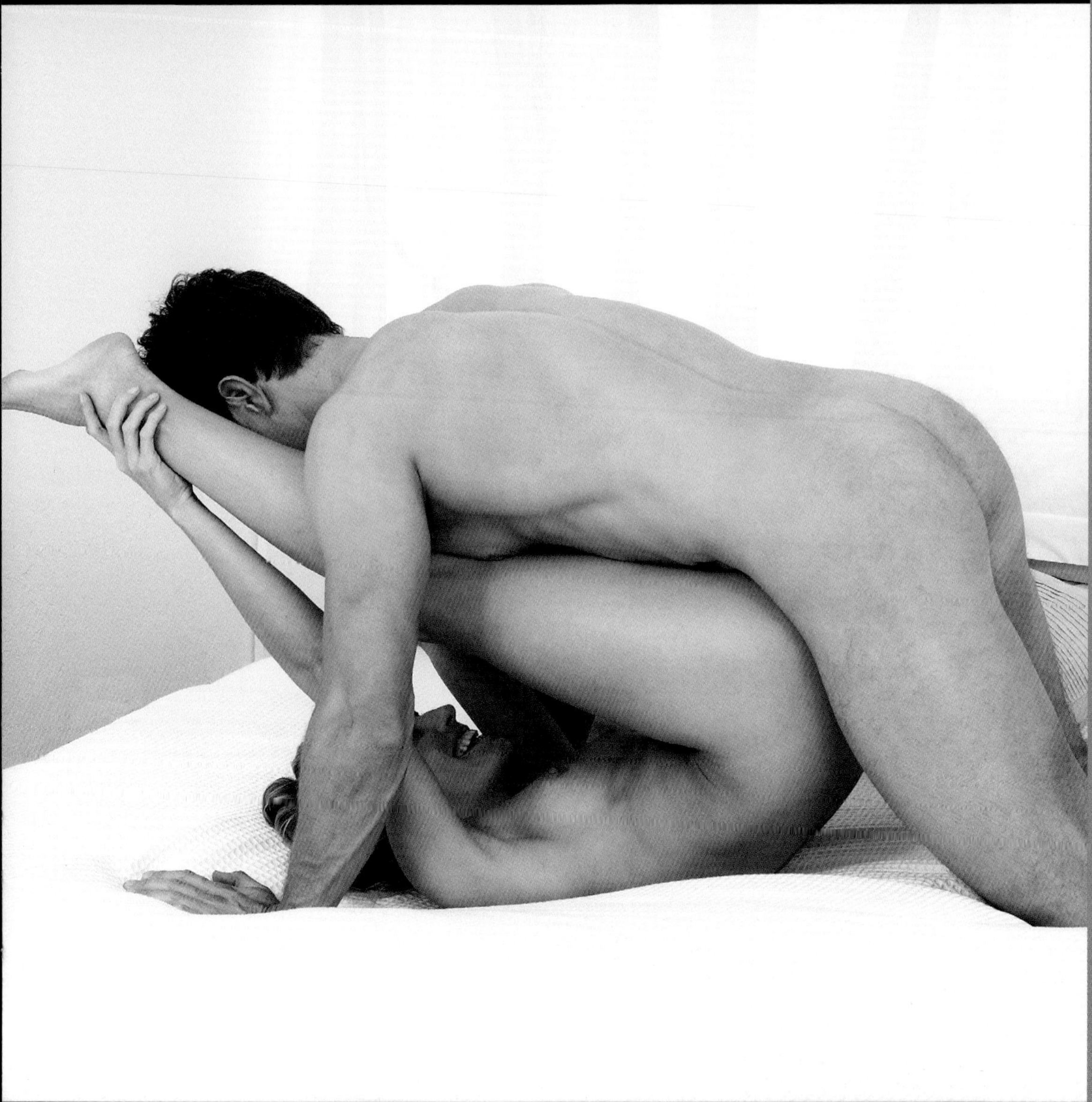

twist and moan

fabulous 5-stepper

1 This part's easy: you're both kneeling on the floor, facing each other and taking a moment simply to hug.

2 He pretty much stays in the same position, while she begins a turn. Putting her left leg over his thighs, he winds an arm around her hips. Pause at this point for him to use his fingers on her clitoris.

3 Continuing her twirl, she's now put her breasts in prime position to be thrust into his eagerly awaiting mouth. Again, stop for a deep, long kiss and to play with what's laid out in front of you.

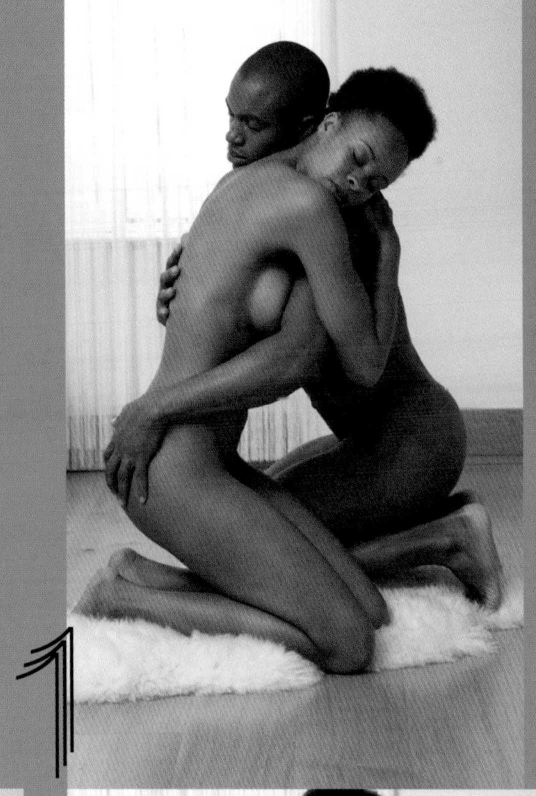

1

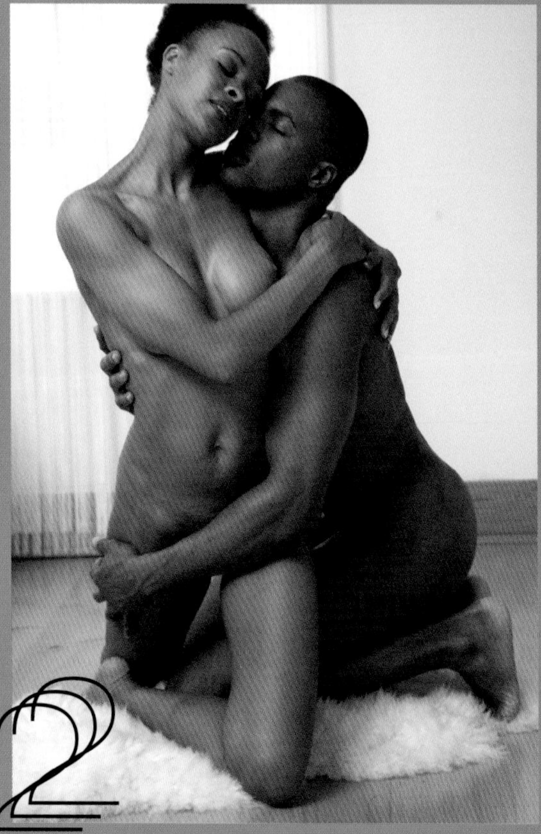

2

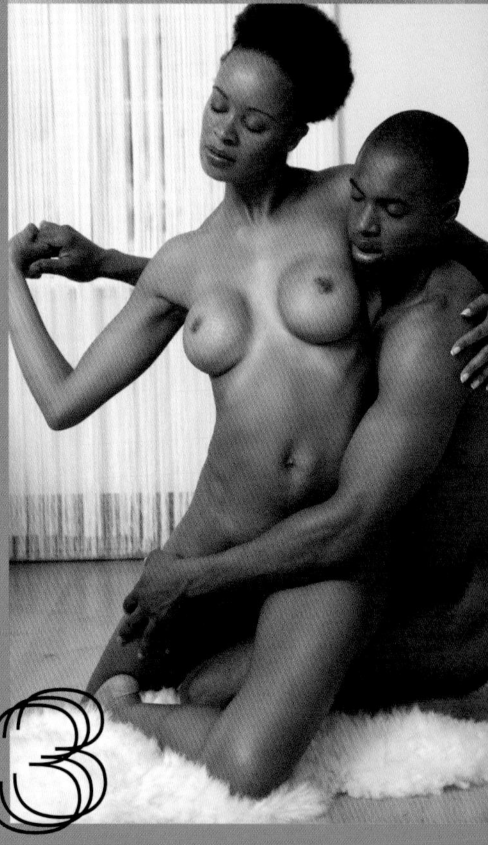

3

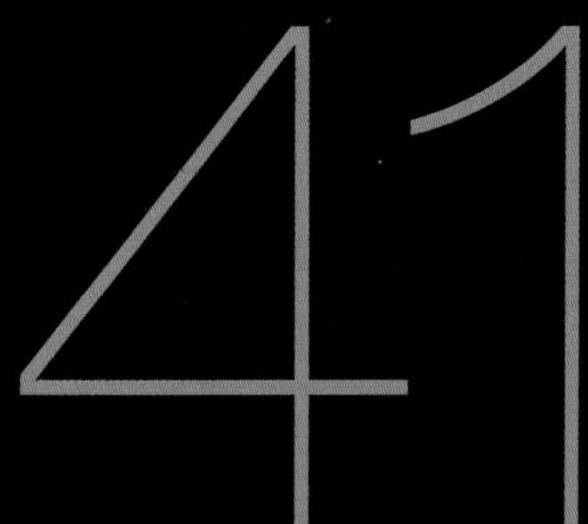

4 How's her back flexibility? You're about to find out, as she twists her spine, pulling her vulva close to his penis and putting herself into a position to allow him to penetrate.

5 Once she's completed her turn, you've both moved into a traditional rear-entry position. In the interests of comfort, it's easier for her to now pull herself up to lean over (and rest!) on a bed or sofa while he kneels behind. Then, let the thrusting begin!

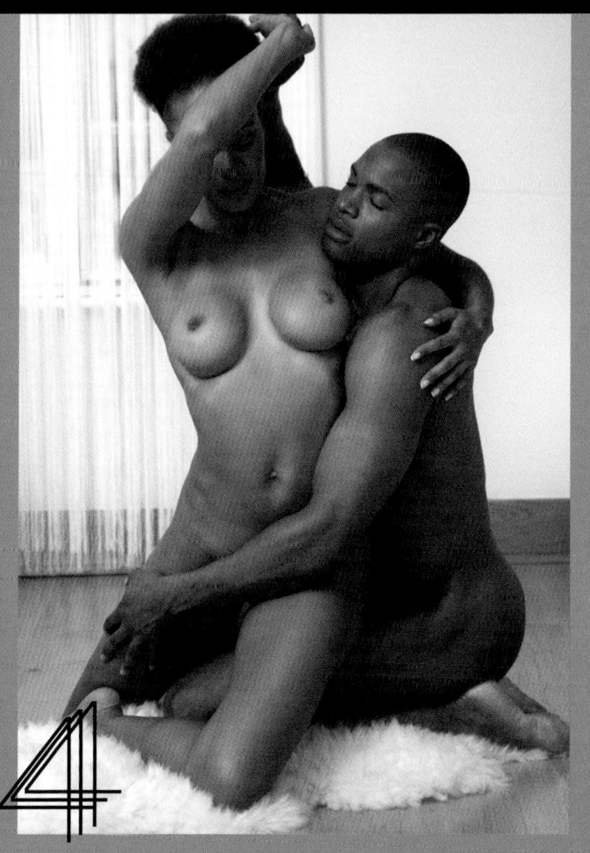

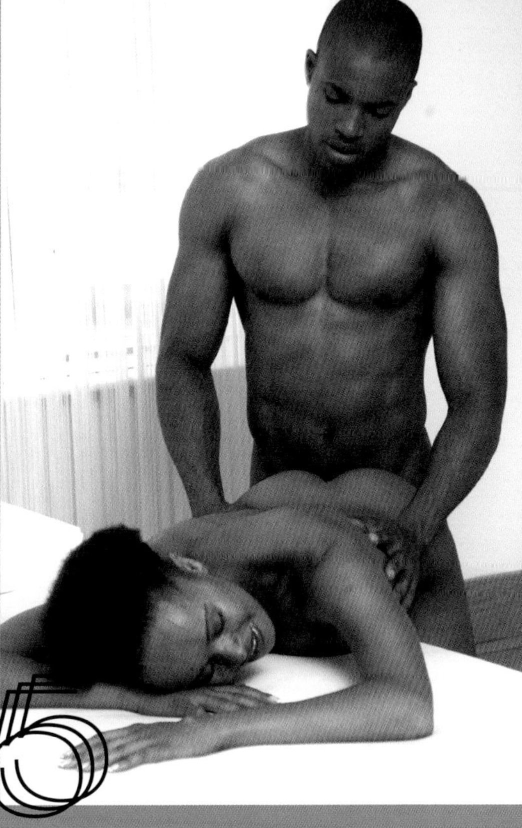

untouchables vs. insatiables

I've said this once and I'll keep on saying it: when you're choosing a partner, if you can possibly swing it, try really hard to choose one with the same sexual appetite as you. Because mismatched libidos—one wanting sex more or less than the other—is one of the main sex problems affecting couples today. For all the Tweedledums who didn't quite manage to match with their sexual Tweedledees, this is for you…

they want it more...

say no nicely Reject sex, not your partner, by making it clear you're not upset just because they want sex when you don't.

take responsibility Don't expect your partner to turn you on, do it yourself! Make it your mission to pinpoint what gets you in the mood for sex, then do more of it.

meet halfway If you don't want intercourse, what about oral sex? If you don't want any sex, do you mind pleasuring them? At the very least, you should be able to offer the intimacy of a cuddle.

masturbate For most people, the more they masturbate, the more their body gets used to having orgasms and the higher their libido. For others, it depletes what little urge they had. What works for you?

know what you want... and need to be satisfied sexually. And I'm talking both in and out of bed. If you need to relax first, ask for a massage. Or for them to do the dishes while you take a bath or shower.

prioritize sex If you're avoiding it or not interested, chances are it's the last thing you do, last thing at night. Well—gosh!—funnily enough, even high-sex-drive people sometimes wonder if it's worth the effort when they're exhausted after a long day at work. Try sex before you start dinner and switch the TV on. Or if you really are too stressed during the week, have breakfast in bed on the weekends and have sex then.

initiate sex even if you're acting. People who have a high sex drive and are always the one asking their partner for sex tend to think of themselves as the "sexy" person. The one who wants it less tends to think they're "less sexy." Initiating sex is a turn-on. It puts you in the sexual power position—and that alone can kick-start a lazy libido. Even if the resulting sex isn't that wonderful, your partner will be thrilled that you're trying or, if they refused, it's given you a taste of what it's like to be in their shoes.

you want it more...

masturbate Take the edge off by having solo sex.

redirect your energy Shift the focus from your sex life to your relationship. Be affectionate and make it blatantly clear you don't just want them for sex.

make sure it's sex you want Don't use sex as a replacement for intimacy, affection, or as a way to de-stress.

accept "no" And do it graciously.

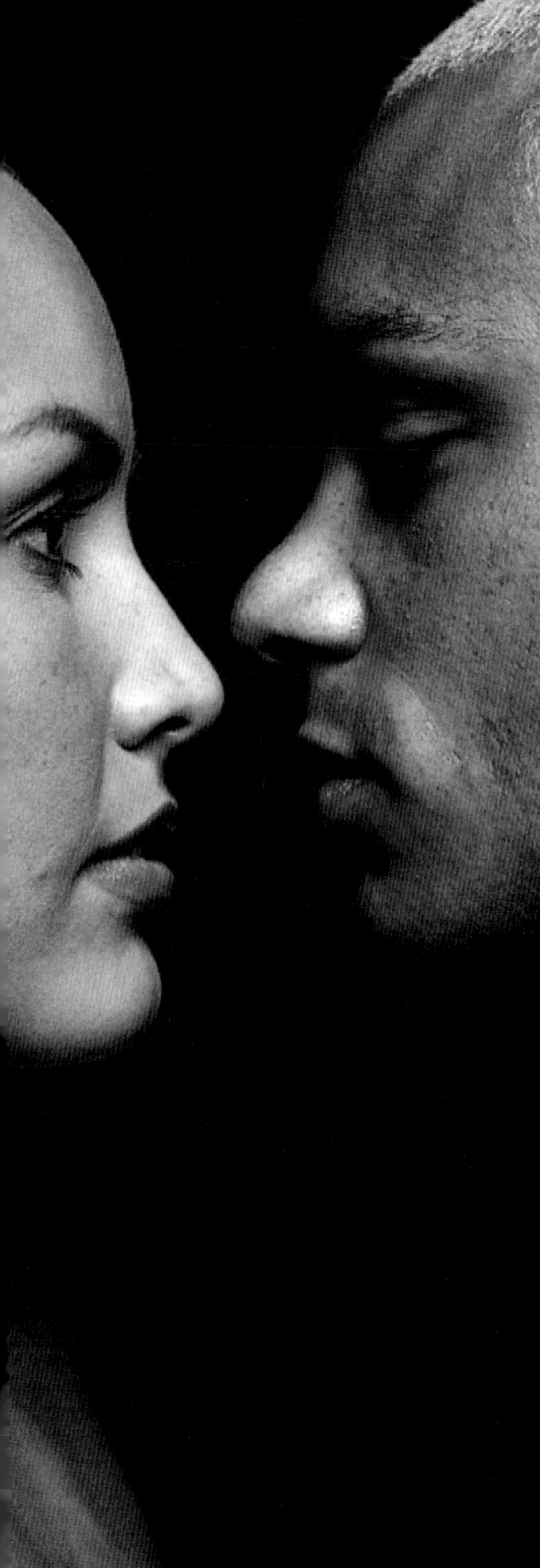

"Initiating sex puts you in the sexual power position."

give them an exit route If your partner agrees to give it a try to see if they can become aroused, let them exit if they want to. If they know they can stop at any stage, they'll be more likely to try in the first place. If they stop early, have a solo orgasm.

don't be greedy Don't demand a smorgasbord of sexual delights when a snack would take away the hunger pangs.

satisfy Know what turns your partner on and off. If oral sex does it for them, explore all possible options. Learn new tricks and tips and broaden your sexual repertoire as much as possible in this area.

don't be insecure Don't confuse love with lust. Just because their tongue's not hanging out from merely looking at you, it doesn't mean they love or want you less than you do them. Your sexual response system works quicker, that's all.

love quickies All sex sessions don't have to be marathons. Use plenty of personal lubricant and make the most of whatever time you do have.

try magnet therapy Put two magnets on the fridge—one each—and agree that you'll each move yours to show how horny you're feeling. The higher the magnet, the more you feel like sex. It's a clear way to let your partner know when you want sex, and removes the pressure of trying to second guess each other—plus the "less sexy" person can take control a little.

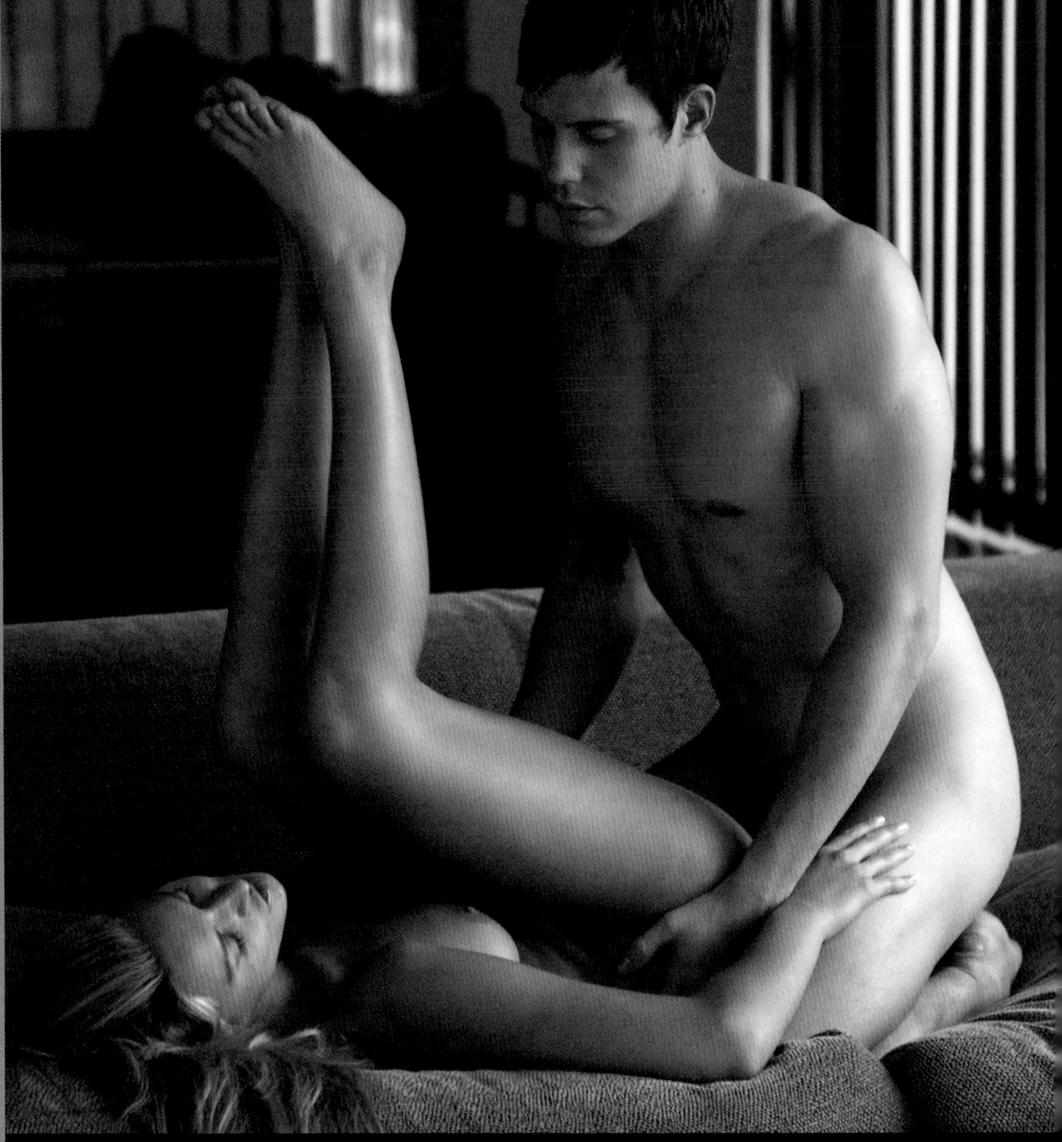

42 steamy seconds

She lies down and drops her legs back toward her head, exposing her vagina and pushing her labia invitingly toward him. If she's aiming to have multiple orgasms in one session, this is a good position to be in because it's easy for him to move from penetration to giving her oral sex and on to anal play and manual stimulation with his fingers. Alternating between different types of stimulation gives her the best chance of climaxing more than once.

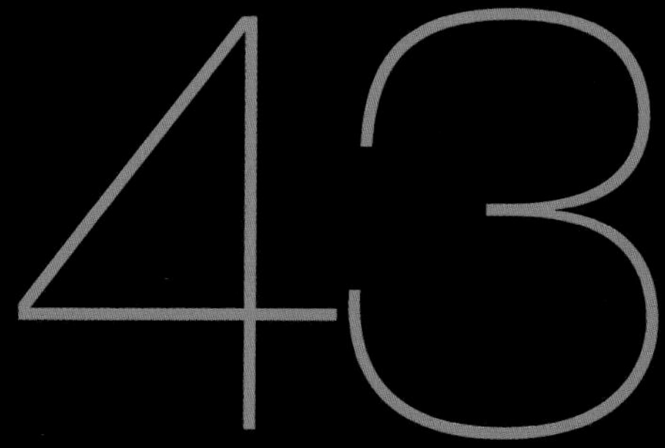

long and lusty

Want to make intercourse last longer? This position is a good option because thrusting is limited. The less intense the friction, the less likely he is to ejaculate early. He lies down and she faces away. There's no eye contact and little body contact, which makes it seem impersonal, but if you're in the mood for living out a fantasy that doesn't revolve around your partner, this becomes a plus. (As I said earlier, it's normal to fantasize about other people—just keep your mouth shut about it!)

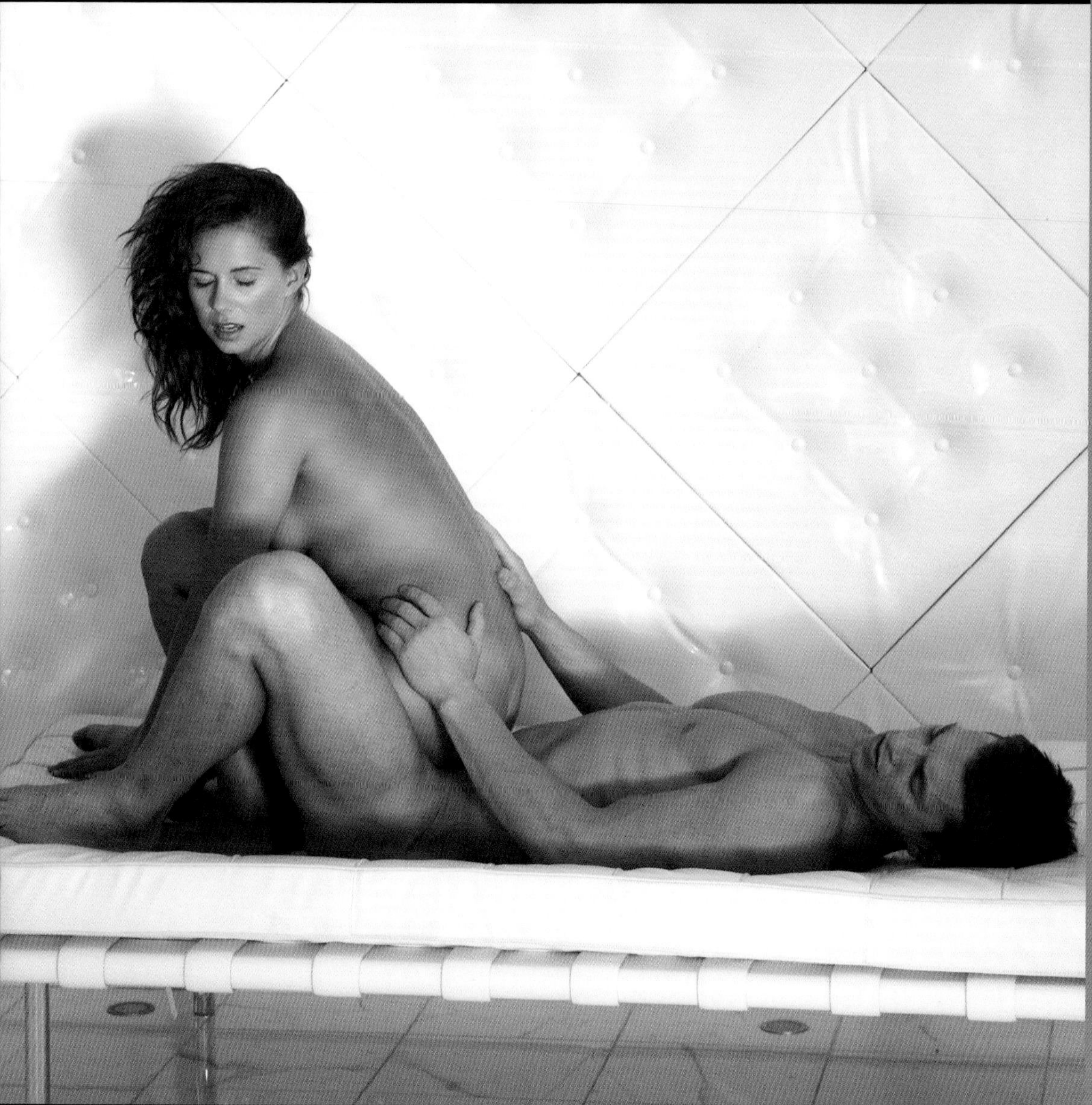

44

the crab

This is satisfyingly show-off-y, but also relatively simple. Send each other into erotic overdrive—in comfort! She lies back and pulls her knees up to her chin. He kneels in front and penetrates, holding on to the front of her calves to hold them together and for balance. She can hold on to his upper thighs to help provide leverage.

This position gives super-super-deep penetration, so make sure it's not a "sensitive cervix" day (don't laugh, it really can be influenced by what time of the month it is!). It's a raw, primitive position, which tends to lead to quick orgasms, hopefully for both of you! Her legs are together, which means a tighter, shallower vaginal canal; he's thrusting straight down instead of at an angle, which directly hits her front vaginal wall.

It's hard work on your legs and you both may feel the need to stretch them out at some point. Use this opportunity to indulge in a little midway oral sex for one or both of you. (If you're squeamish, take a break and wash off in between.) Because it's a "good time, not a long time" position, switch to it when you're both on the edge or use it as an erotic appetizer.

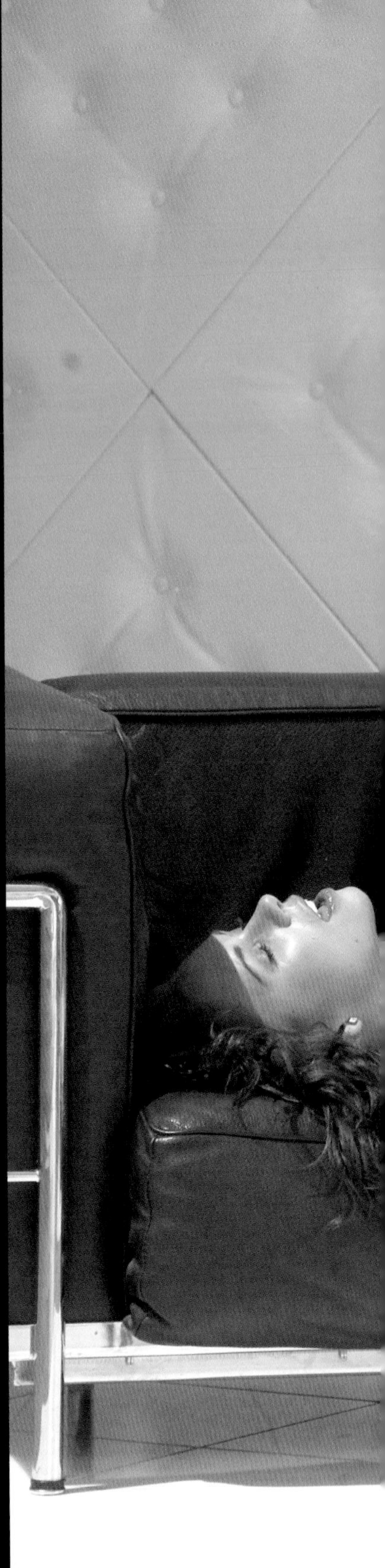

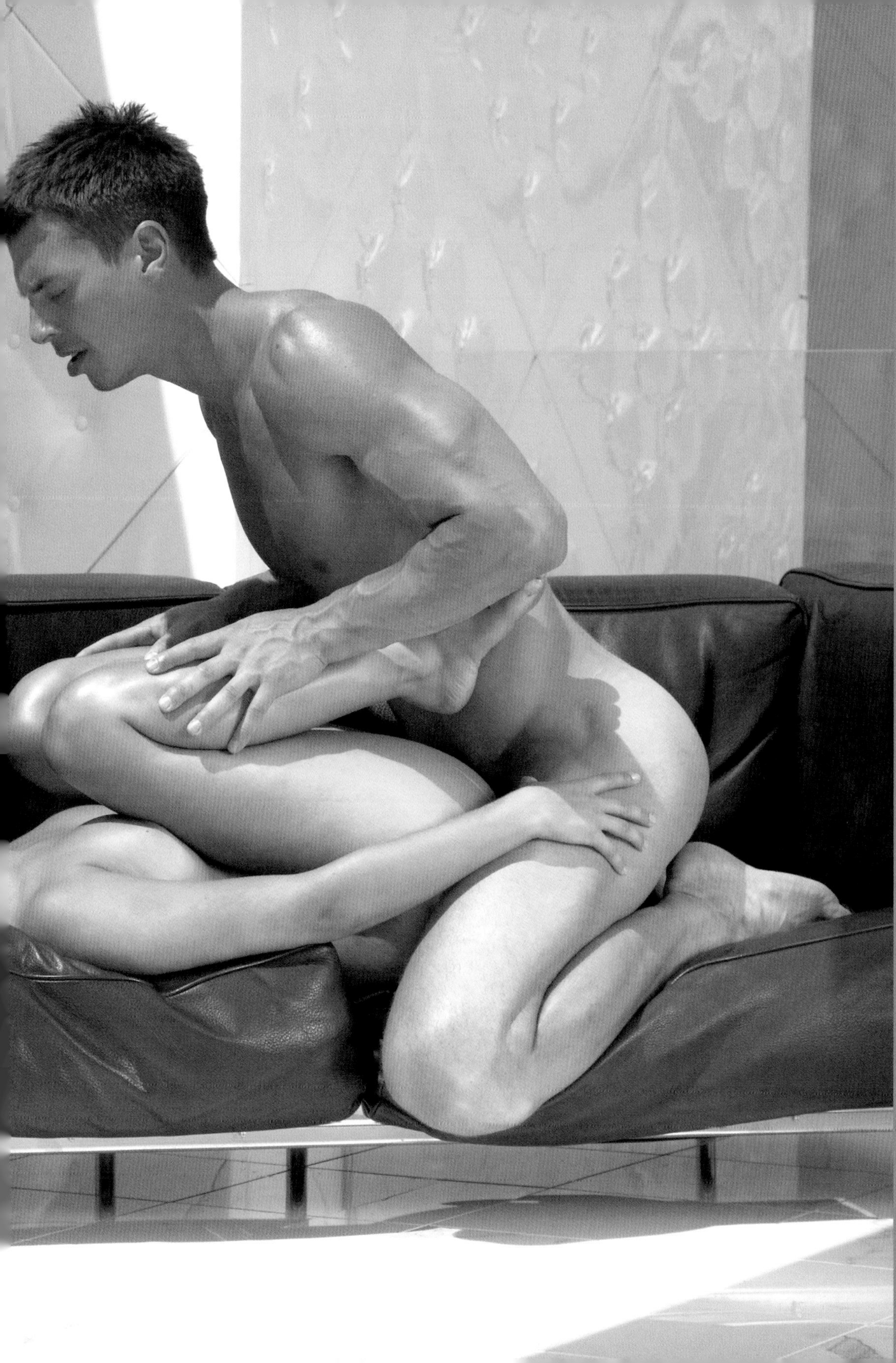

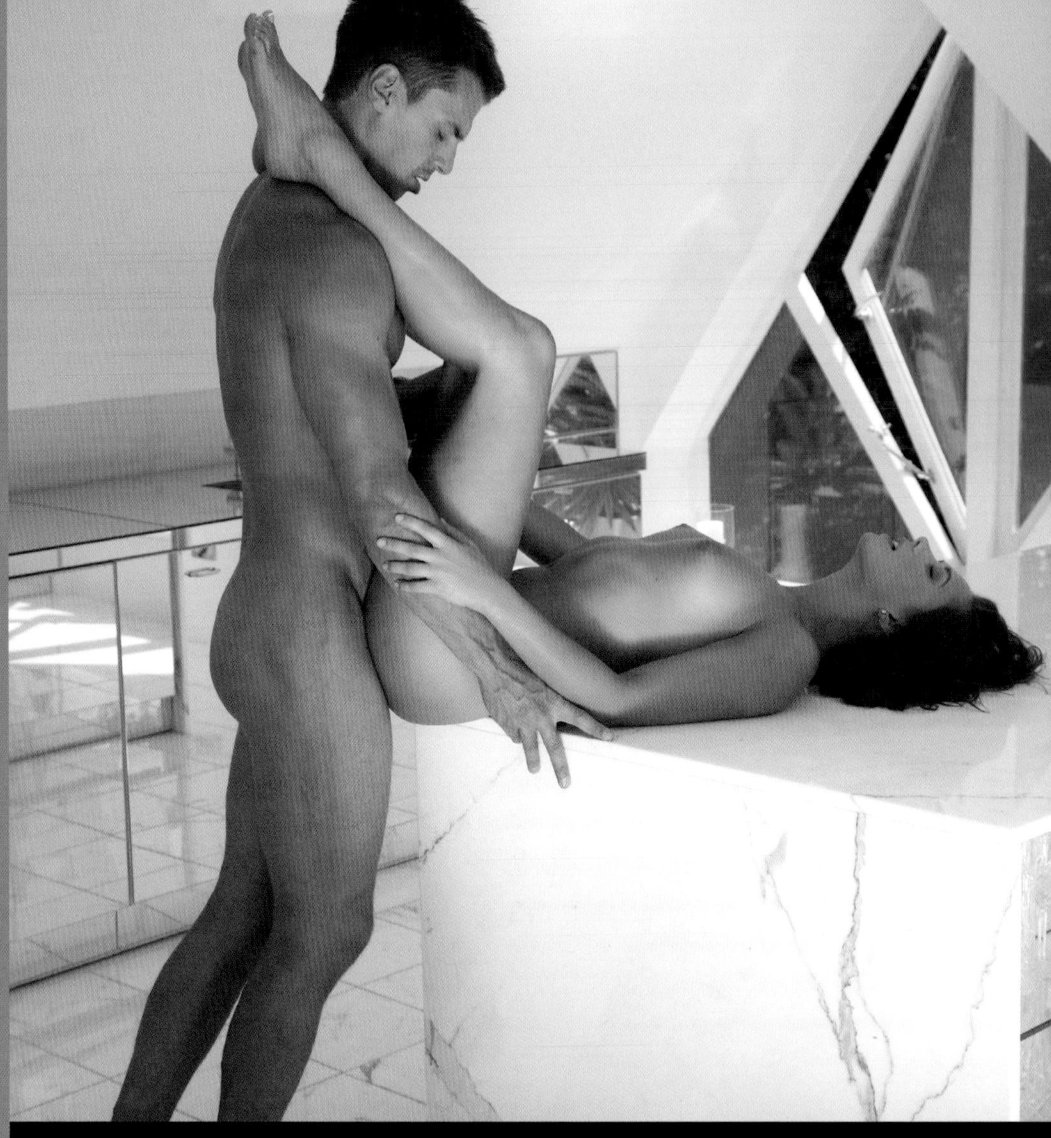

45 beats cooking

At the risk of giving you far too much information, this is one of my favorites. For some reason, I often end up having sex in my kitchen (yes, I am now expecting lots of polite refusals to my dinner parties!) and this one's made for the kitchen counter! It's simple: she lies back, with her feet on his shoulders. He stands and, holding onto the bench or her hips, enters her. Penetration is deep, traditional thrusting is easy, and it's primitive enough to satisfy spontaneous erotic urges.

46 down and dirty

Doing it "like they do on the Discovery Channel" makes for detached sex. But it's the anonymity and crude, primative element that makes it so erotic, causing men to orgasm much faster when doing it doggy style than in any other position. This may be a good or a bad thing, depending on what mood she's in. How quick is quick? Well, research says 1.8 minutes...

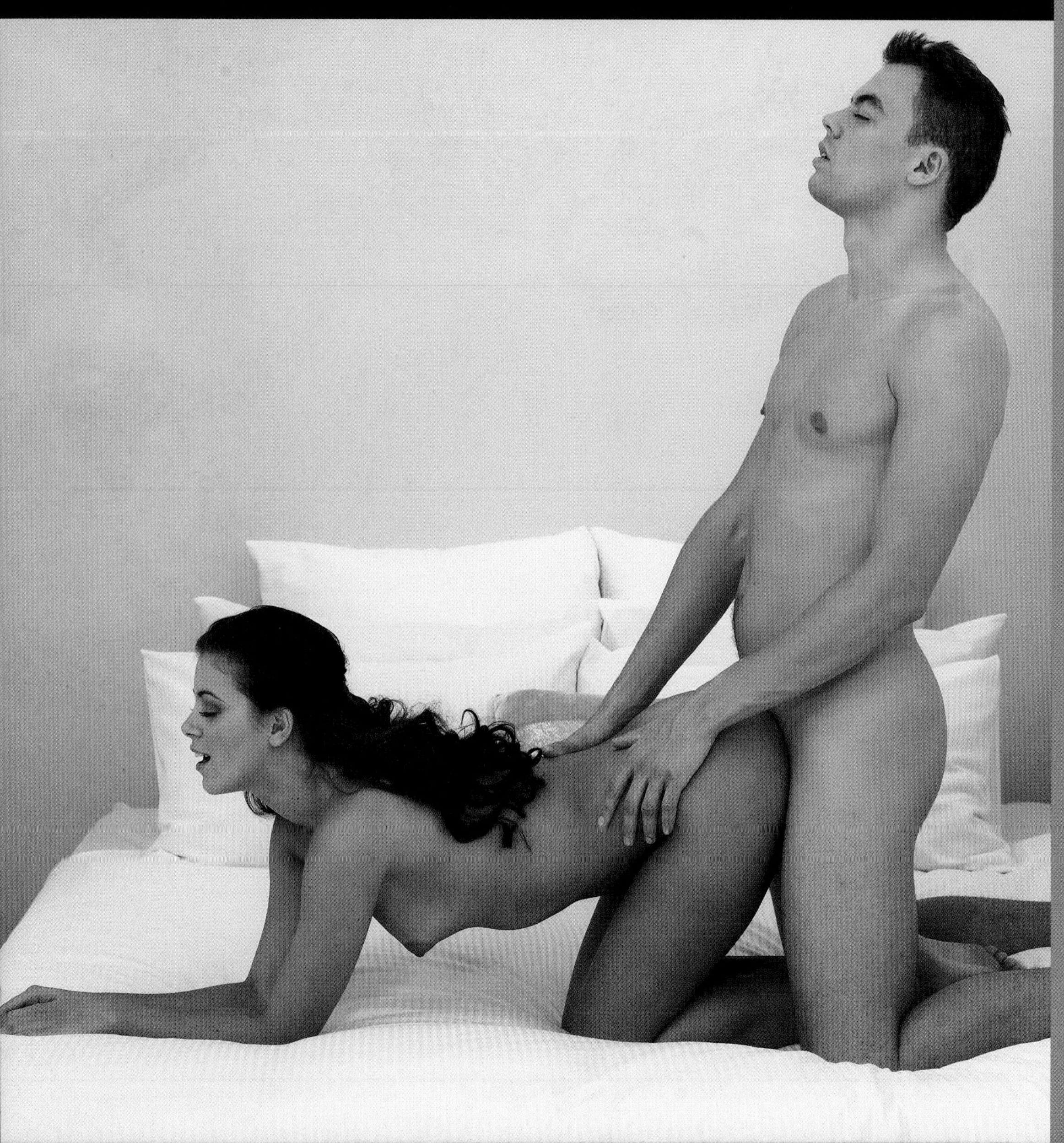

ant meets elephant

There's only one instance when a small penis or large vagina can cause problems: when the owner is so insecure about it that they're constantly apologizing and are inhibited in bed as a result. Now *that's* boring. Lopsided love isn't a problem if it's confined to the genital area. So whether Cupid's aimed his arrow to link a small penis with a large vagina or matched petite with jumbo the other way around, there are ways to even it up. Here's how…

he's big/she's small

she should Make sure you're fully aroused before he penetrates, so that the vagina expands and lubricates. Spend plenty of time on foreplay so that you can accommodate him, and while he's penetrating, push down with your vaginal muscles. Comfort yourself with logic: your vaginal muscles are elastic enough to take the biggest penis—after all, you can deliver a baby from the same place! Use water-based lubricant and get him to gently thrust his fingers inside you for at least a few minutes before intercourse.

he should Squeeze that tube of lube—even if she's wet to start with. Penetrate slowly, and stop each step of the way so that your bodies become accustomed to each other. Let her control the insertion. Try penetrating from different angles to see which feels comfortable. If you're really big, she might not want full penetration. Keep thrusting shallow and gentle. Have intercourse just before she's about to have an orgasm from oral sex or manual masturbation so that she's as lubricated and expanded as possible.

prime positions Choose positions that don't allow deep penetration: her on top, so she can control the depth of his thrusts; or side by side facing each other, her resting her upper leg over his hips; or missionary with a twist: she tightly closes her legs to minimize access as he thrusts—this not only helps control the depth of penetration, but it also feels better for him.

"Shift focus and don't make intercourse the main event."

he's small/she's big

she should Have a non-penetrative orgasm first so intercourse isn't the main event. Get in the habit of doing lots of pelvic floor exercises (see page 67).

he should Not get too hung up about it. Placing two pillows under her bottom will make her feel tighter and you bigger. Also try putting your legs on either side of hers, rather than getting her to open hers wide.

prime positions She lies on her back and wraps her legs over his shoulders, narrowing the vaginal canal and allowing him deep access; or she kneels on all fours and he penetrates from behind; or she lies on her back and brings her knees up to her chest, and he penetrates from on top with her feet resting on his shoulders.

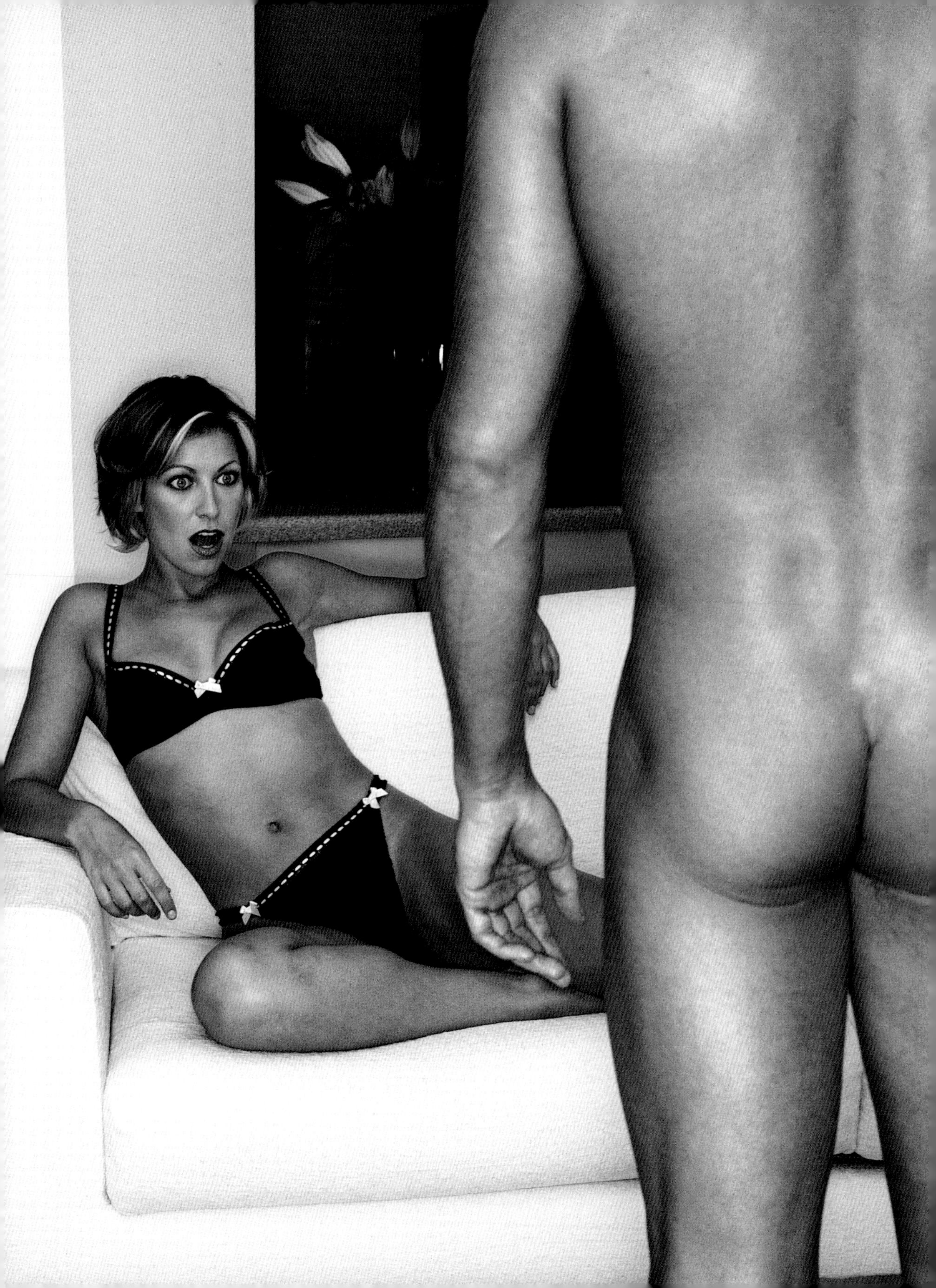

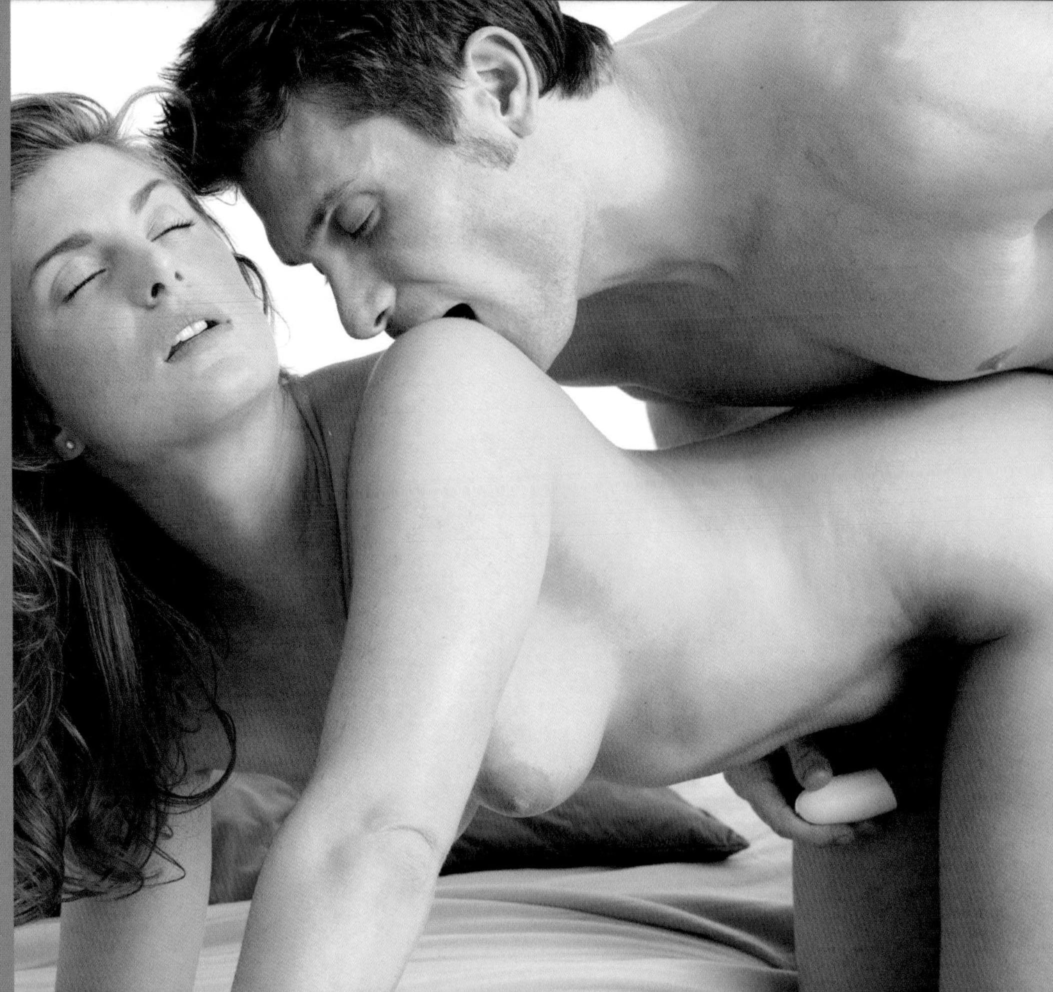

47

look, no hands!

The best way to up her orgasms during intercourse is to have a threesome—with her vibrator. This is a great position for him to stimulate her, or opt for a "no hands" couple-friendly alternative. My favorite is a new invention called a "We-Vibe." It's small, C-shaped, and worn by her. Turn it on, insert one end up to the bend, and it opens to an L shape. The clitoral pad sits against the labia and clitoris, the other end works on the G-spot. It flattens out so he can't feel it during sex, but he will still feel a pleasant little buzz.

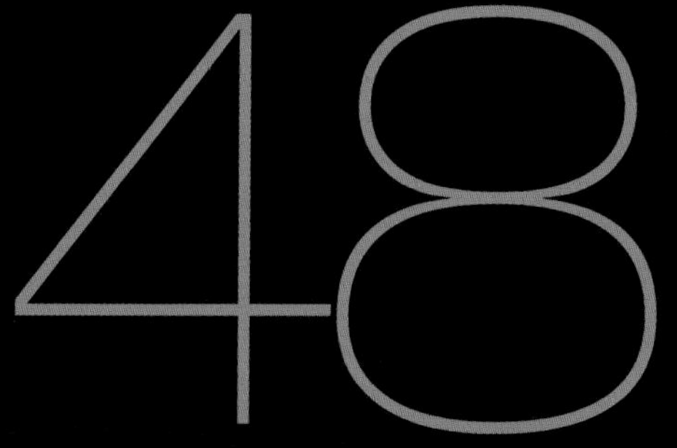

the butterfly

The full name of this position is "Butterflies in Flight"—the outspread arms resemble wings and she's on top with him, well, pinned below. It perfectly reflects the Taoist belief that life is a balance and everything has an equal and opposite reaction. Needless to say, she's the boss, completely controlling the rhythm. Movement is limited, and yes, you'll spend a lot of time saying "Oops, it slipped out again," but get it right and it's unrivaled for sensual full-body contact.

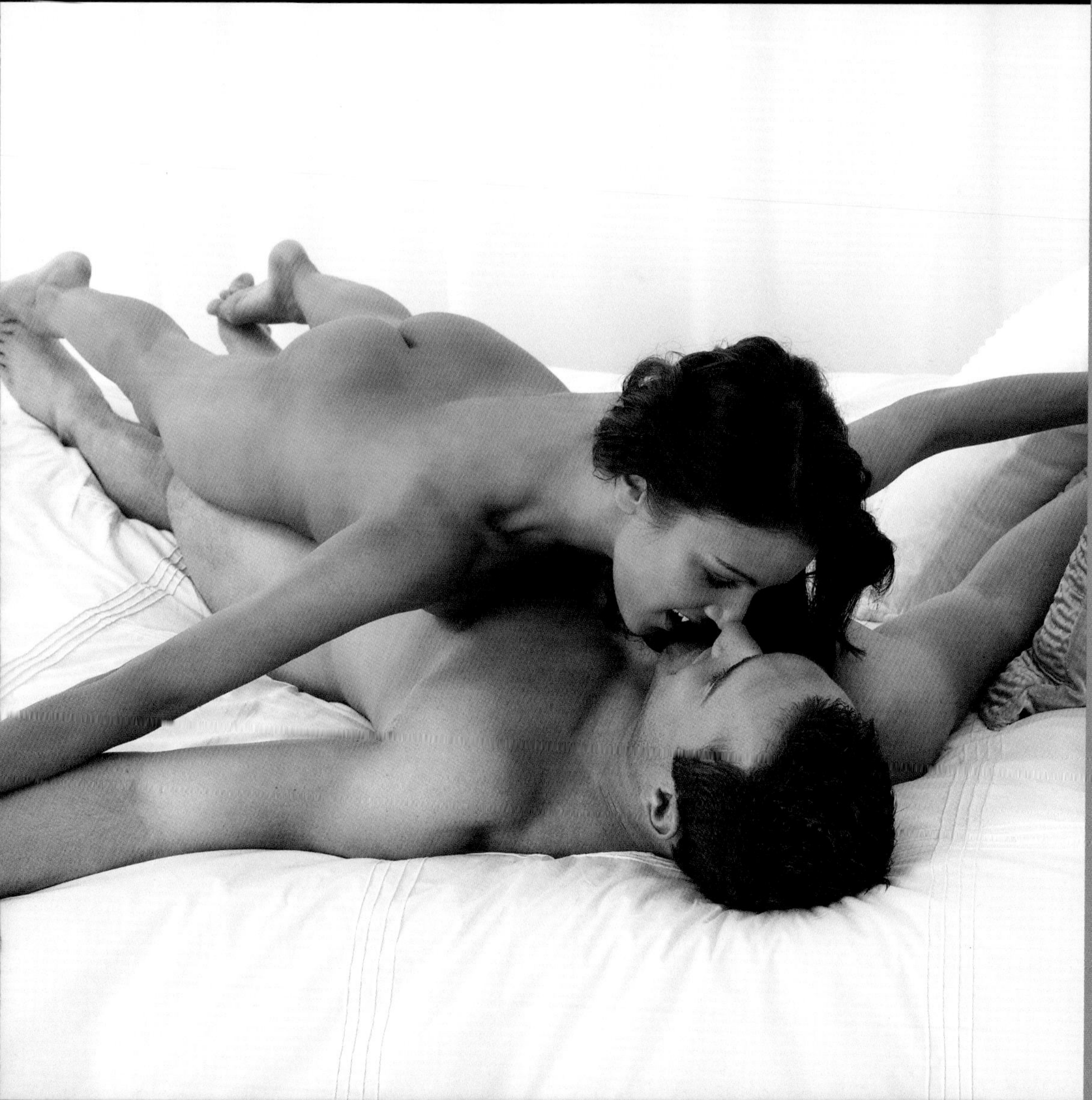

on the edge

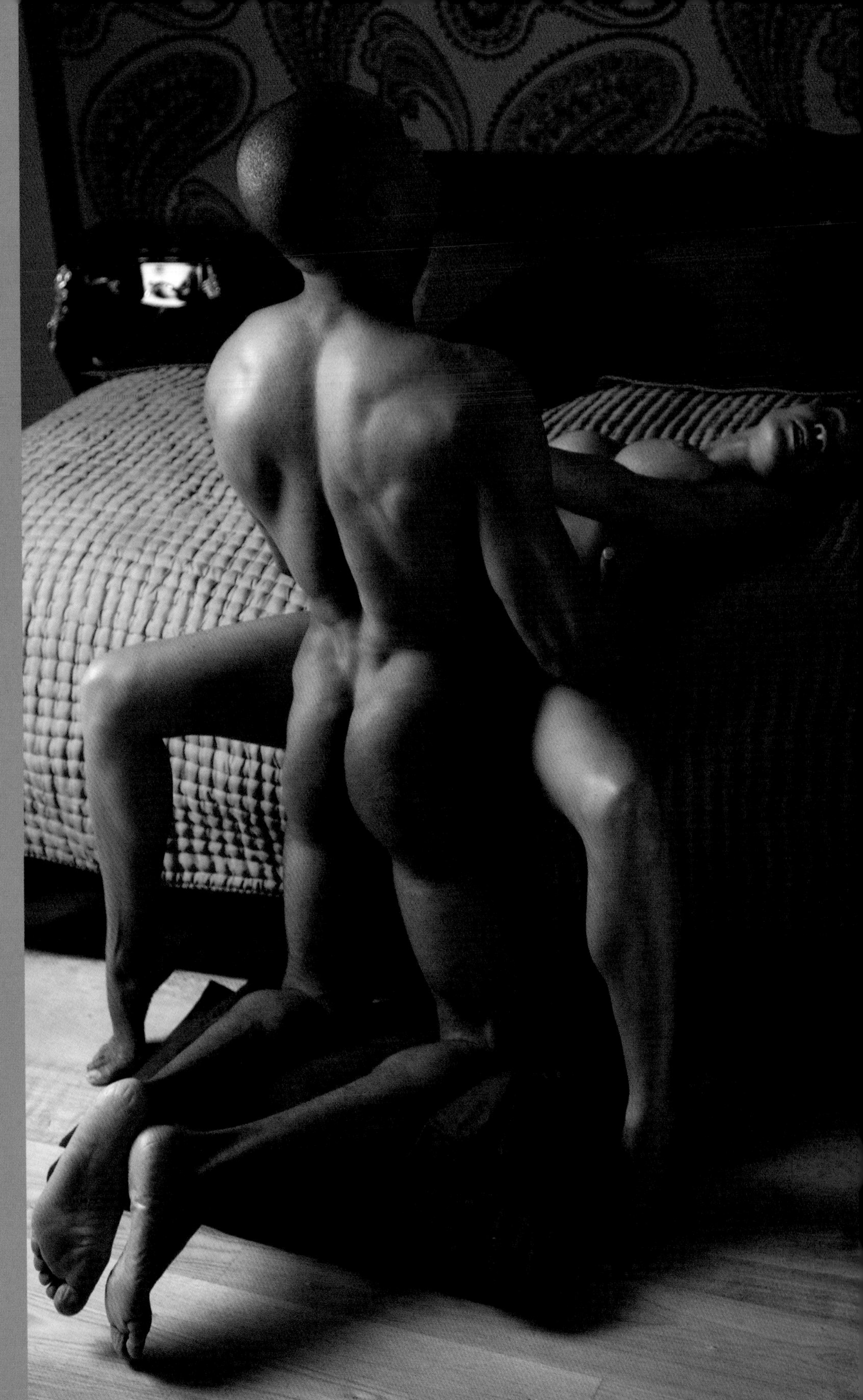

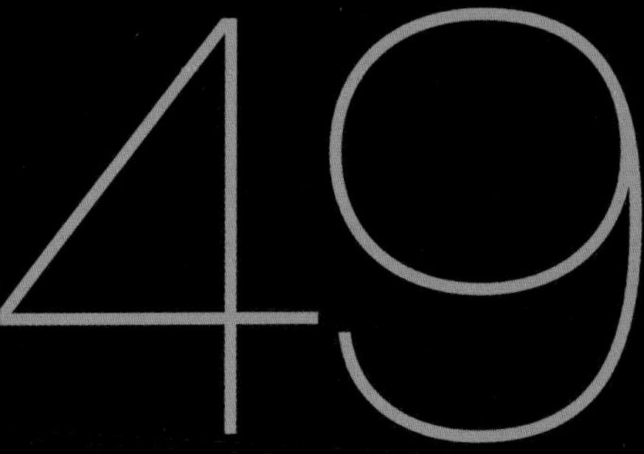

racy recliner

This is inspired by a Tao position, but it's already a favorite for lots of couples because it manages to satisfy two appetites simultaneously: the need for both hot sex and comfort!

He kneels on something soft, she positions herself on the edge of the bed and opens her legs wide so he can enter her. He takes firm hold of her hips and moves her up and down on his penis. Simple. And oh so effective. The edge of the bed isn't just great for intercourse—it's also a far more versatile (and comfy!) position for giving and receiving oral sex as well, allowing easy access for hands and tongues.

beg for it

Nothing, but nothing, will make more difference to your sex life than you initiating sex more often. But if you're constantly being hassled for sex, you don't get chance to miss it. It's the "seesaw" phenomenon: the more often they initiate sex, the less often you will. Never getting the chance to say "How about it?" is tedious, demeaning—and deeply unsexy. Time to redress the imbalance!

my turn, honey

✻ Say you miss initiating sex. I guarantee that this alone will get an extraordinary reaction. "I'm always the one doing the asking" is a common couple complaint.
✻ Make a pact that they stop making any sexual overtures for two weeks to give you the chance to approach them. Wait for a bit, then—around day 10—pounce!
✻ Be obvious, direct, assertive. Rolling over and kissing once you're in bed is OK but not terribly original. Think "If I don't have sex with him now, I'll die."

it's OK to fake it

✻ Even if your first approach is a bit forced—you're not exactly foaming at the mouth, but it might be OK [illegible] pretend. Pack the kids off to your mom's, grab your partner, push them against the door, and make out like teenagers.
✻ "Pretending" passion creates it. Power is a massive turn-on, and if you're the one who's suddenly up for it and making all the moves, you'll be surprised by how turned on you'll feel.

50

the tongs

Nothing too fancy about this one—it's your basic woman-on-top! He lies back and relaxes (bliss, since he's normally the one doing all the work), she straddles him, knees bent. This is one of two or three positions the majority of couples use regularly—for good reason. His hands are totally free to ravish her—and it's all laid out in front of him, including a bird's-eye view of her breasts, pleasantly jiggling away. She's in complete control of penetration and can easily reach down to touch her clitoris or hold a wand vibrator for extra stimulation.

But here's the secret to turning it from satisfying to sizzling: her pelvic floor muscles. In the *Kama Sutra*, this position is called "The Tongs" because instead of lifting herself up and down, the woman squeezes his penis repeatedly with her vaginal muscles only, moving it in and out rather like someone using a pair of tongs! If her muscles aren't strong enough to do the job on their own, she can easily grind with controlled, circular movements. It feels incredibly intense at his end and she gets the clitoral pressure she needs to orgasm.

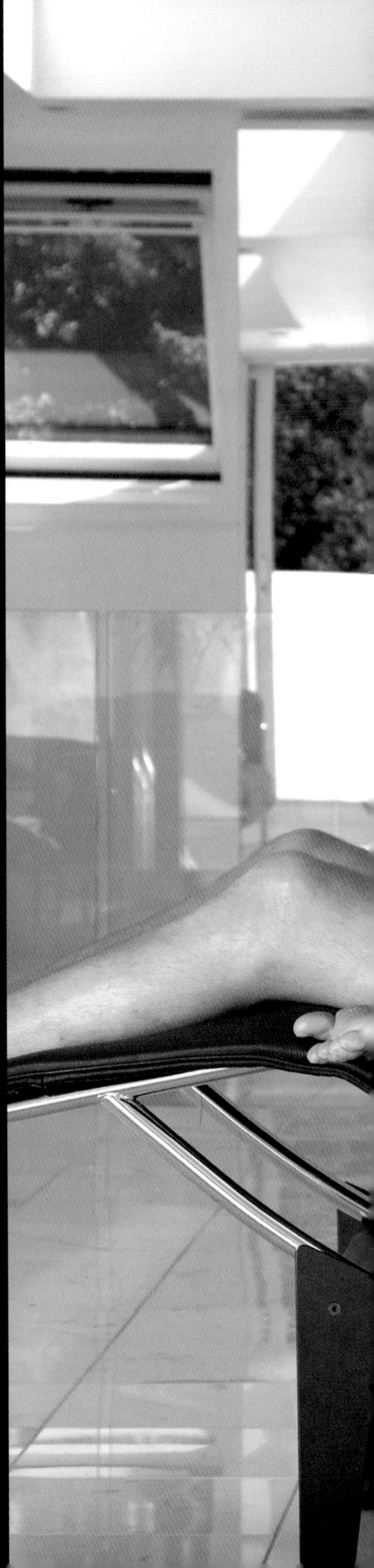

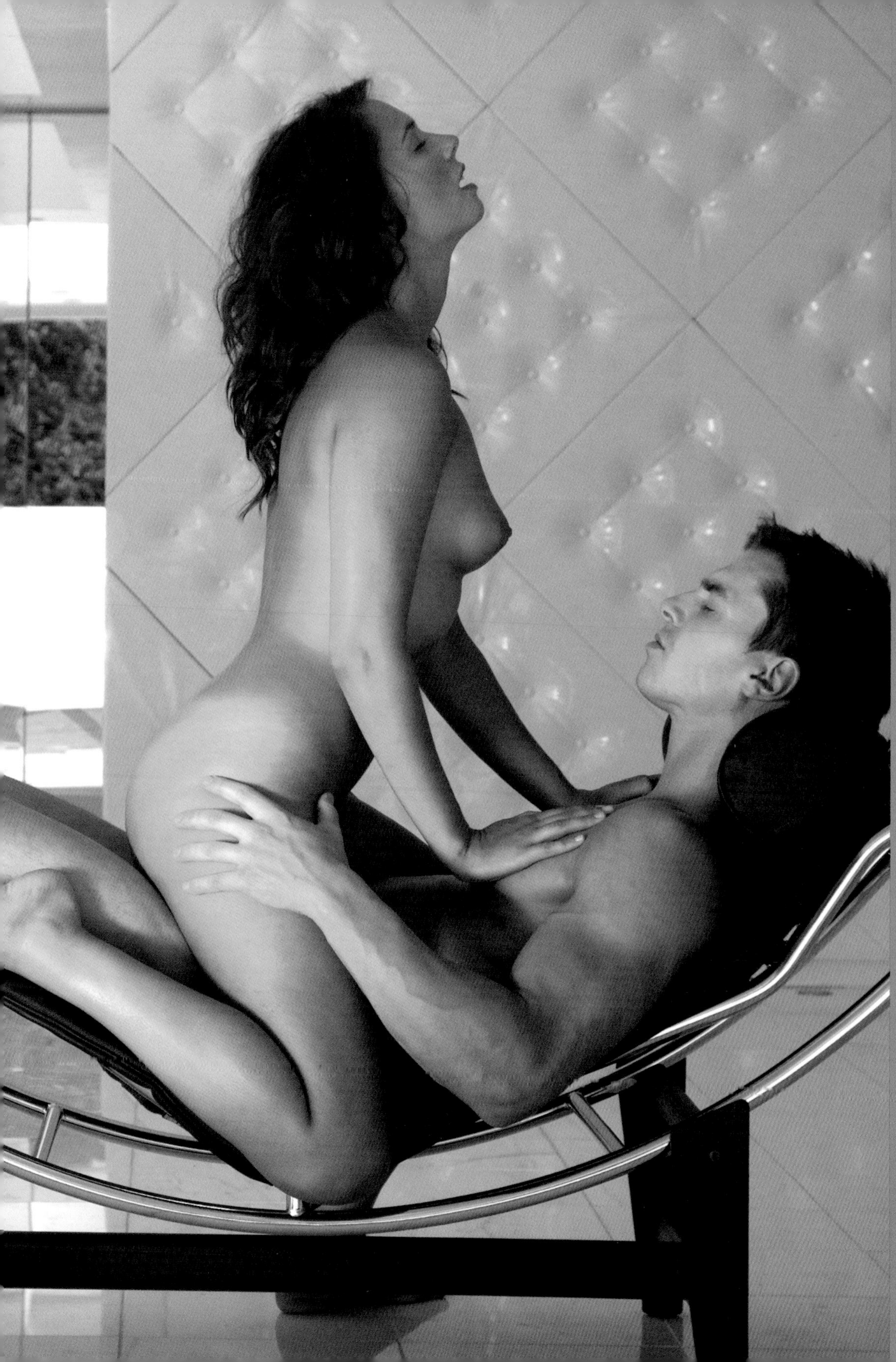

chapter

3

head games

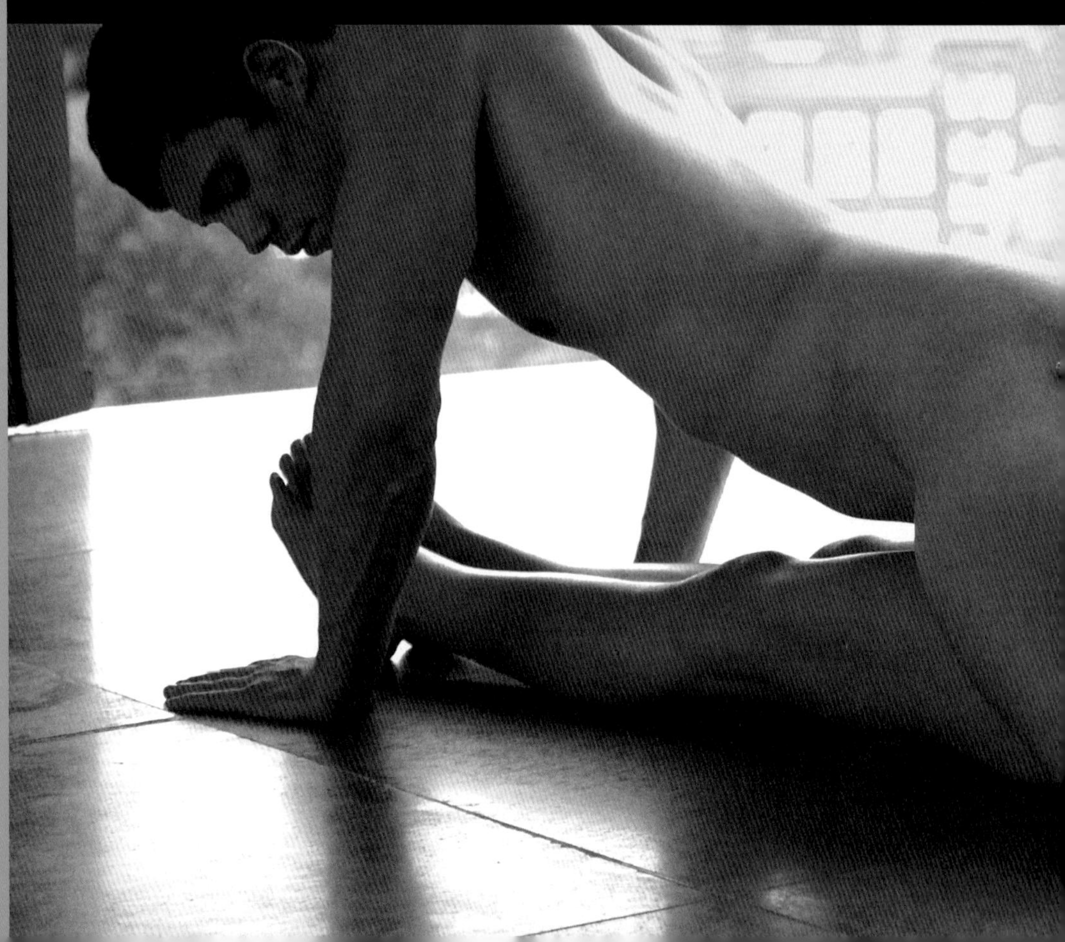

Advanced and adventurous for when you're energized, up for a challenge, and craving a torrid tangle of limbs.

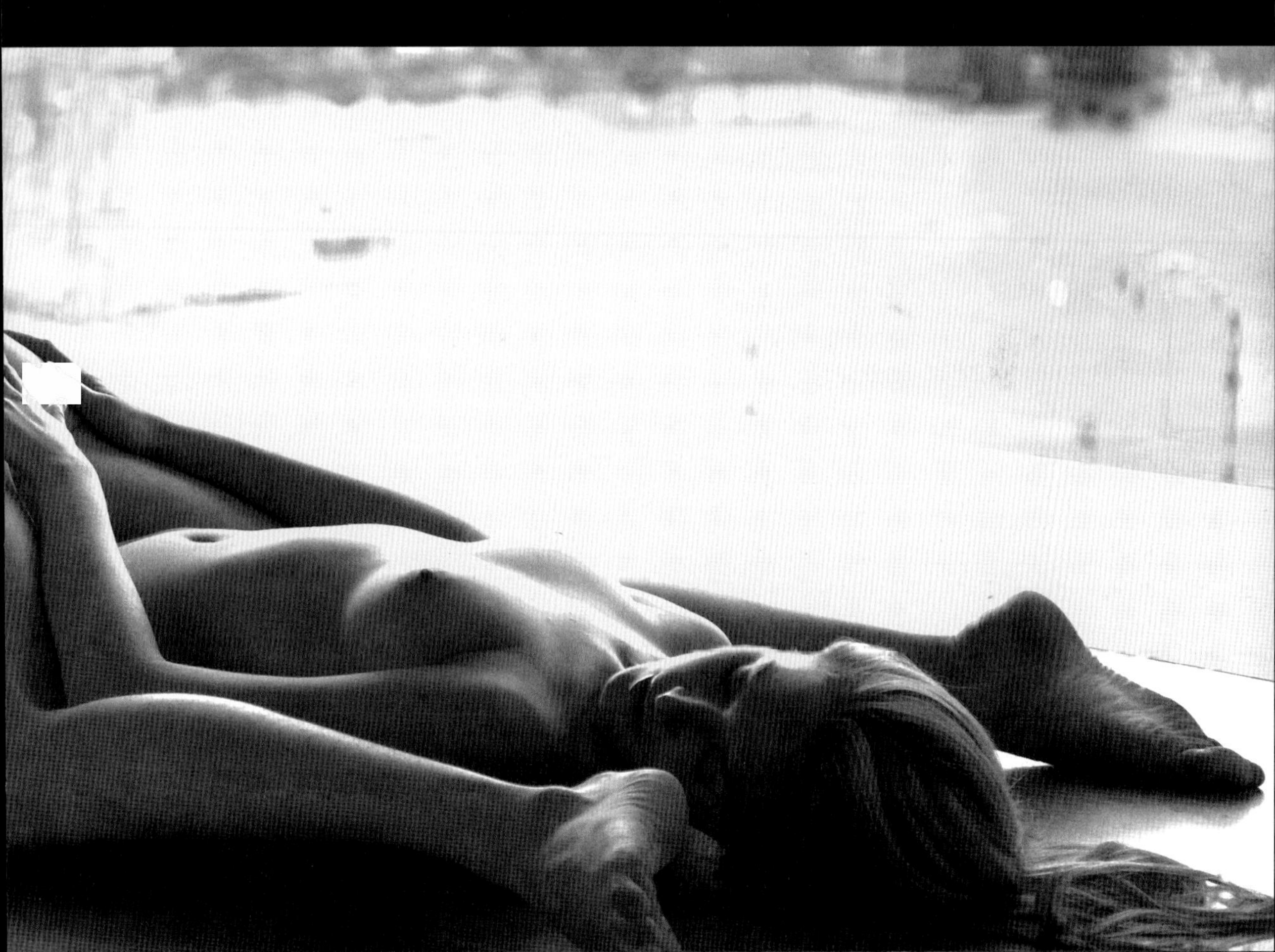

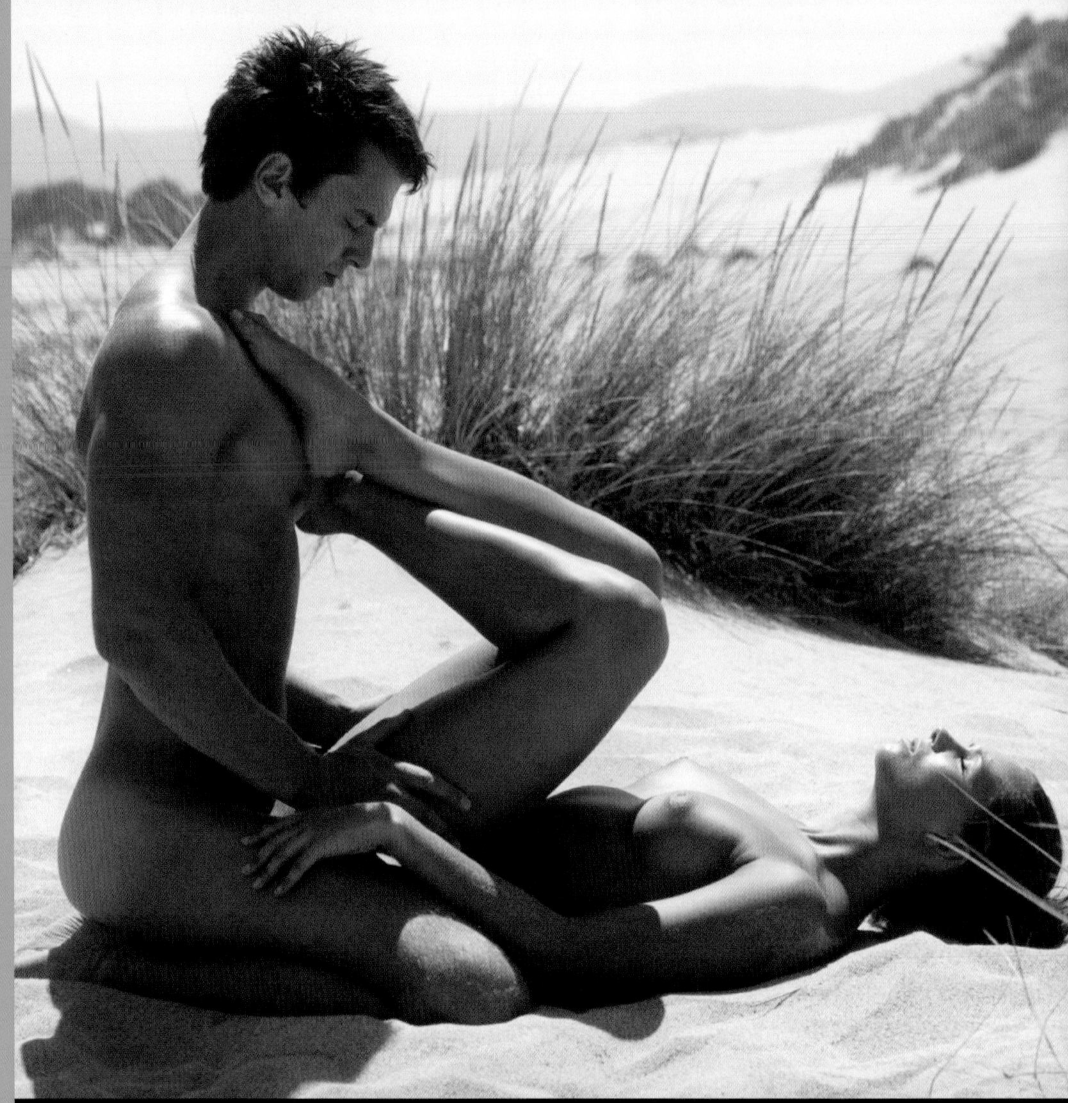

51

deep plunge

Inspired by the *Kama Sutra*, this position is suitable for the "highest congress"—meaning the vagina is fully open to allow for maximum penetration. She is fully exposed, showing her "wet and longing" parts to her partner, which can be one hell of a turn-on for both of you. He has a great view, watching his penis move in and out. You can't kiss because your faces can't get close, which ups the erotic tension and makes you concentrate solely on penetration.

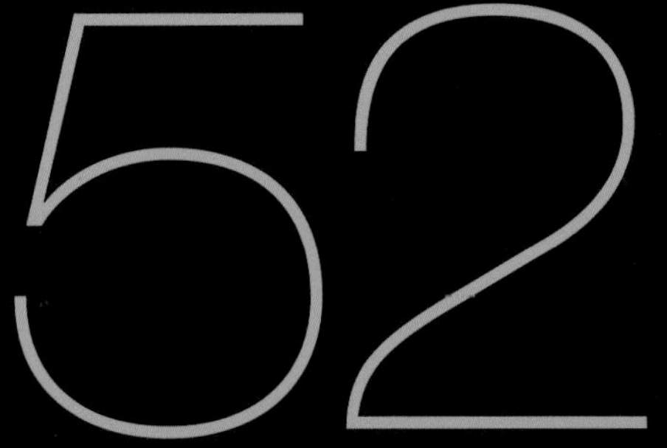

be as one

A version of a Tantric sitting posture, this ensures you'll "dissolve" into each other. Eye contact combined with close torsos makes it intimate and you can practice synchronizing breathing (if that appeals). You both have power in this—she's on top, so can control the rhythm, speed, and depth of thrusting, but she's also sitting in his lap, a traditionally submissive female pose. If she sat higher, resting her thighs in the crook of his elbow, he could lift her up to take complete control.

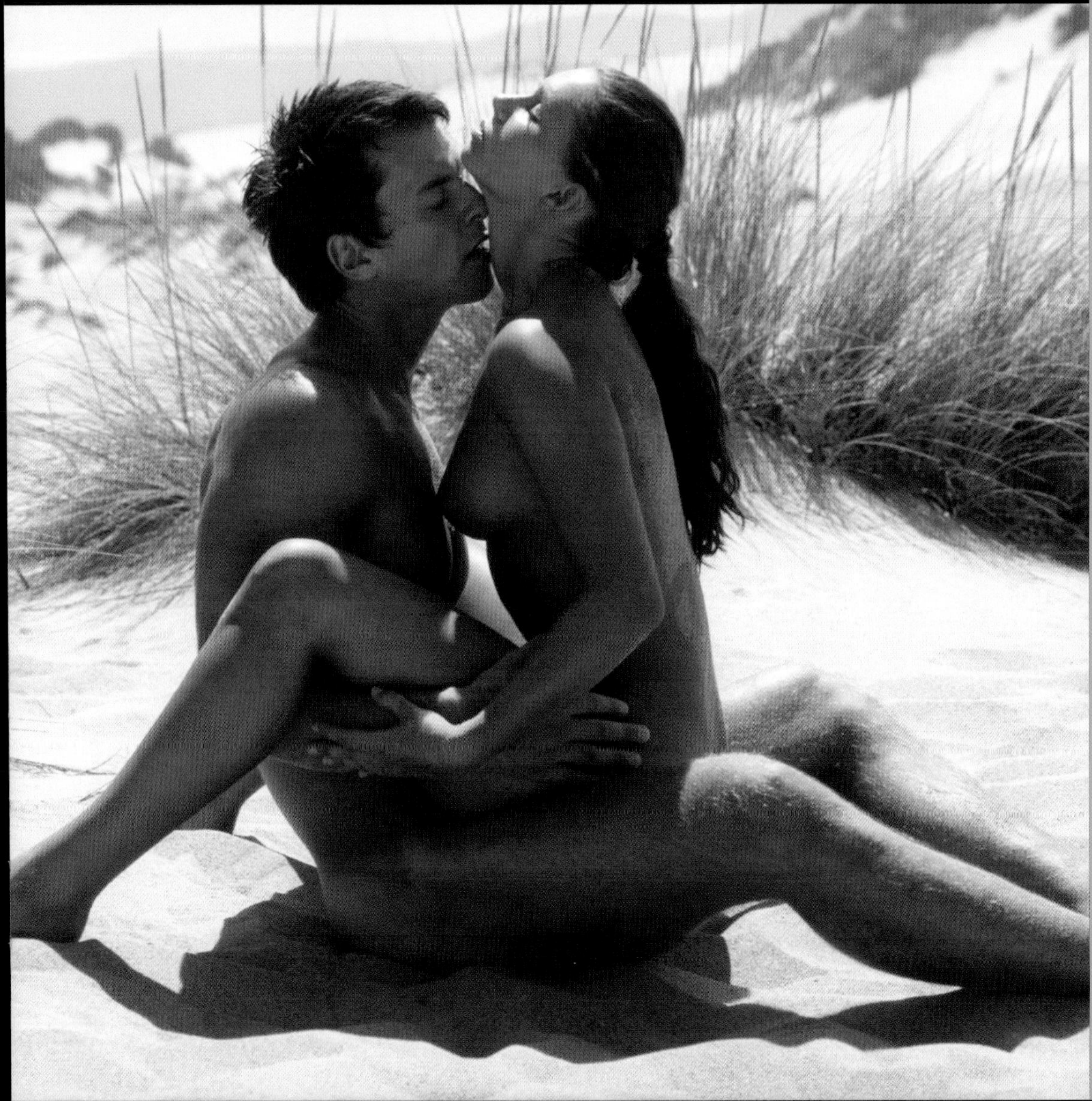

rocking horse

1 He sits with legs stretched out; she sits sideways in between them, with her legs over his thigh. Both hug and enjoy the flesh-to-flesh contact. There's no action yet, but be patient: this is a spiritual sex position that's not just about passionate pounding!

2 She provocatively places her ankle on his shoulder and holds her calf muscle. The point of this? Flexibility can be super-sexy! He's impressed by her sensual stretch and gets a view of her private parts, making him fully aroused.

3 Hurrah! He can penetrate once she gives the secret signal (lets go of her leg). She leans back, keeping her leg on his shoulder. Still no thrusting—simply enjoy the moment.

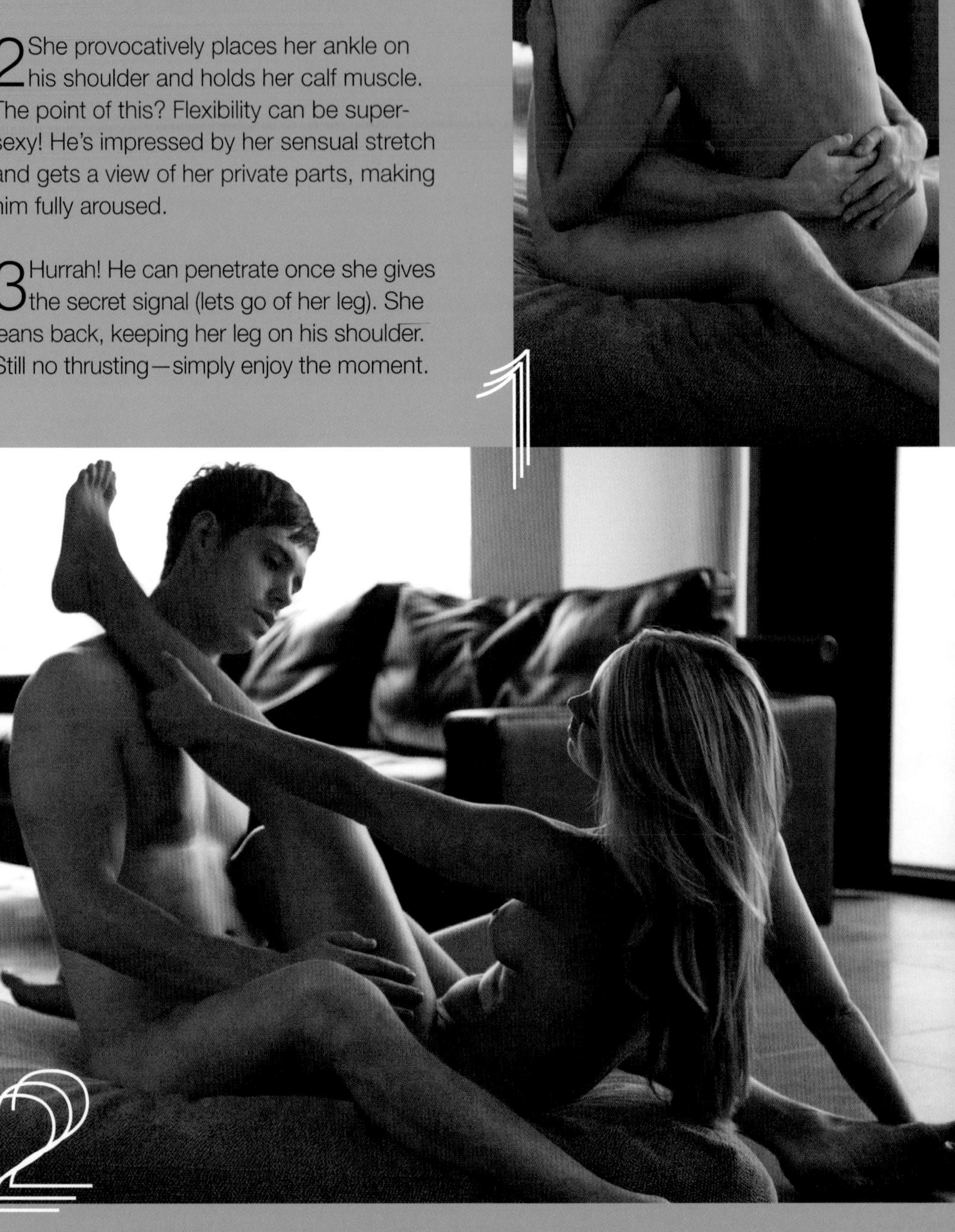

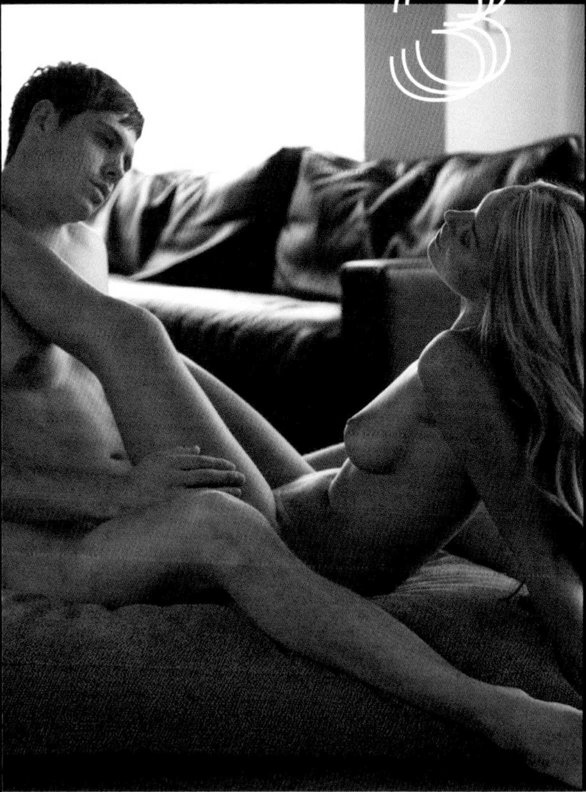

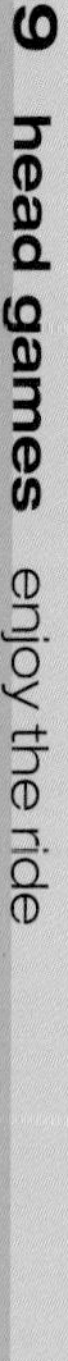

53

4 Clasp each other's wrists, then both lean backward, before moving into a rocking-horse motion where one leans back as the other leans forward, pulling each other up with your arms. It's a sexual seesaw, with the erotic focus on watching each other's faces as you experience pleasure.

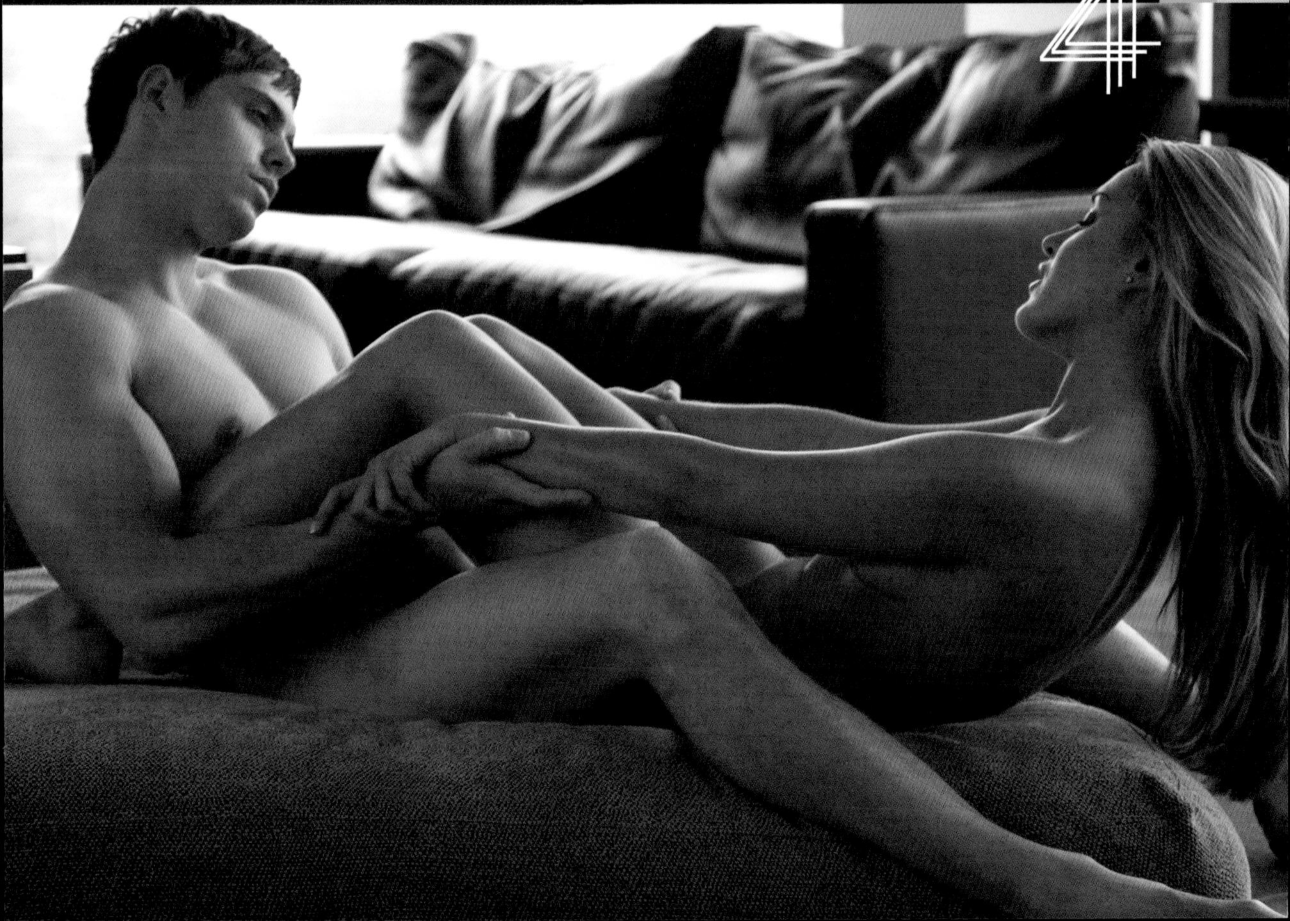

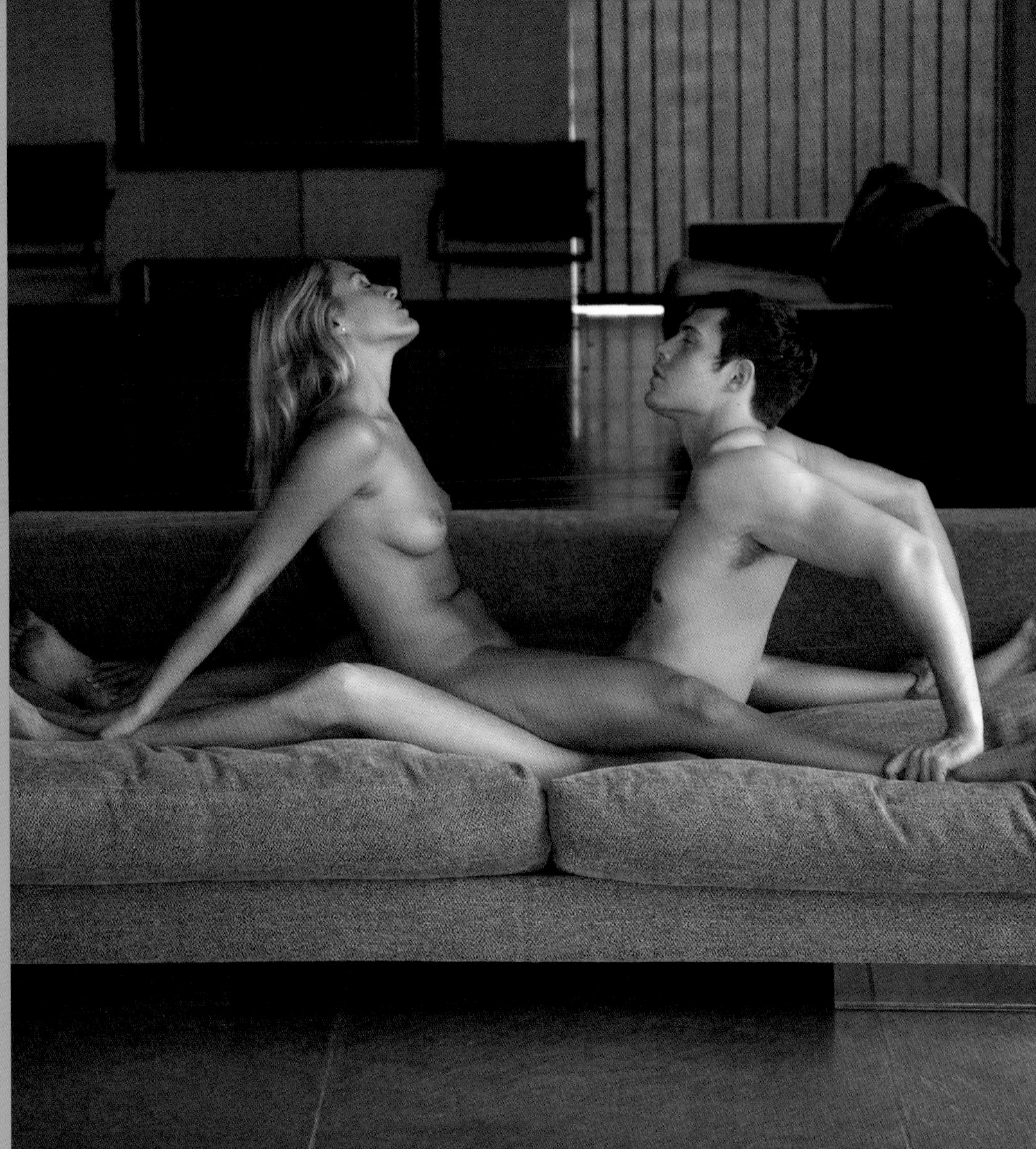

54

sex reflex

Feet are seen as highly erotic in many cultures—ever seen those infamous ancient drawings of men satisfying women by using their big toes to stimulate the clitoris? This position allows you to hold and massage each other's feet, and provides a tranquil pose for you to lie still and/or circulate the sexual energy that's passing between you. (If, instead, you start pondering what colour to repaint the walls, it's time to move on...)

55 randy robot

Yes, this is a particularly odd position. First, it's unusual for her to lie flat on top of him. But that's not nearly as strange as her holding her arms by her sides in such a robotic fashion. (Like, if you don't feel like it, just say so!) The *Kama Sutra* suggests this pose puts her in the steering position. I have to be honest, this isn't a runaway favorite of mine, because it can feel dispassionate. Others get off on that very fact: forbidding each other to get turned on can have the opposite effect!

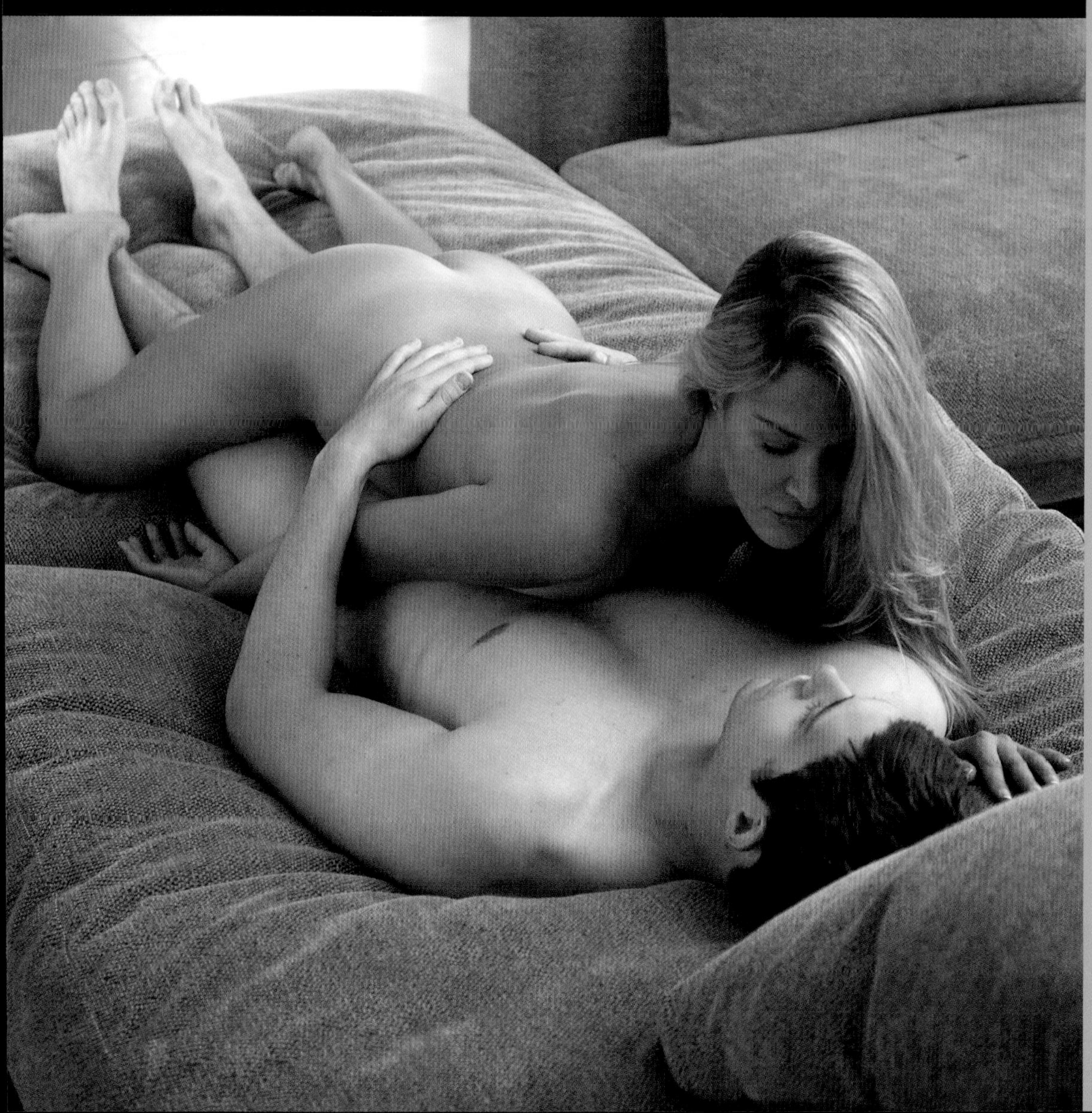

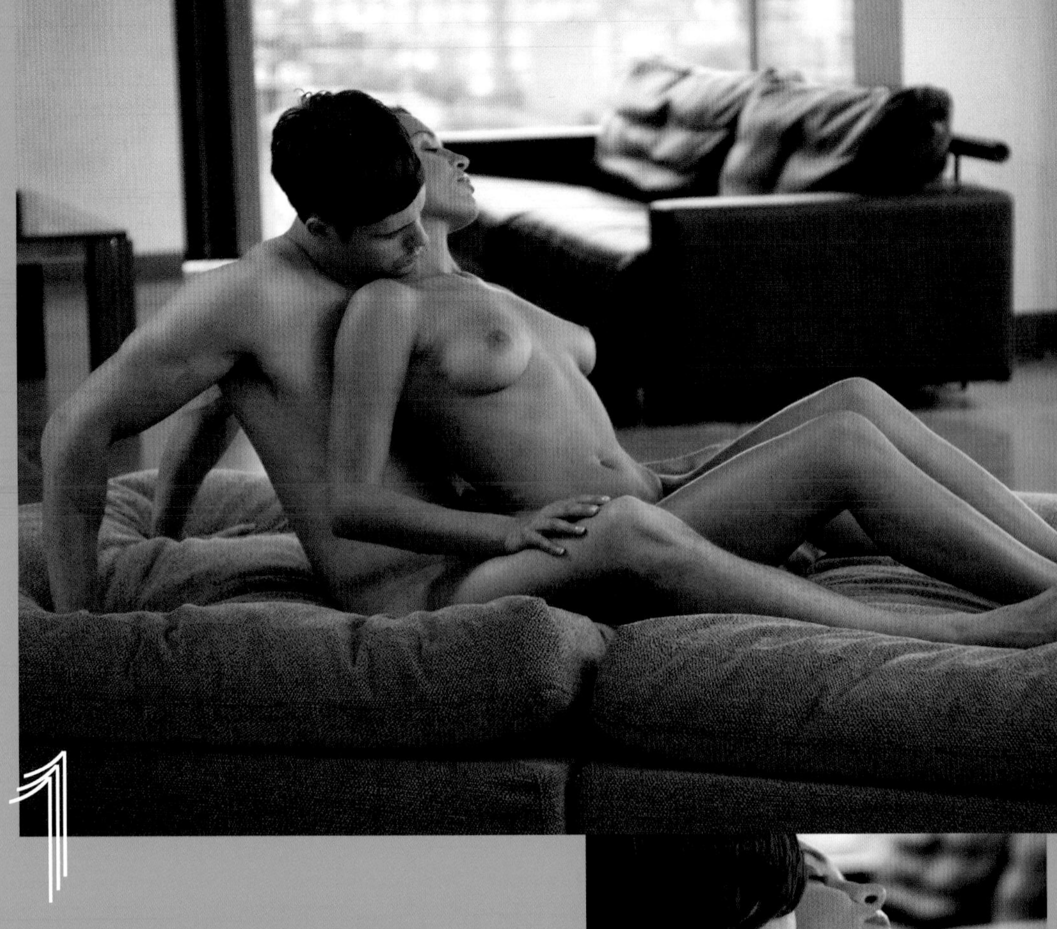

clench tightly

1 He lies back, legs stretched out and apart, and supports his weight on his outstretched arms. She lies back against his chest and, pushing back against him for leverage, lifts her bottom and uses her hands to help him penetrate before settling into his lap and relaxing against him.

2 By alternately arching her back then relaxing against him, she creates enough friction to stimulate both of them. He's in a prime position to nibble her neck and whisper horribly filthy things into her ear—or sweet soulful somethings, which is probably more what the inventors intended!

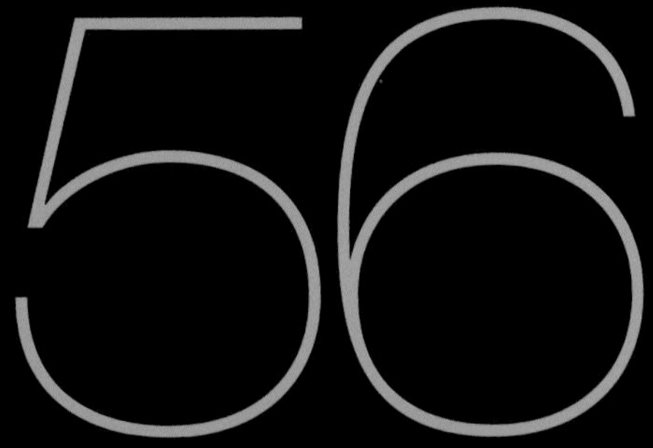

3 Squeezing her legs together, she leans forward and puts her hands on her ankles to hold herself there. (The truly flexible will put palms flat on the bed.) This squeezes his penis. He, meanwhile, clenches his thighs around her buttock cheeks as both rock to and fro. For men who sometimes (OK, often) enjoy a rear view, this could well become a sexy new staple to add to your erotic repertoire.

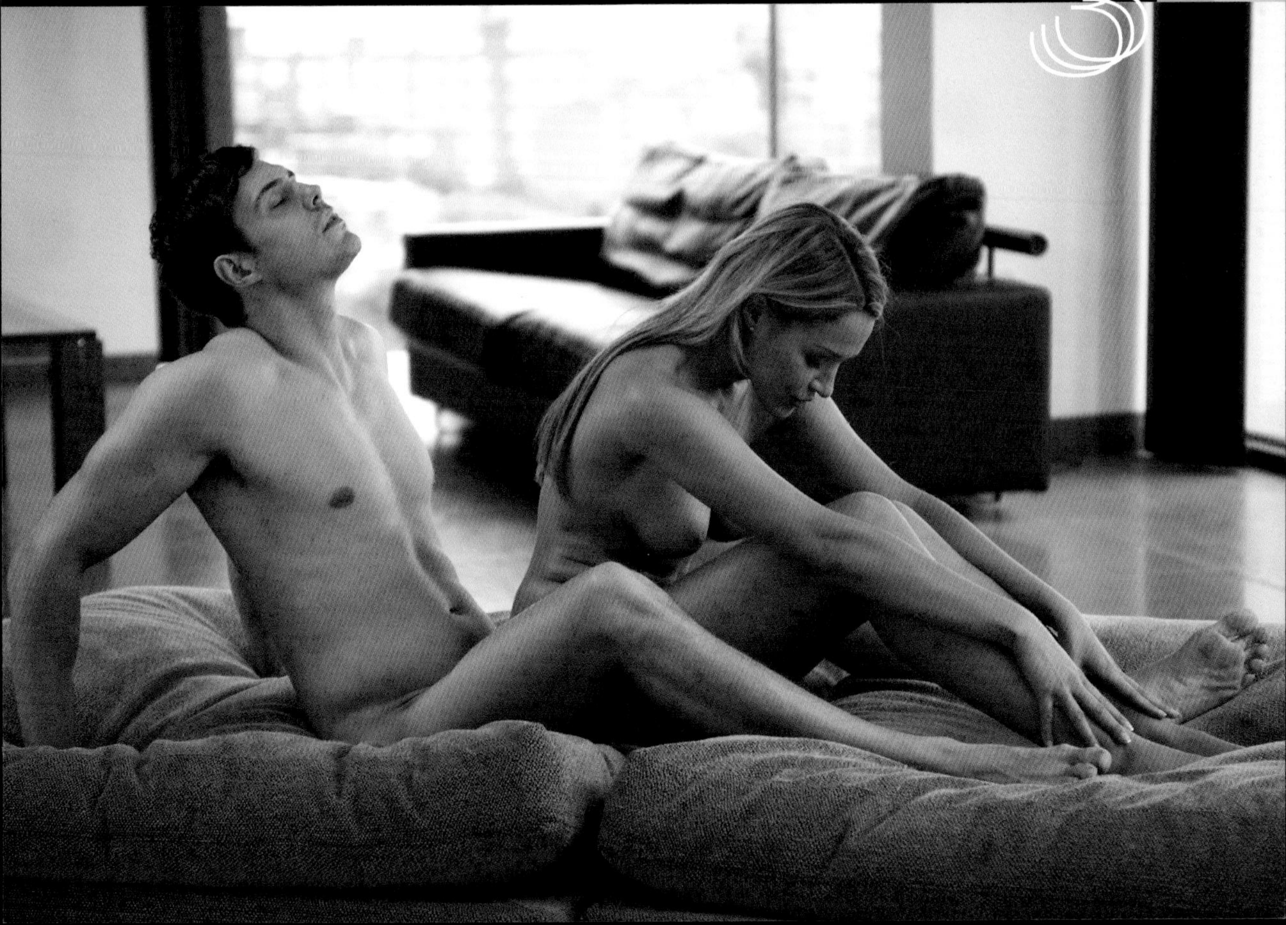

3

hippy trippy sex

A spiritual sex fan, I wasn't; let's be honest—some of it really is a crock. But then I began reading in earnest and if you can get past the let's-all-pretend-we're-little-flowers-growing-in-the-wild stuff, there's actually some really good, sound advice there. I emerged from the research pleasantly surprised and, dare I say, a tad converted! Here's what I think are the best parts...

tantra

basic principles Sex is slowed down. There's gradual, controlled thrusting, rather than a frenetic free-for-all. This enables women to use techniques like vaginal tensing and flexing—a posh version of pelvic-floor exercises. Tantric sex can go on for one or two hours, but the jury's still out on whether longer sessions lead to more enjoyable sex.

If you're the type to drift off while your partner's thrusting away ("Have I got time for the gym tomorrow?"), "connecting" exercises could be useful. Traditional sex therapy encourages people to lose themselves in the experience; Tantra is about staying fully aware and present. Breathing exercises help to improve sexual tone and prolong intercourse.

lessons to learn Tantra encourages couples to stop being time- or orgasm-focused and to involve the heart as well as other body parts. There's no place in it for lovers to be selfish—it's all about giving.

kama sutra

basic principles Interestingly, all the complex seduction and sexual techniques actually aren't aimed at couples in love. If you love each other, you just need to "let yourselves go and be led by instinct." (Oh, really?) The techniques are designed to help you achieve this state. Some positions seem yogalike because they're designed to facilitate meditation as a couple and are intended to allow you to have sex for one or two hours with minimal movement. During this time, you will exchange vital energies—or fall asleep. (It's appealing or *soooo* not.)

"There's no place for lovers to be selfish—it's all about giving."

lessons to learn The *Kama Sutra* recognized female orgasm in a time when others thought there was no such thing, and recommends the man ensures she climaxes before he does. Sexual boredom and monotony are seen as the reason why couples split up. (In some parts of India, men are encouraged to read the *Kama Sutra* before marrying. If everyone enforced this kind of premarital sex research, I think affairs and divorce rates would fall dramatically!)

taoism

basic principles Taoism recognizes men can have multiple orgasms because orgasm and ejaculation are separate events. Using long, involved "Stinglike" processes, men are taught to train their brain and body to separate orgasm from ejaculation. There's a focus on lots of foreplay and nine types of thrusting to try—the goal being to achieve 81 thrusts (one set of nine of each type)!

lessons to learn Taoism recognizes that male desire is easy to ignite and quick to burn out, while female arousal takes longer but lasts longer. Foreplay is prolonged, with lots of finger and mouth action for her.

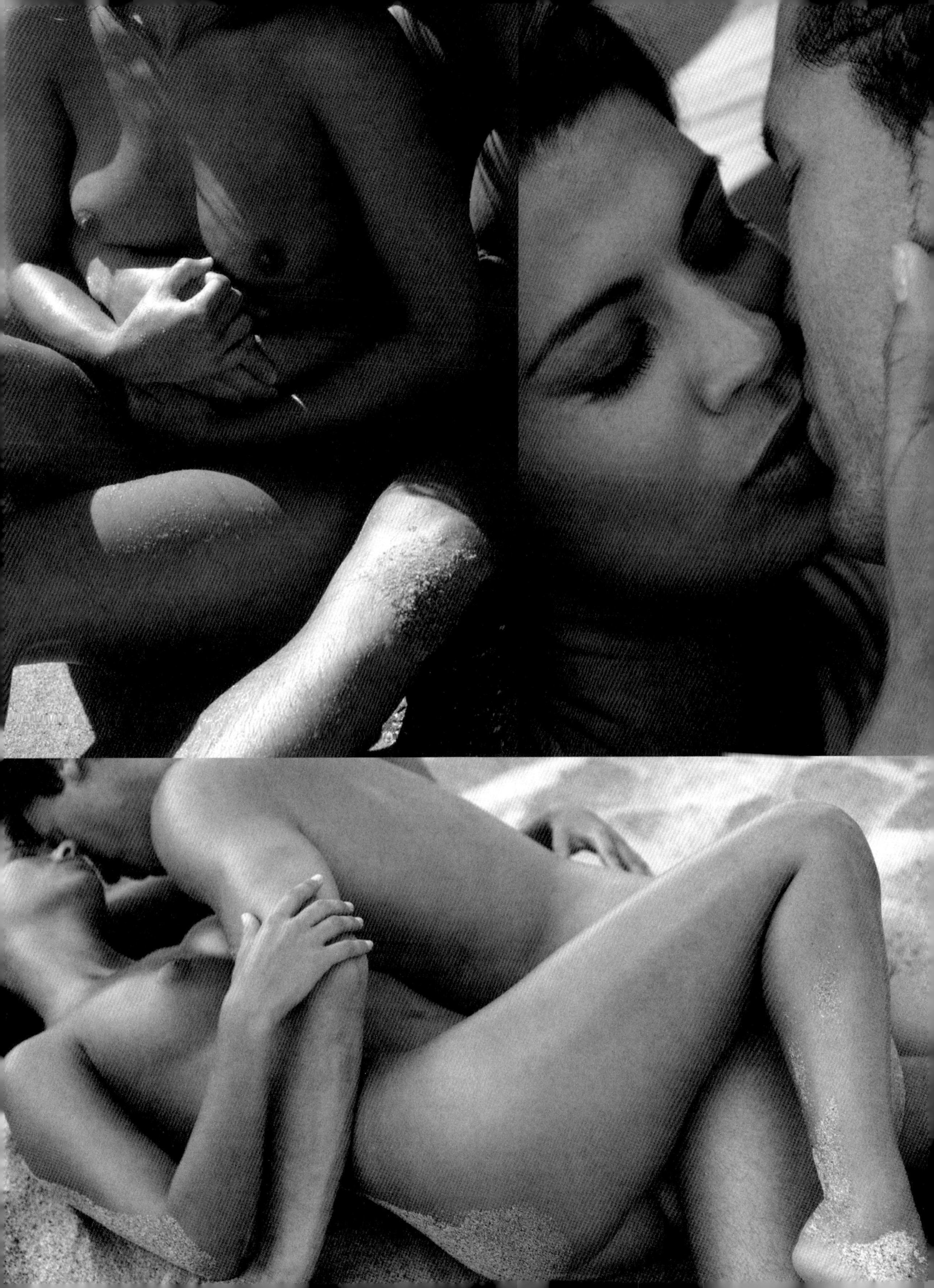

57

worldwide favorite

Ever tried this one? Hah! Of course, you have: the good old missionary position is a favorite for couples worldwide.

When you want to get up close and personal, you can't beat him just climbing on top! Which is basically what's happening here: she lies flat on her back, he jumps on top and enters and—*voila!*—you've just assumed the staple sex position for pretty much every couple on the planet.

There's a reason why it's so popular: you can lick, bite, and kiss each other, watch each other's expressions, fondle breasts

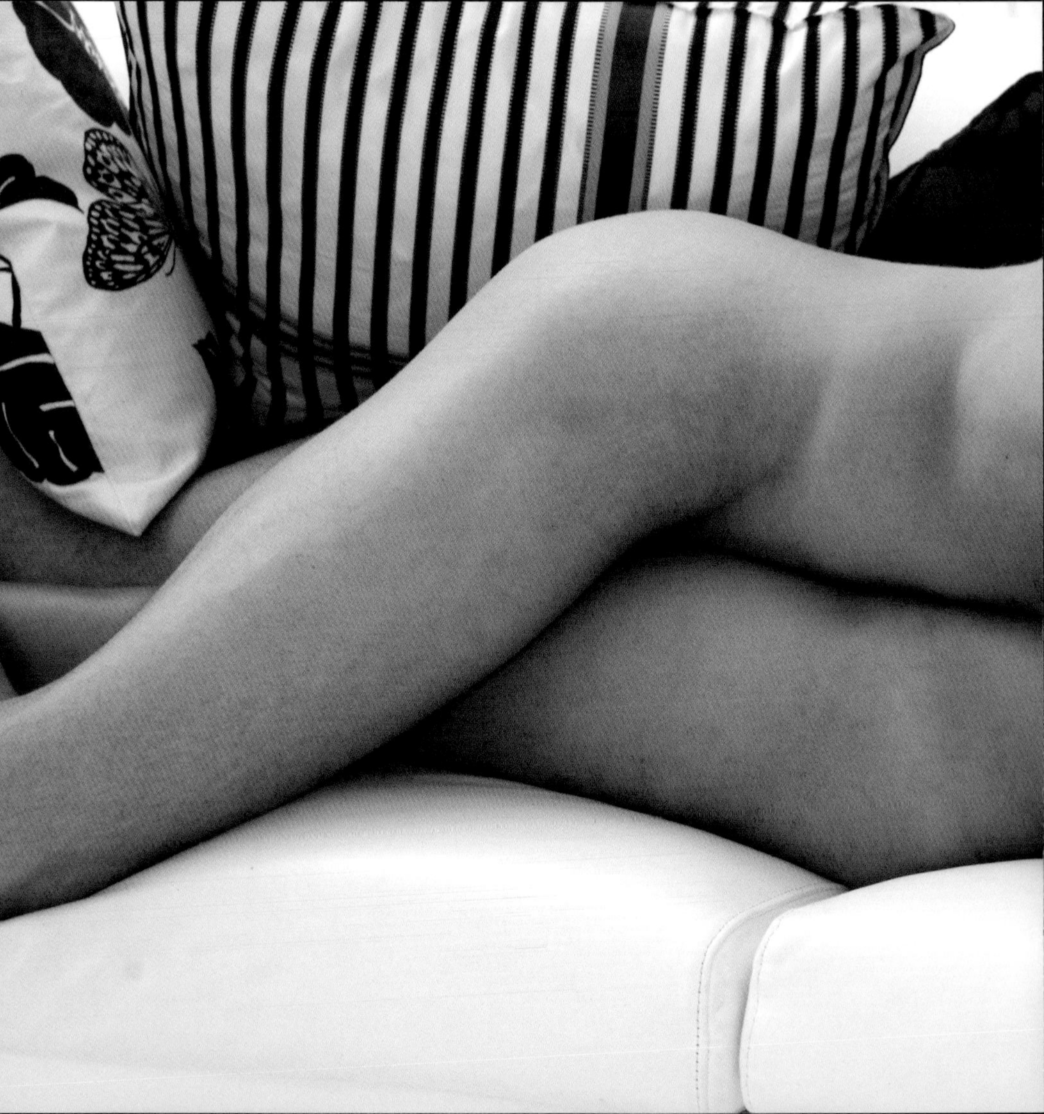

and bottoms, and whisper wicked things. Another reason why it's so well liked? It's versatile enough to do just about anywhere. On the floor, the table, the sofa, the outdoor furniture, your parents' bed…

The slow and soulful sex positions in this chapter can feel a little tame, but I'm trying to introduce a spiritual element along with a feisty frisson, and face-to-face favorites like this one help you stay in the moment. For a varied pace, move from a position in this chapter to a more adventurous one from elsewhere in this book in the same session.

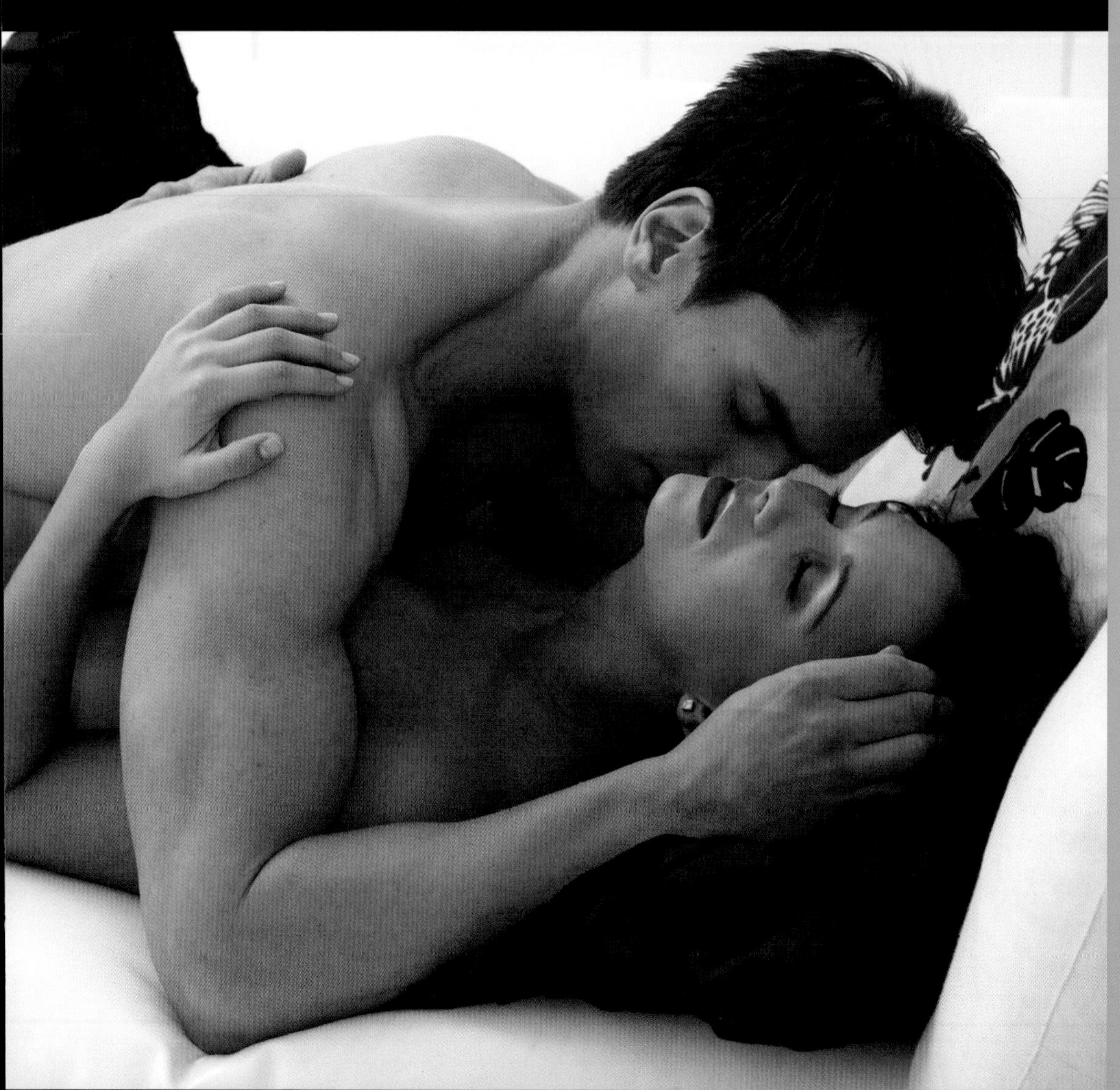

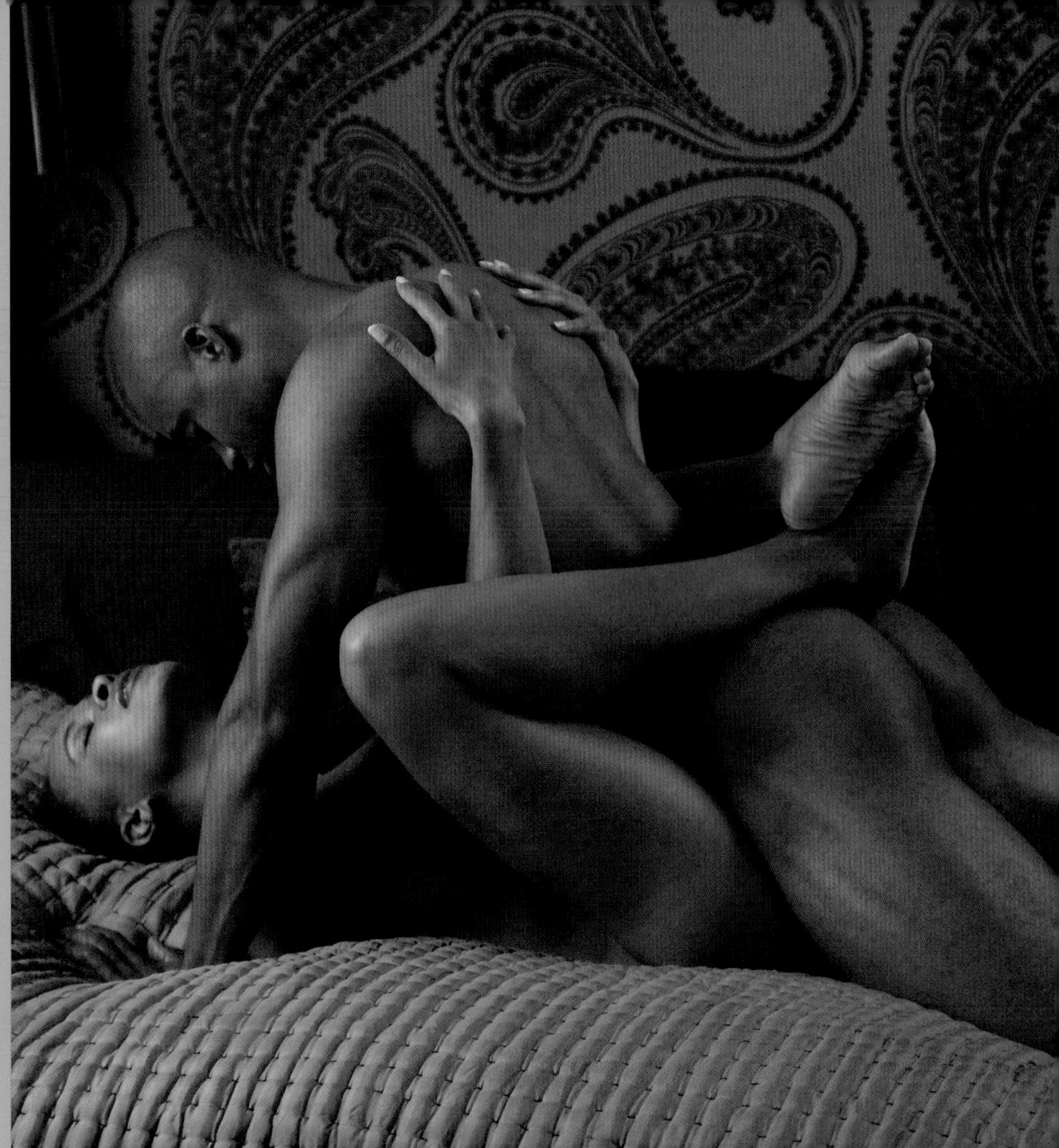

58

sexual healing

Start in the missionary position, with him supporting his weight on his hands. She wraps her legs around his waist, crossing her ankles in the small of his back. He climbs "up" her and rides her so high, her pelvis rolls back to put the penis and vagina in perfect alignment. He then stays completely still as she rolls her hips in small circles, first one way, then the other. The purpose of this is to "heal" and stimulate her sexual organs. Not feeling sick? Try it anyway—it feels fab!

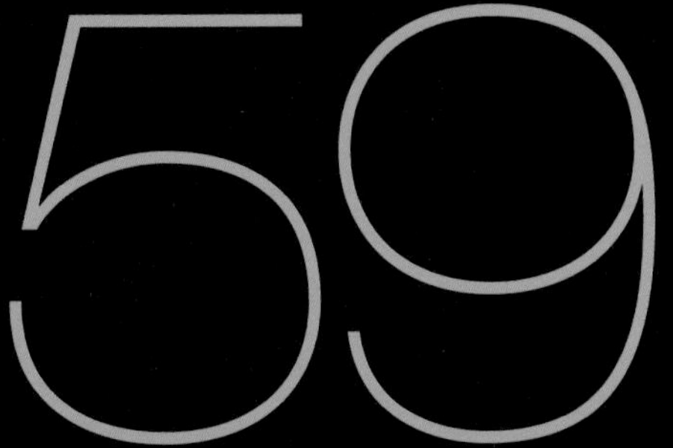

sexy snooze

This handy little number is designed to be used as a “breather” position, slipped in between more dextrous and demanding ones. You’re even allowed to have a little nap if you choose (which is pretty likely if he’s already had an orgasm, has his head on a comfy pillow, and is being flooded by Mother Nature’s sleepy post-orgasm hormones). In theory, his penis would stay inside her as you both sleep. In reality, it will sneak out to snuggle up against his thigh and join you!

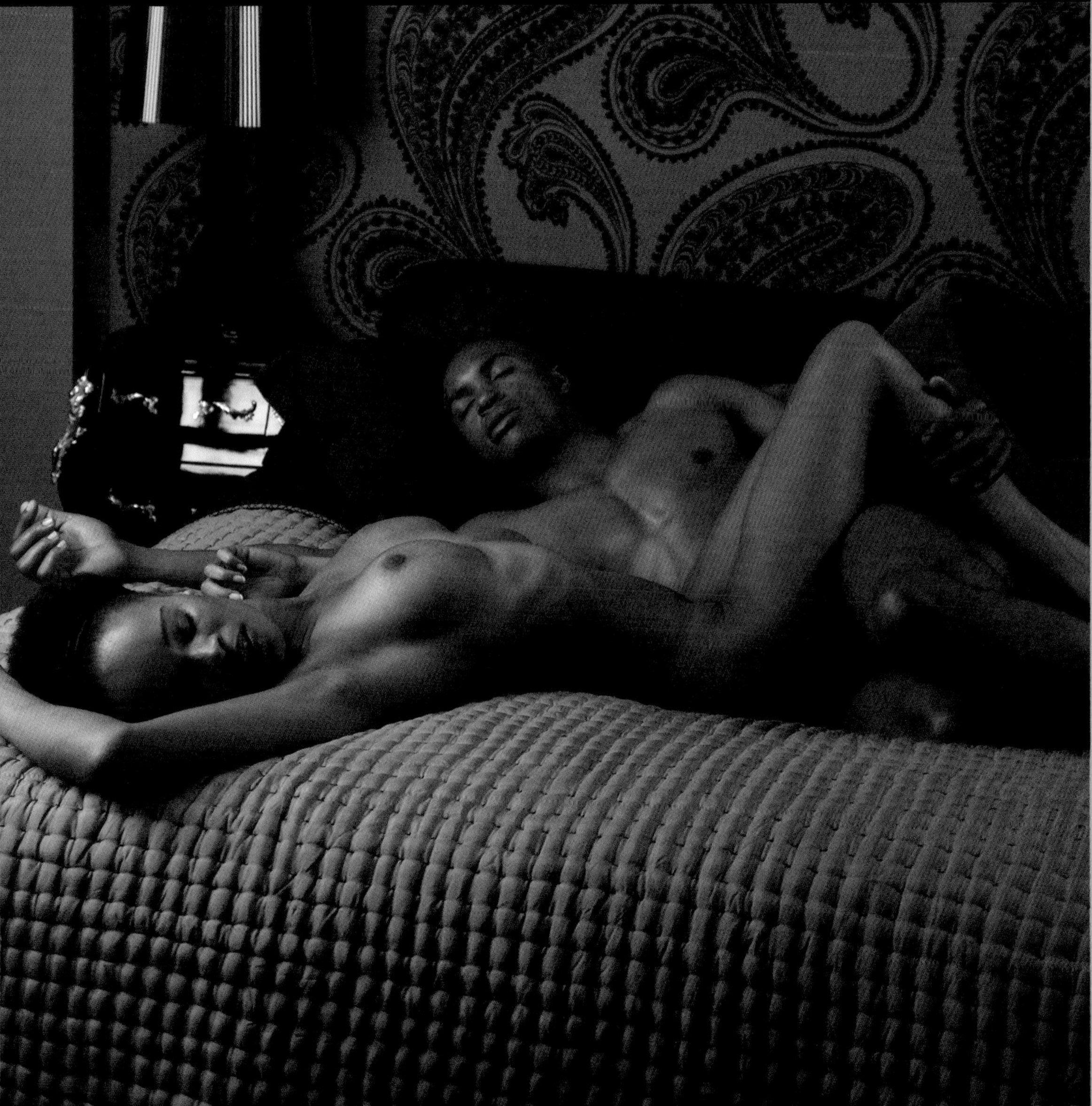

standing ovation

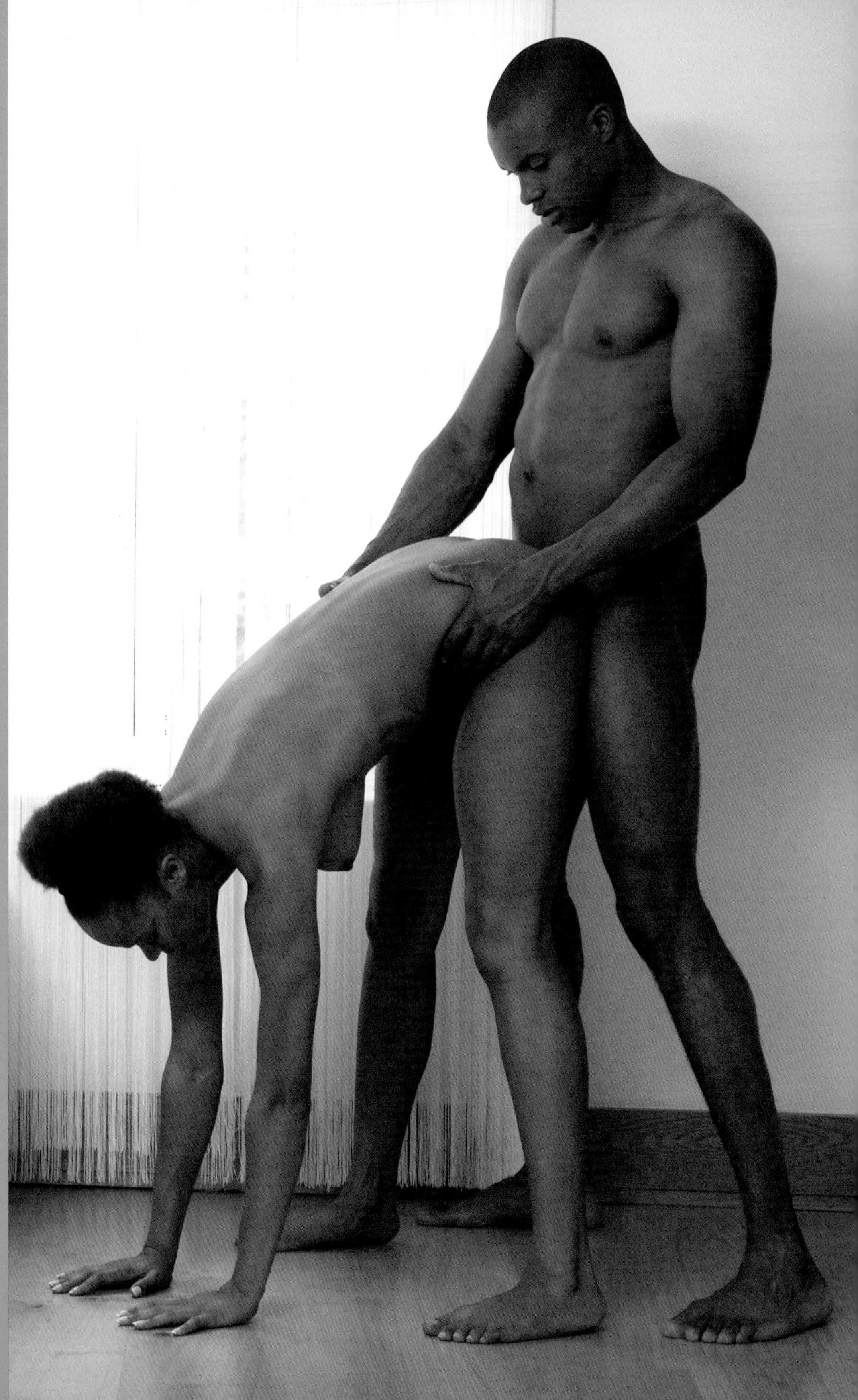

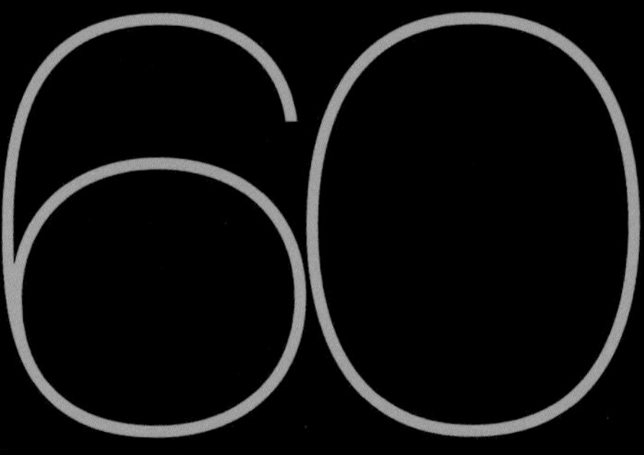

the cow

Desperately dying to boff each other, but there's no bed in sight? Enter "The Cow"—and you, in an impromptu fashion. This is a perfect position for spontaneous sex—and great for feeding those naughty, anonymous stranger fantasies.

She plants her feet wide apart for balance and bends over until both her hands are flat on the floor. He enters from behind and holds her by the hips to enable him to thrust. He's dominant and she's vulnerable, which equals hot sex. Yes, it's challenging, but with his pelvis pounding against her bottom, thrusting downward to make a beeline for her G-spot, it's so worth the effort. Once you both feel stable, he can also use his hand to stimulate her clitoris.

the orgasm argument

We're humans, not machines and yet we tend to judge the success of our sexual encounters by who came and who didn't. Instead of counting orgasms, aim to keep your libidos nice and high so you feel like sex regularly.

be realistic

* To expect an orgasm every time you touch each other is both unrealistic and restrictive. Instead, aim to keep both of you permanently on sexual simmer: warm up, but don't always allow yourselves to boil over.
* Do this by having sessions that don't end in orgasm. Just because neither of you climaxed doesn't mean it didn't rate as a hot, sheet-clutching experience. And not being fulfilled leaves you wanting more.

libido lifters

* Have quickies. The more quick sex encounters you have, the higher your libido will soar. The more orgasms you have, the more easily orgasmic you will become.
* Masturbate frequently. No one can give you a better orgasm than one you give yourself, and the more of them you have, the more you will want.

know your triggers

* Most of us have a surefire position or technique that usually guarantees orgasm. Know yours, know your partner's, and when you're both dying for release, shamelessly press all the right buttons.

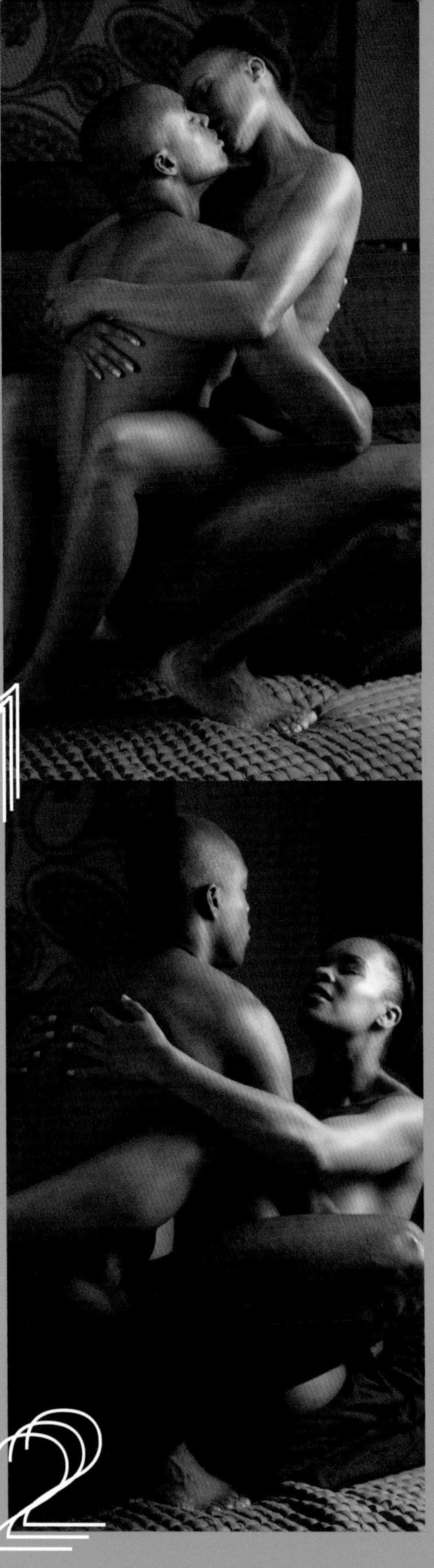

the chariot

1 Even though it's harder to balance on a cushy surface, it'll pay off later… believe me! He squats, she lowers herself onto his penis to sit in his lap and kiss him senseless.

2 Staying inside her, he tips her backward. She supports herself by holding on to his back, and he also holds on tight. The tipping action changes the feeling for both of them, since it dramatically alters the angle of her vagina.

3 Dropping onto the soft surface, still connected, this time you both extend your legs, placing them near or on each other's shoulders, supporting your own weight on your elbows. The angle of the vaginal canal alters again, providing another novel sensation.

4 Sitting up to move closer, he widens his thighs as you both link arms underneath his knees. His feet are on the floor to steady you as you both move into a rocking motion. It's a balancing act—and can quickly reach the point where the effort of maintaining the pose outweighs the pleasure.

5 And that's the moment when it makes perfect sense to shift into the infinitely more relaxing final position. Erotically knitted together, it's time to seesaw your way to orgasm. Open your eyes and watch each other climax if you want to up the intensity.

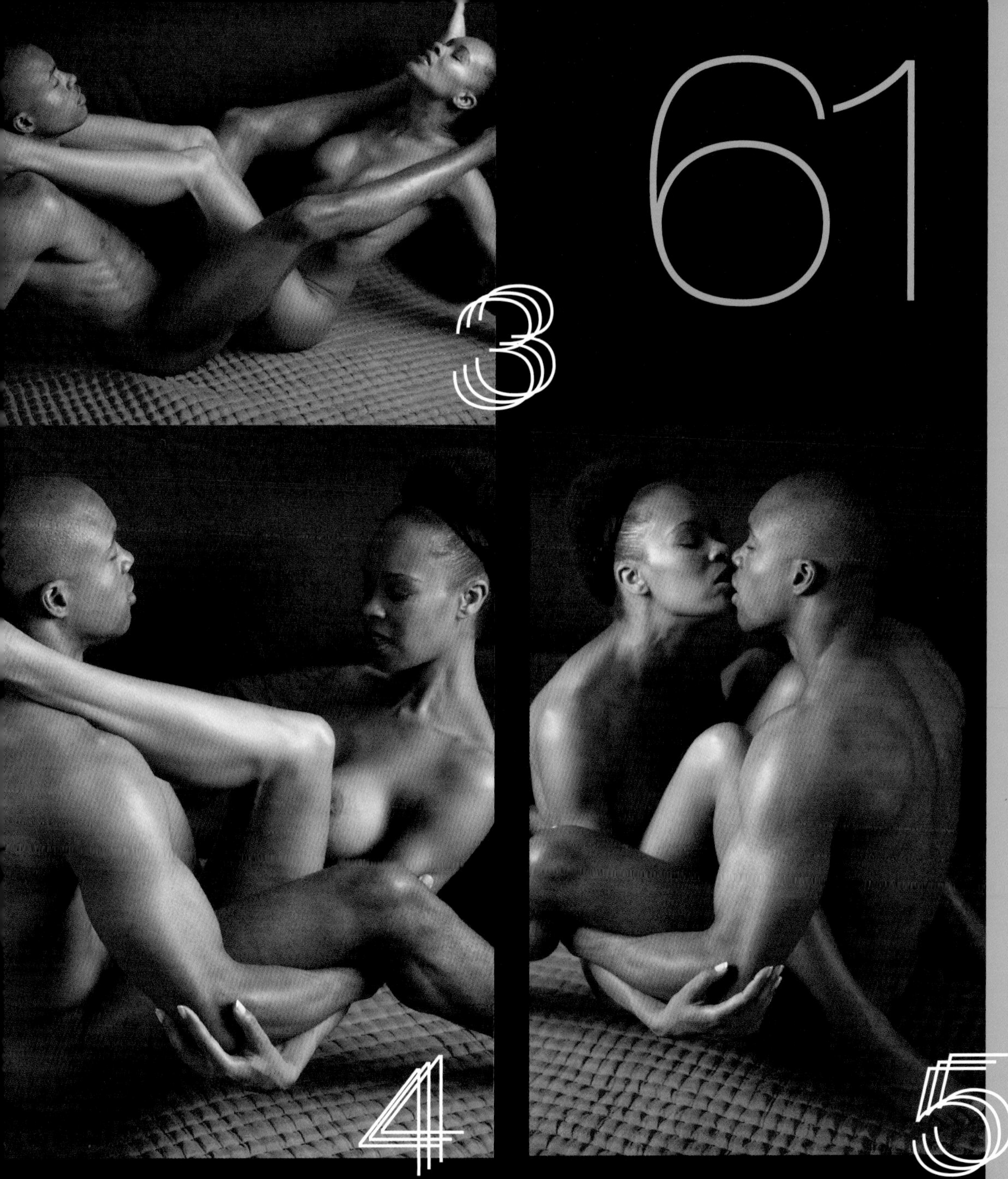
61
3
4
5

62 goddess

He sits back with lots of cushions propping him up so he can comfortably see what's about to be laid out in front of him. She straddles him, but instead of leaning forward, she reaches behind to grip his knees. This has the effect of lifting her breasts—and exposing her entire front torso for him to visually feast on. This is a very equal position, since you can take turns with the thrusting: either he can lift her up and down or she can move her hips in a circular motion.

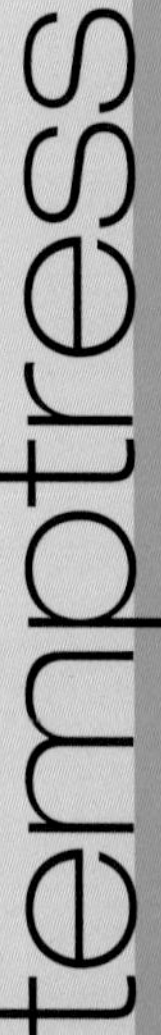

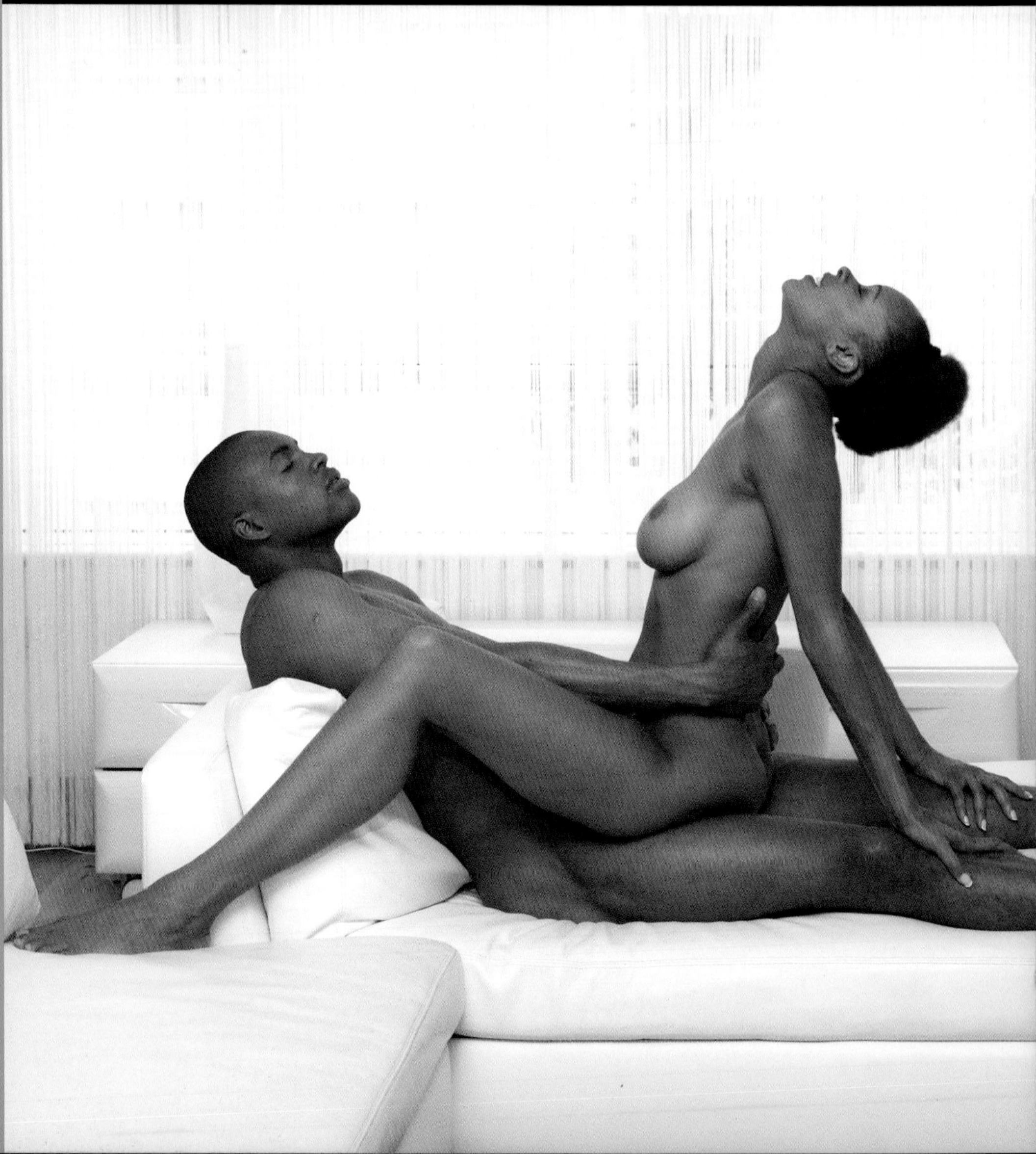

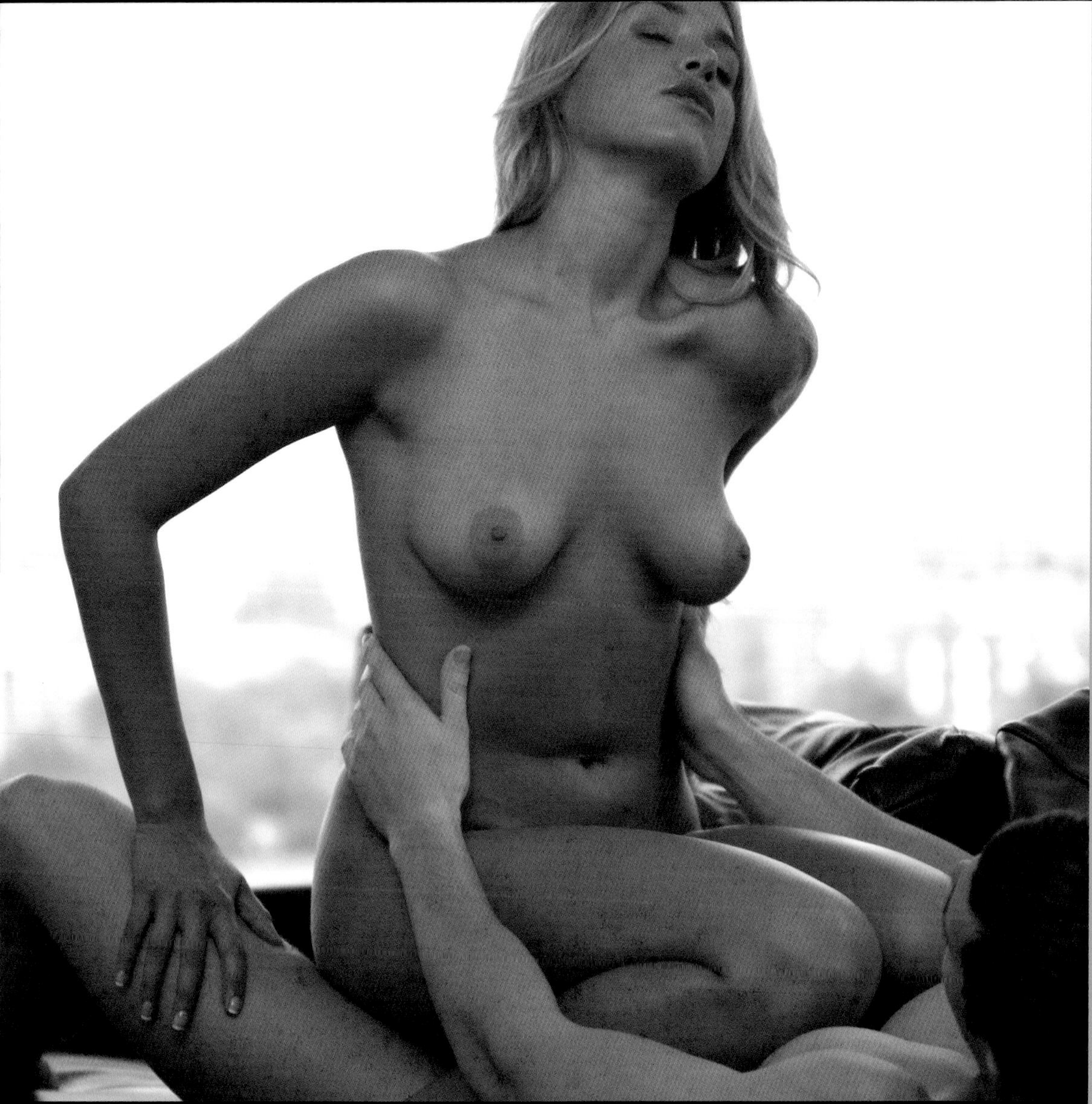

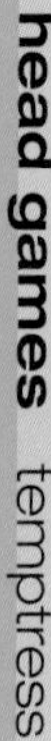

63

sensual hover

Feeling particularly strong? This one looks deceptively easy, but you need both strength and practice to master it. He lies on his back and she jumps on top, feet flat on the bed beside his hips, then, holding his thighs for support and leverage, she swings her hips both left and right over his penis, hovering in sensual circles, just as a bee floats above a flower. It's all about varying her movements to produce exquisite sensations.

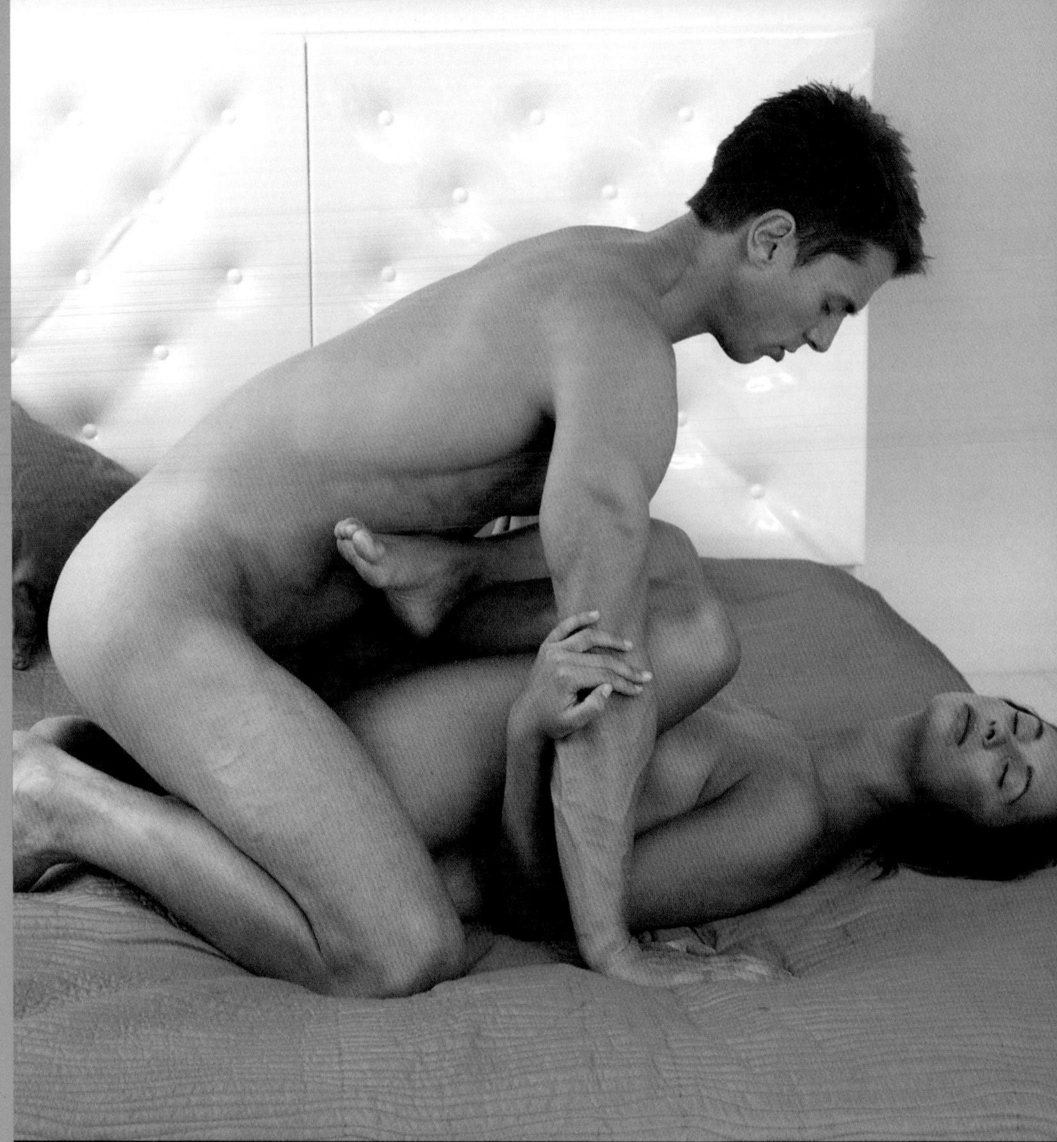

64

lotus

A sexy staple for spiritual devotees, this is classic *Kama Sutra*, so well worth trying for that reason. "Trying," however, is the operative word, because staying in position is more likely to make her grit her teeth than grunt with orgasmic bliss. She lies back, crosses her legs, and draws them up to her chest. He kneels and penetrates. It's designed to draw the vagina up to meet the penis. But unless you're the star of your yoga class (show off), penis and vagina only wave at each other.

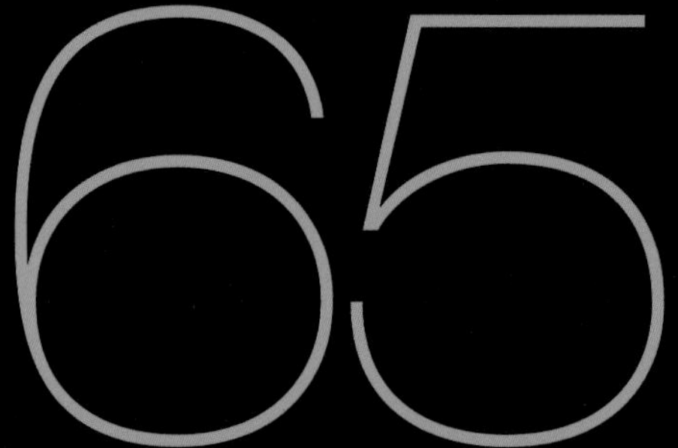

high rider

It's standard side-by-side, but small alterations make a dramatic difference. Altering the position of her legs changes the fit and feel. She might feel like a twit with her leg in the air, but it means his penis is likely to hit a hot spot. If she raises her legs, he can thrust deeper. Keep them straight, with his legs outside hers, and her vagina tightens, allowing him to grind against the clitoris. Wrapping her legs around his back suits "rock 'n' roll"-style thrusting, again providing clitoral stimulation.

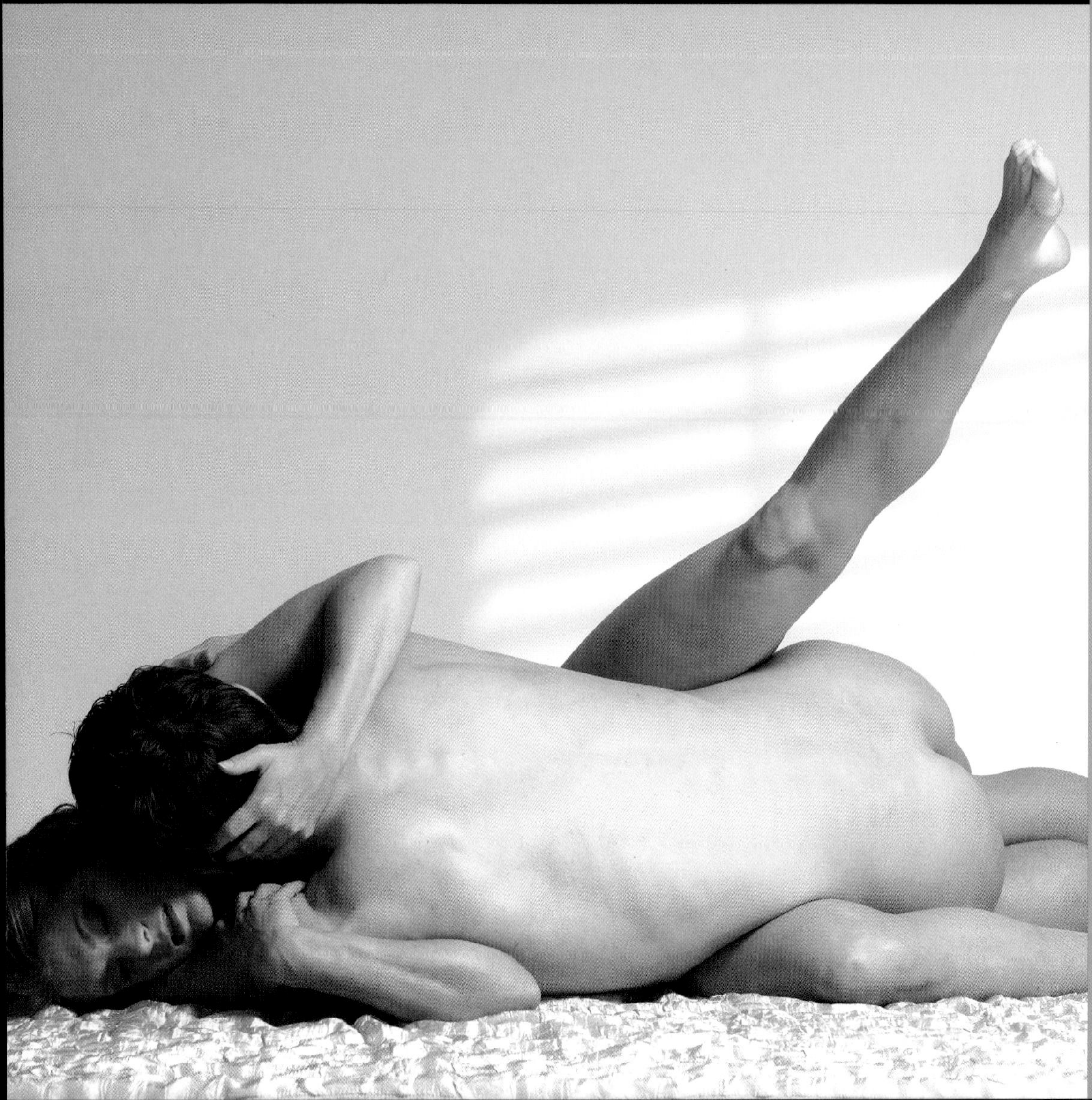

picture perfect

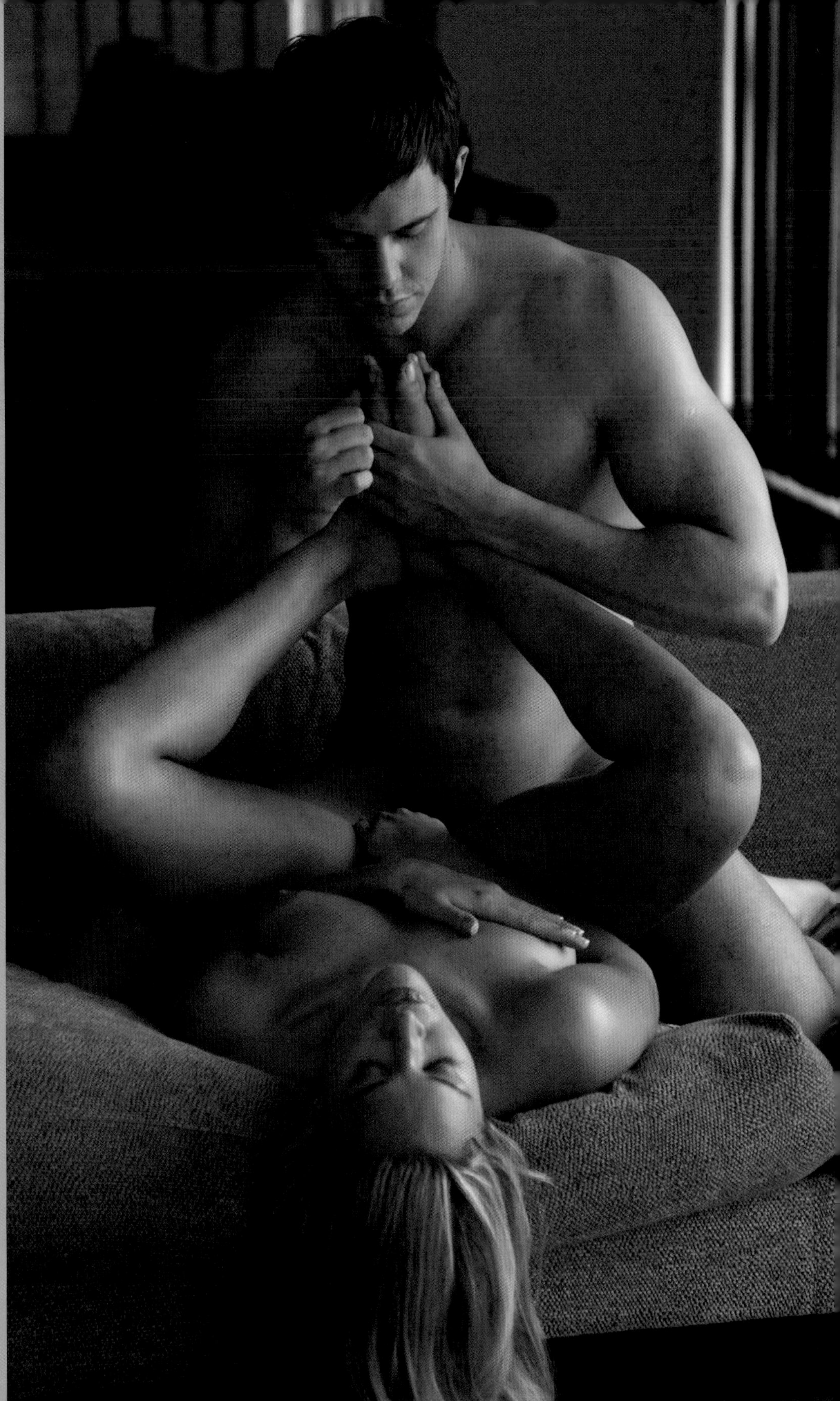

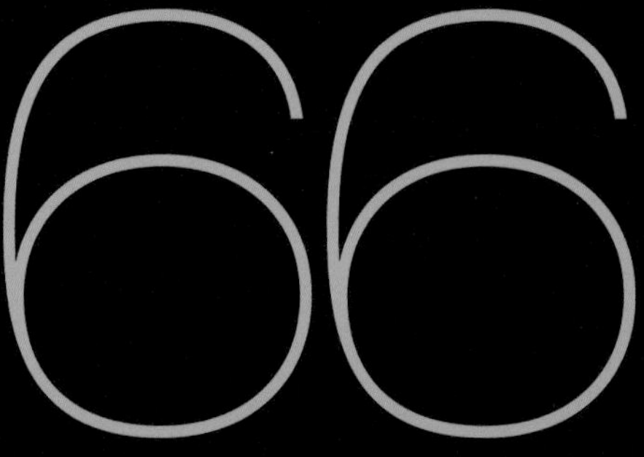

love triangle

She lies back and he kneels in front of her. He takes hold of her feet and brings the soles together, pushing her legs back toward her chest. Her legs then form a triangular shape, forming a "frame" around both genital areas.

It's sweet and spiritually significant—but there are some purely practical reasons for giving this one a try. For a start, it gives her easy access to her clitoris, upping the odds of her climaxing in this position. Second, she can play with her own breasts, making his day!

simple sex treats

The small things tend to make the most difference in life, so it's better to do lots of little things often, than plan one grand sex gesture a month. Think simple, saucy, daily.

effortless

✻ Run her a bubble bath, fetch two glasses of wine, then jump right in there.
✻ Wake him up on the weekend by putting his sleepy or erect penis in your mouth.
✻ Sleep naked—always. But especially if you're going through a low- or no-sex period. Skin-to-skin snuggling at least satisfies the cuddle craving.

out and about

✻ Play in public. Discreetly suck his finger like it's a small penis. Pull her palm to your mouth and bury your tongue in it.
✻ Park the car and have sex in the garage.

dare to do the clichés

✻ Buy some chocolate body paint, pour it on, and lick it off; or dress up as a French Maid. These clichés survive because they're often what people want to do, but don't want to risk appearing ridiculous by asking.
✻ Start a "sex jar": each write down 10 things you'd like to try. Rip into separate pieces, fold, and put all of them into a jar. Pick out one a week to try. (Insist on pre-approval before you pop them in if you think "Lure the hot 18-year-old next door in for a threesome" will simply be repeated 10 times by your partner.)

67 crouching tigress

He lies on his back, she turns her back on him and lowers herself onto his penis in a sitting position. Grasping her feet, she then pulls herself upward so her torso is as straight as possible. Back in *Kama Sutra* times, the man would have admired her elegance, flexibility, and superior posture. Today, he's more likely to be checking out how good her bottom looks going up and down. She's supposed to do the thrusting, but he can help by lifting her at the hips.

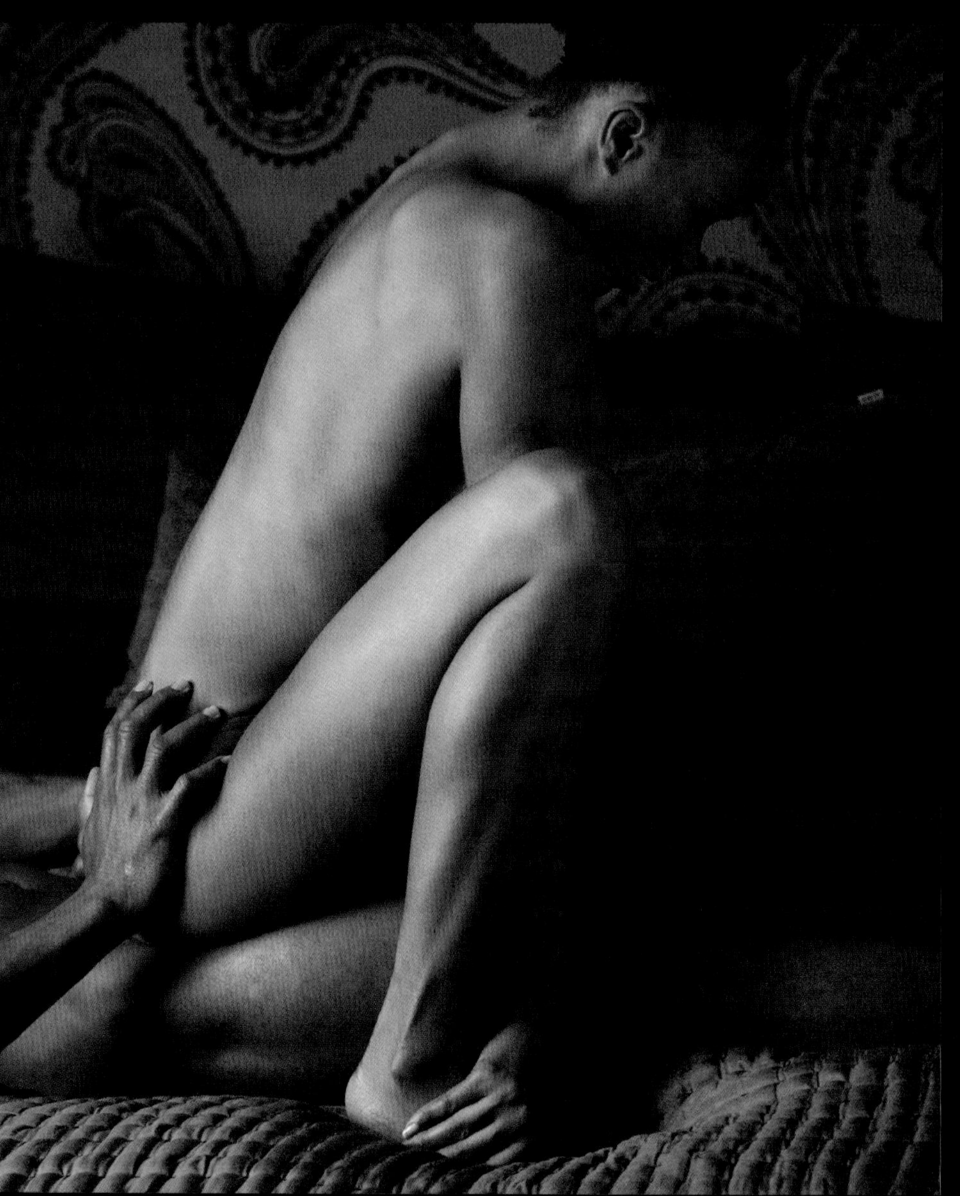

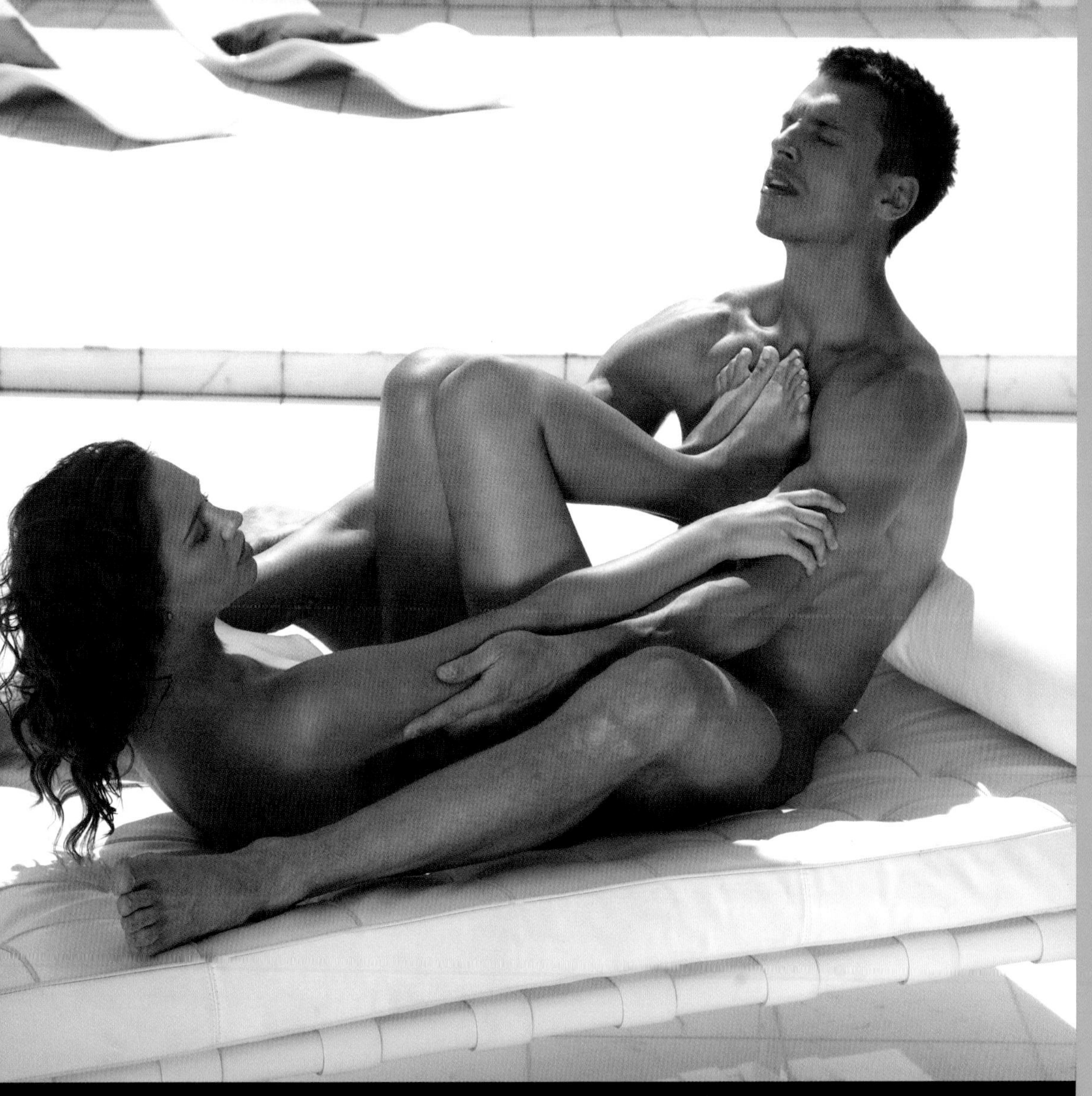

68

tug of war

Start with both of you sitting up straight. She puts her feet on his chest and leans back to allow him to penetrate, then both of you hold on to each other's arms and lean backward. If you were to do this one strictly by the book, he'd also put his feet on her chest. (If you manage to do this, contact the *Guinness Book of Records* immediately!) Not surprisingly, the only "thrusting" option you have in this position is to rock back and forth.

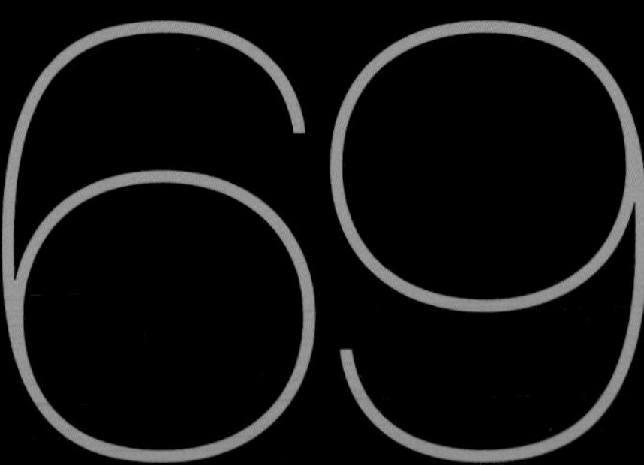

the nail

More playful than passionate, this is perfect for a light-hearted romp. Try taking sex seriously with someone's foot on your head!

Officially called "Fixing A Nail," the name is inspired by her placing her heel on his forehead—the idea being her calf and foot look like a hammer, his head resembles the head of a nail. Hmmm. Sounds al pretty dangerous to me, but I'm liking the leg in the air bit! It's cute, quirky, and simple: she lies flat, he kneels astride her and penetrates. She then stretches one leg out and lifts the other, putting her foot into position.

The thrusting has to be slow and controlled, which can be unbearably sexy. To up the erotic tension, he can put his hand on her breastbone and pretend to hold her down. Be forewarned, though: while some women find this a deliciously "dangerous" turn-on, others may feel uncomfortable.

As he thrusts, her leg moves. If the thought of her kicking you in the face doesn't really appeal, get her to put her leg to the side. Even better, suck her toes, or instead, use your mouth to tell her how breathtaking the view is from up there.

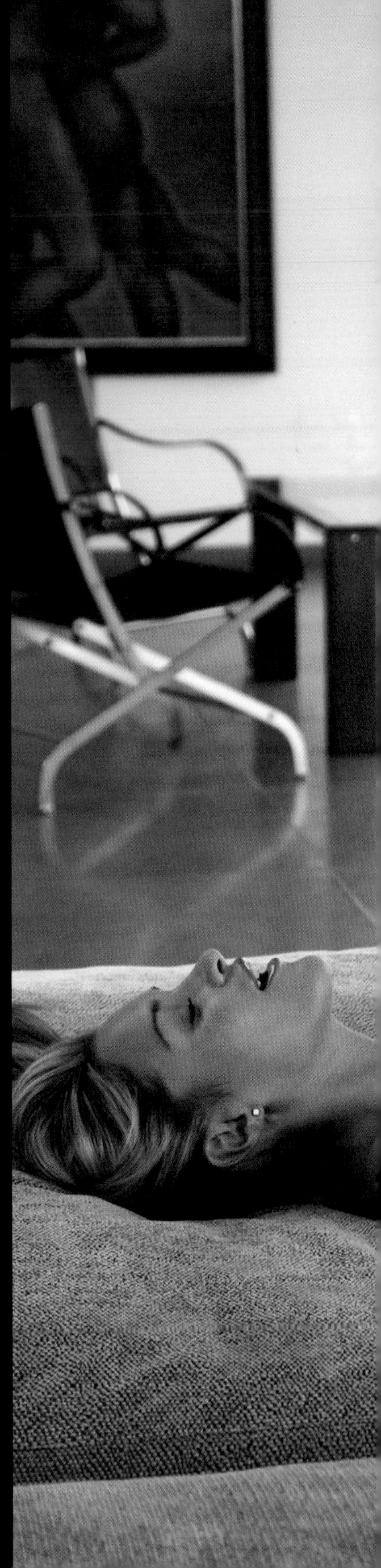

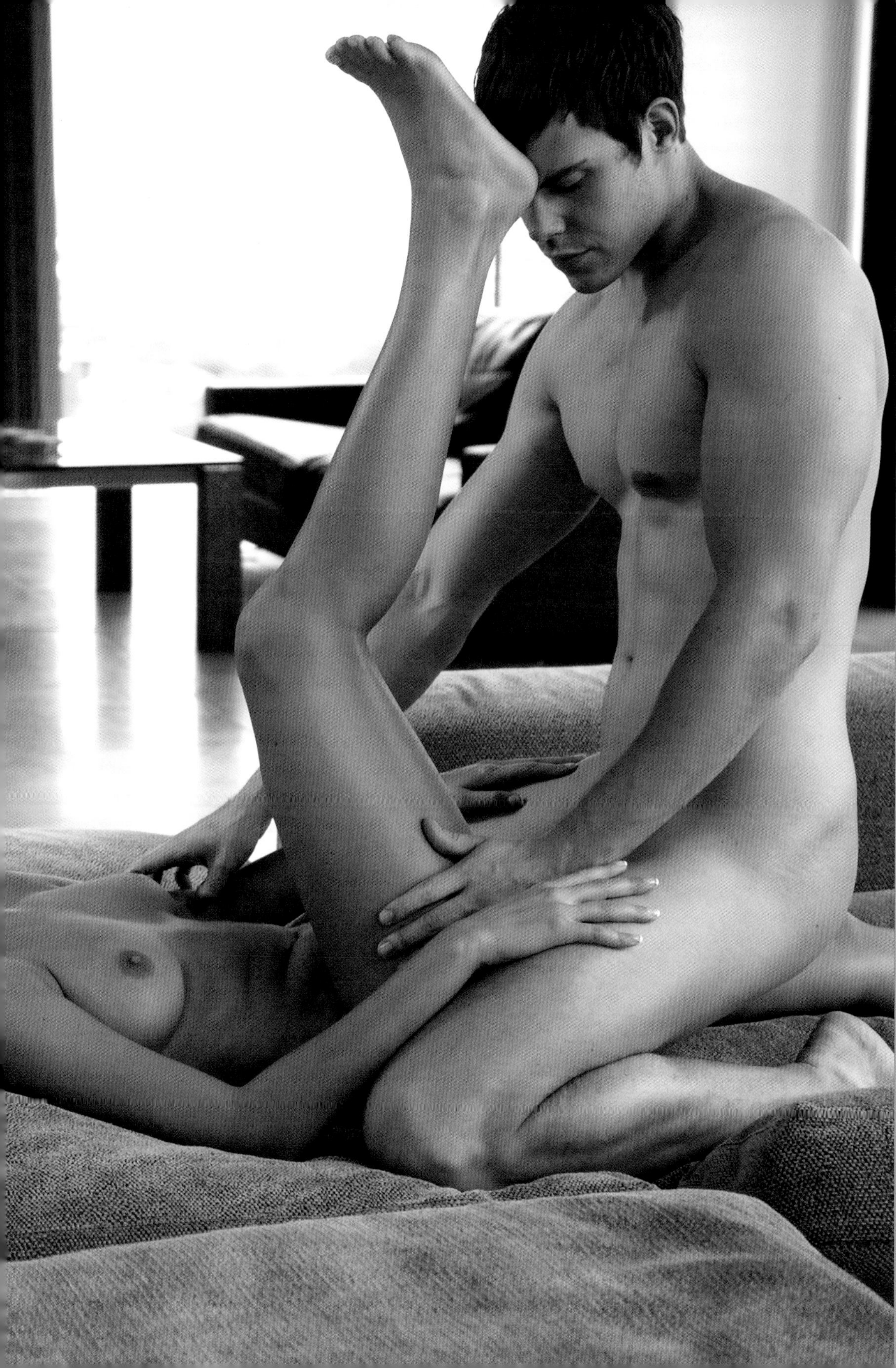

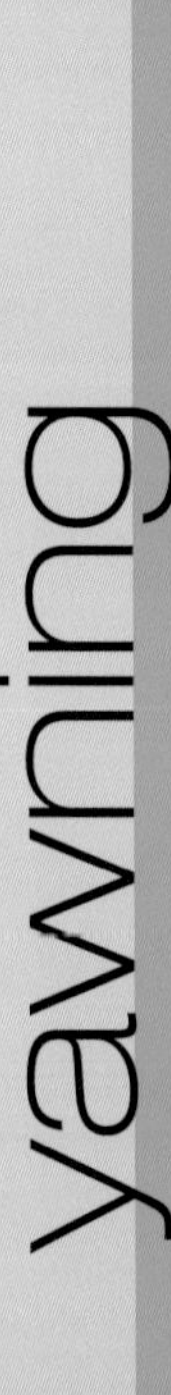
yawning

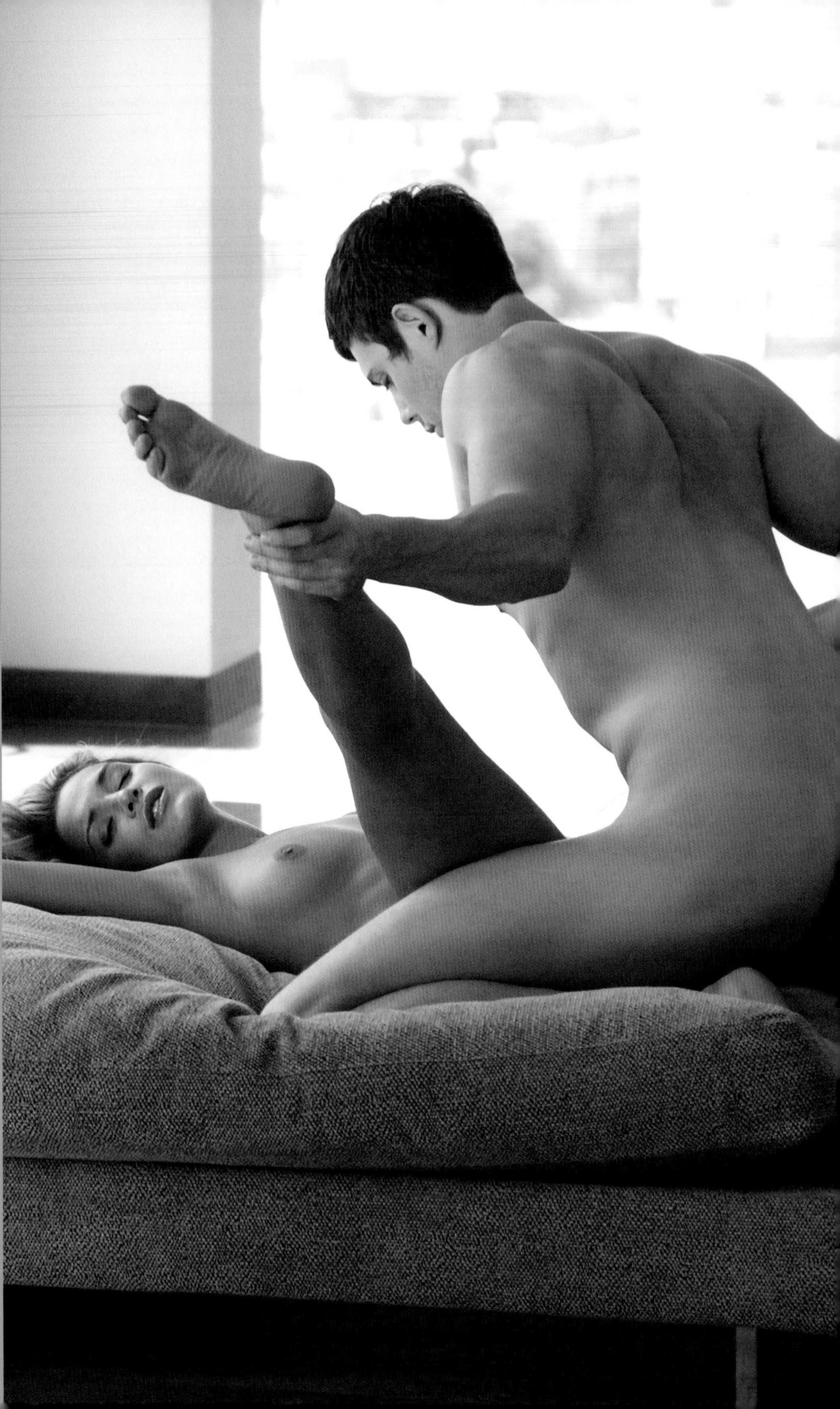

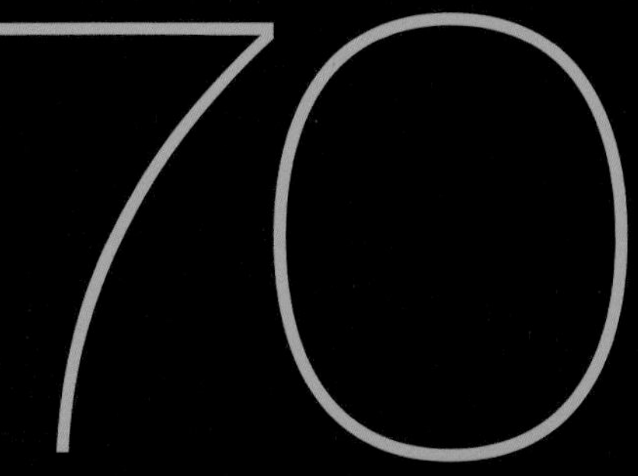

wishbone

This is a *Kama Sutra* favourite originally called "yawning"—but it's likely to do everything *but* inspire boredom! She lies back and spreads her legs as far apart as possible. He kneels in front and penetrates, holding her ankles to hold her legs wide (and make it even sexier!).

To the average Western philistine (that's us), the pay-off is penetration. According to more ethereal types, the wider she opens herself, the more a woman exposes her sexual soul to her lover. It's a visual vulval feast for him and it also lends itself to intense eye-gazing. He can stop thrusting occasionally to lean forward and kiss her deeply; she can vary the sensation by moving the position of each leg one at a time.

Think of this one as more of a treat for the imagination than the body. There's no clitoral stimulation, but it's such an erotic pose you'll be happy to relinquish it. She needs to be fairly supple in the groin and hips.

your toy chest

Trying new positions is a great way to maintain variety. Another trick of lusty long-term lovers: a well-stocked toy box. Here's what to throw in yours:

the basics

* Condoms, lube, scarves and stockings to use for blindfolds and tie-ups, gorgeous lingerie (slutty and sweet), erotic magazines and DVDs, massage oils, and candles.
* Vibes to hold on her clitoris during penetration or to add an extra buzz (sorry, couldn't resist) to oral sex. Finger vibes are great for nipples, clitorises, and around the outside of bottom openings. Also try a "classic vibe"—a slim cylinder, which is a good size to hang on to but not too intrusive.

added extras

* Love eggs: slip these smooth, super-effective egg-shaped vibrators inside her for deliciously discreet vibrations. Double the pleasure by using fingers (or his tongue) simultaneously on the clitoris.
* Vibrating penis rings: these slide over an erect penis and sit snugly at the base. Position the vibrator to make contact with the clitoris once you've penetrated. Maintain pressure with a grinding, circular motion.

the couple's toy

* Hands-free "intercourse" vibes: insert the slender end of the C-shaped vibe into the vagina and it opens into an "L" shape with the clitoral pad against the clitoris. He then penetrates. Fab for her, it provides vibration on the clitoris and front vaginal wall as well as penetrative stimulation as he thrusts.

sex with soul

Just as falling in love lifts us above the mundanity of real life, the thought that sex could do the same—and not just in the beginning, but for a lifetime—is awfully appealing. Achieving this requires a change in attitude, but the key elements are simple: reacquaint those old friends love and sex, and give your love life the most precious gift: time. Here's how to turn wham-bam-thank-you-ma'am sex into something with a bit more depth and feeling.

get connected Stop thinking of sex as a physical activity. Instead, think of it as a way of connecting your minds and souls as well as your bodies.

imagine exchanging energy Even if you don't believe you can move sexual energy around your body at will, you can't argue with the concept of it. It's really just another term to describe being aware of which part of your body is most aroused.

maintain eye contact Most of us close our eyes during sex to concentrate on the sensations of what's happening to our body. Others do it because they feel faintly embarrassed looking at each other, convinced a fit of the giggles is a heartbeat away. Eye contact might feel a bit weird and over-intimate at the start, but once you get past the initial discomfort, it's deeply sexy and you do feel a lot more connected.

If you can't maintain eye contact the whole way through, take baby steps and try it for short bursts of time. (You're supposed to continue the "eye lock" during kissing. But if you're like me, seeing two eyes weirdly morph into one is likely to spark musings of alien invasions rather than tender thoughts!)

match your breathing While exchanging breaths—you inhale what they're exhaling and vice versa—doesn't appeal to the squeamish (or sensible, if it's the morning after the night before and he's had pizza and beer), breathing in time is simple and effective. It's calming, slows you down, and does make you feel more "as one."

have sex without a goal Stop judging the success of your sex sessions by how many or how intense your orgasms were or how many positions you tried. Stop thinking of sex as having a beginning (foreplay), a middle (intercourse), and an end (orgasm). Instead, think of it as a time when you're going to pleasure each other and be connected.

be present in the moment This isn't just a spiritual sex rule—it's something almost all therapists get couples to work on. It's way, way too easy during sex to let the voices in your head hijack you: "Yuk, look at the dimpling on my thigh!/Is she enjoying this? Bet her ex was better at it./Oh my God, is that the time? The kids are going to be home any minute. And what the hell do I give them for dinner? Maybe I should defrost something from the freezer." While you're mentally reaching for the fishsticks, your poor partner's killing themselves, trying to come up with the carnal equivalent of Beethoven's Fifth with whatever body part they've got their hands, tongue, or parts attached to. During sex, try to stop thinking

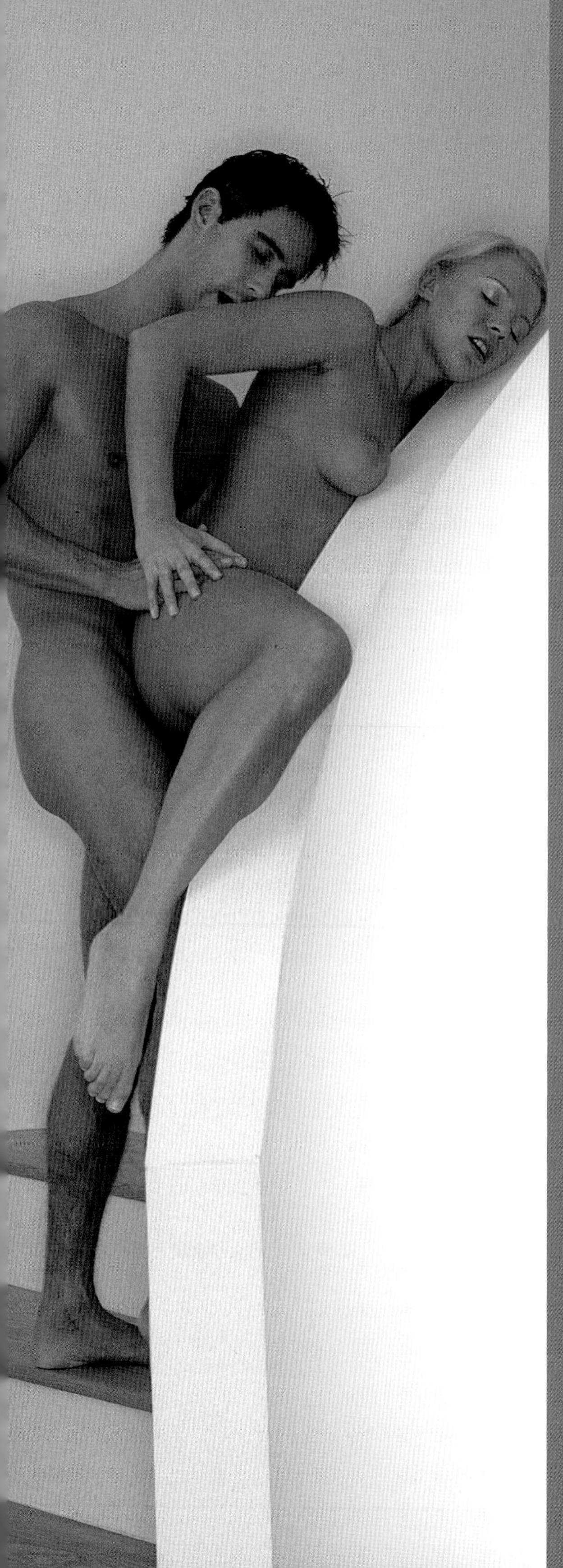

“Sex slowed down can be unbearably, tortuously erotic.”

and start feeling. Be in the room, in the here and now. Do this by keeping your eyes open and focused on what's happening. Concentrate on all your senses: what you are smelling, feeling, seeing, and hearing. If you feel your thoughts pulling you away, drag yourself back.

go slowly At times you'll want to dispense with the niceties, rip each other's clothes off, and have furious, frenzied, lusty sex. I'm not suggesting for a moment that you don't (God forbid!), just that you stop thinking of those sessions as the “hot” ones and slower, more soulful sex as the “romantic” version. Sex slowed down can be unbearably, tortuously erotic. It just means paying attention to more subtle sensations.

Looking in, a couple doing Kabazzah, a Tantric technique, won't appear to be having much fun. He's inside her, but they're completely still with no movement from the waist down. What you can't see is her “milking” him—squeezing her pelvic-floor muscles to massage his penis.

While I'm a huge fan of quick sex, there's a biological reason to slow sex down. Touch and arousal sets off the secretion of natural hormones. Some sexologists believe quick sex isn't emotionally satisfying because there's not enough time for these to be released into the bloodstream. The post-coital “feel-good” factor is short-circuited.

If you want to make her feel super-connected, choose a position where there's full body contact that's maintained for at least 20 seconds at a time. This stimulates production of oxytocin, the “cuddle hormone,” which is stimulated via touch.

the swivel

1 Want to really impress her the first time you have sex? Pull this one off and she'll be on the phone to her girlfriends seconds after you're gone! Be forewarned though: even the *Kama Sutra* advises it takes a lot of practice! Start in the basic missionary position, but just as she's starting to think (yawn) "How predictable," you pull back, look deep into her eyes… and prepare to move.

2 Lift one leg, then the other so both your legs are on one side of her, taking care that your penis doesn't pop out. Keep your legs slightly apart to prevent this from happening. Work yourself around by moving your hands and feet until your body lies sideways across hers. Continually support your weight on your hands.

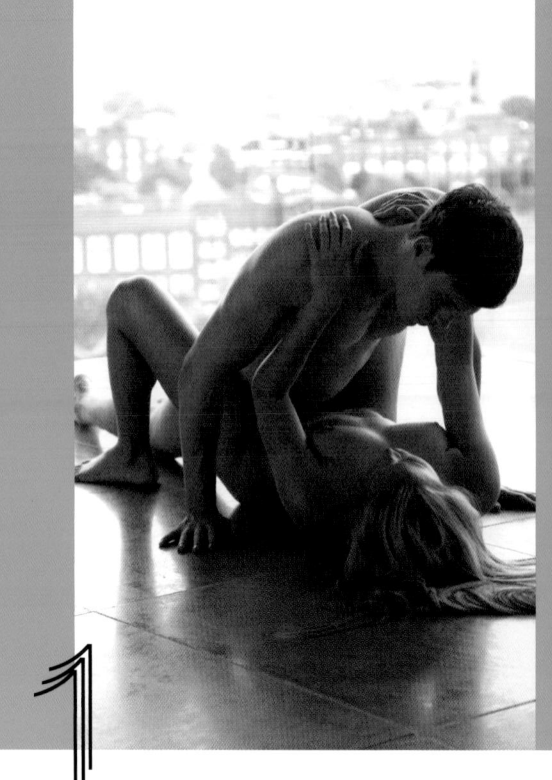

1

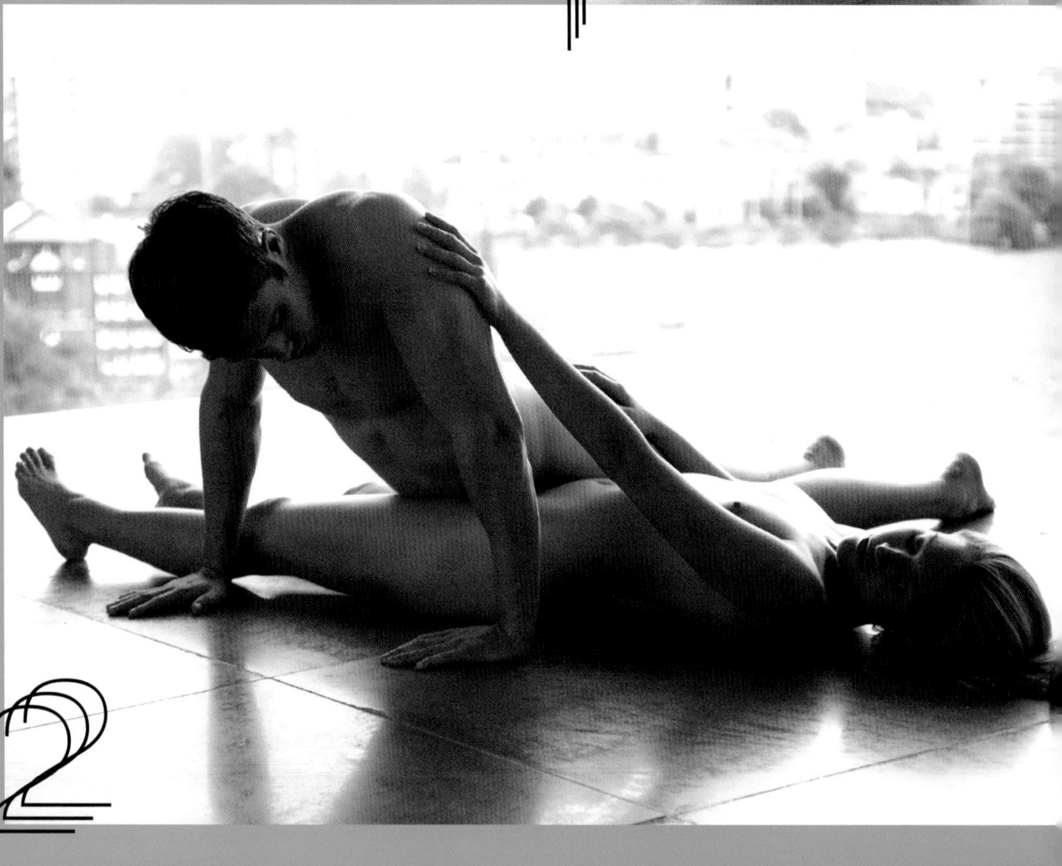

2

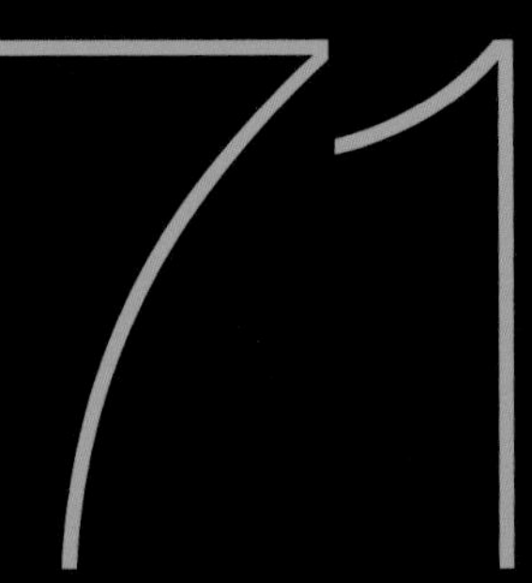

3 Keep moving around until you're facing her toes, very carefully lifting one leg over her face into position. (Pray she's not squeamish, because she now has a prime view of a very private part!) You didn't quite get there or (worse) accidentally kicked her/fell over/fell out? Hopefully she's got a sense of humor. It's best to save this one until you've got it down pat.

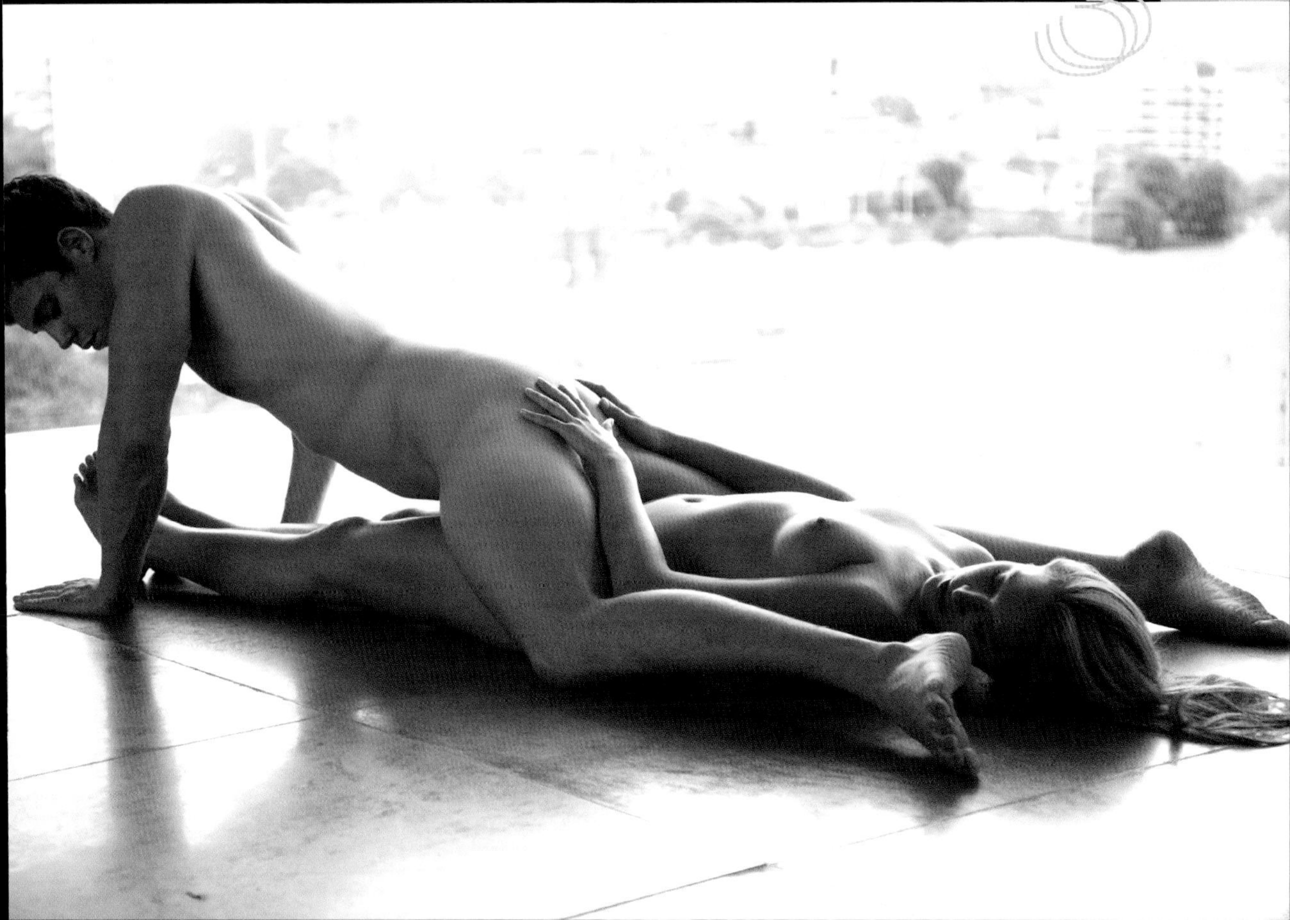

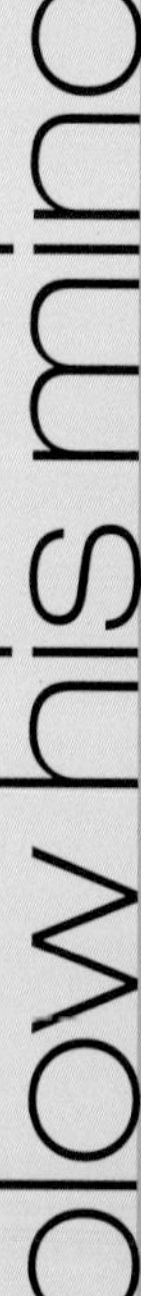
blow his mind

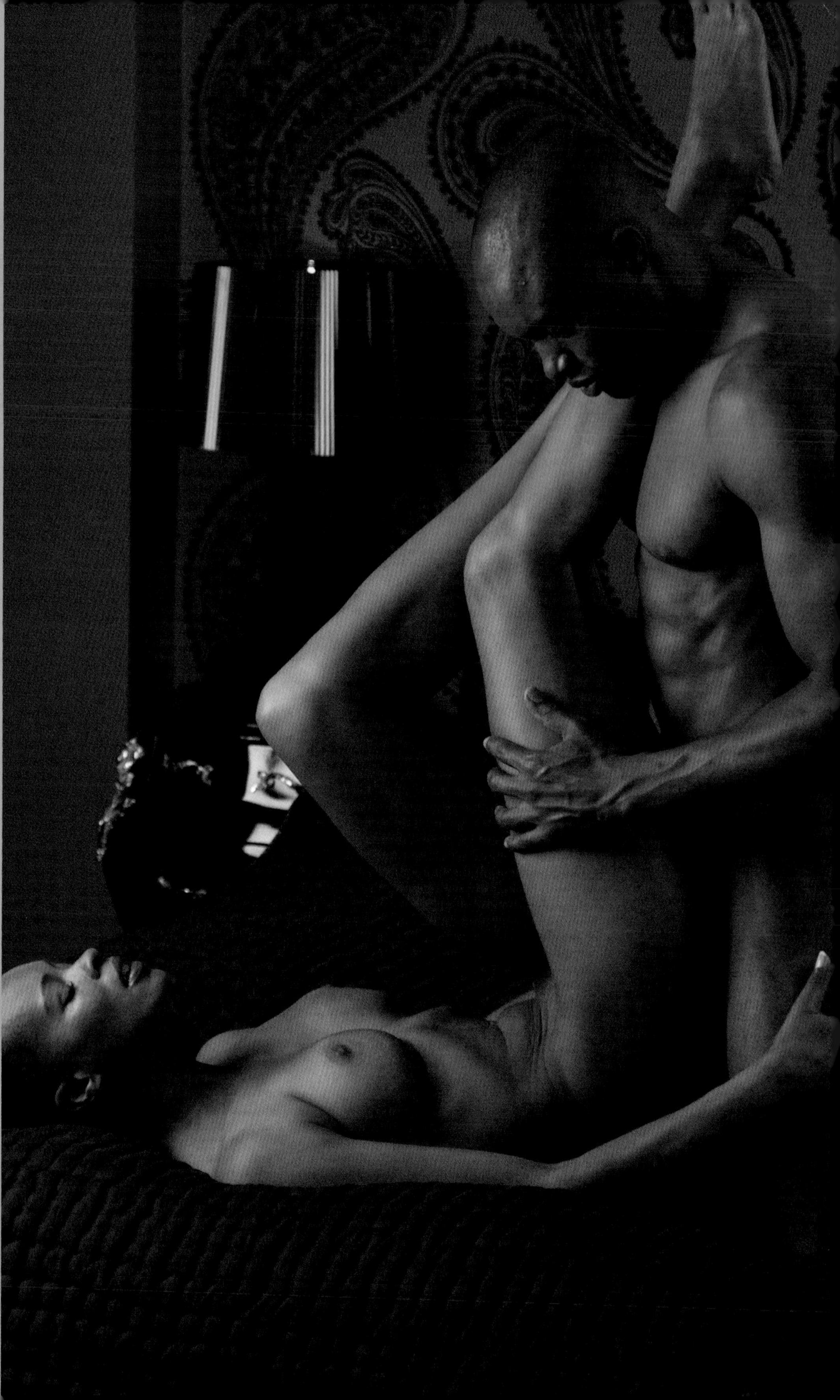

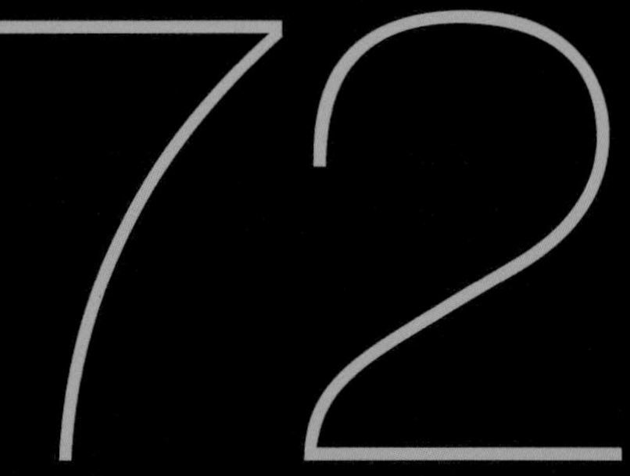

privates dancer

In a beautifully choreographed lusty leg lift, she performs an erotic dance for his penis. She lies face up and brings her knees up to her chin. He kneels in front and penetrates, she then straightens her legs and rests them on one shoulder, pulling one leg back so it's bent. She holds on to the back of his thighs and he grips hers for balance then she "dances": alternating her leg position frequently throughout.

Her vagina is shortened, so it's a tight fit for him. As she alternates the position of her legs, this massages his penis with a unique rolling sensation. He looks manly, and has a great view of her breasts.

on the side

Adventurous positions are more likely to be attempted by new lovers… or those having an affair. Why? Because we make far more effort sexually when we're playing away than we do with our live-in lovers. Want to affair-proof your relationship? Here's how:

know your enemy

* It's long-term laziness that makes us susceptible to an affair in the first place. Affairs provide exciting sex. Long-term couples have cuddly sex, familiar sex, satisfying sex—but the adjective that disappears the most rapidly is "exciting."
* Familiarity makes you shy: it's easy to say, "While you're down there, put this in your mouth" to your new girlfriend. Not so easy when your wife is on her knees picking up the kids' toys. Force yourselves to see each other as you were. Find a photo of the two of you when you were in lust and put it on the fridge.

recreate the turn-ons

* Intensity is often caused by time limitations: enforce deadlines on sex sessions and you'll achieve a similar effect.
* Rediscover technology as the sexy stimulator it can be. When those in an affair text, email, or phone, the communication is lustful and longing. Long-term lovers use electronics for mundane purposes ("pick up the milk on your way home"). Change. Now.
* Leave home: a coffee at lunchtime, when you both have to get back to work, makes us listen more and engage with our partners. Sex on vacation or in a hotel is nearly always better than sex at home.

73

top to toe

This looks damn impressive, but the truth is, if you've had side-by-side sex, you've probably done a similar version without even realizing it. It's just that no one took a picture of you at the time (or at least you hope they didn't).

The only difference is, instead of facing the same way, you're lying in opposite directions (heads pointed toward each other's feet). Thing is, most women move down the bed to make penetration easier anyway, and this position simply exaggerates that natural movement.

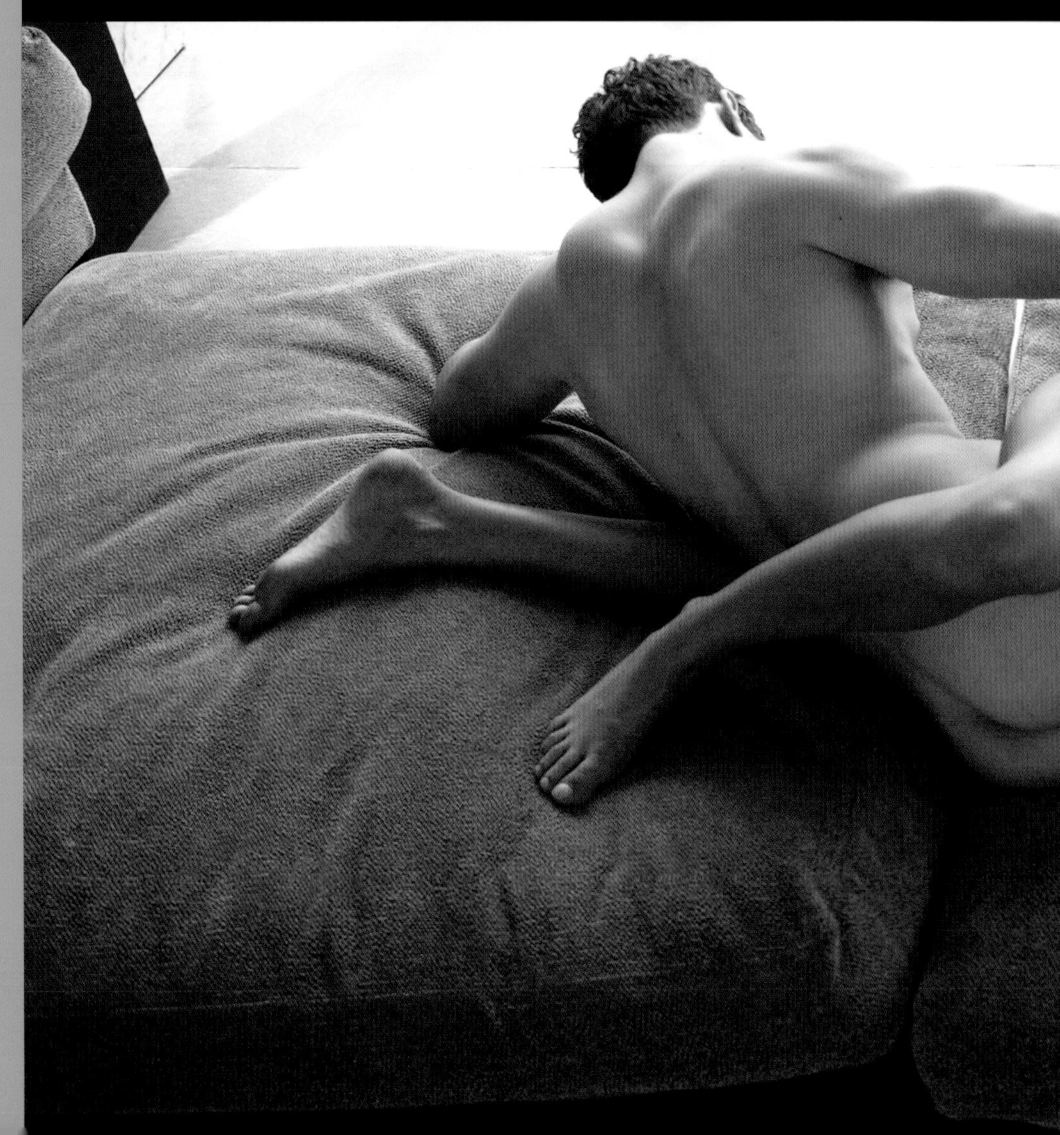

It's easy. It's fun. It's familiar. Do you need any more good reasons to go for it? How about this one: it's something new. Try to get into the habit of trying something different every single time you have sex, and you'll avoid falling into that would-rather-do-my-tax-return-than-have-sex-with-you thing that lots of long-term couples get stuck in. It's easy to do, just change one of the following elements for each session: the time of day you do it, which room you do it in, what you're wearing, what position you choose, who initiates, and what the focus of the session is (hand-job, oral, intercourse, etc.).

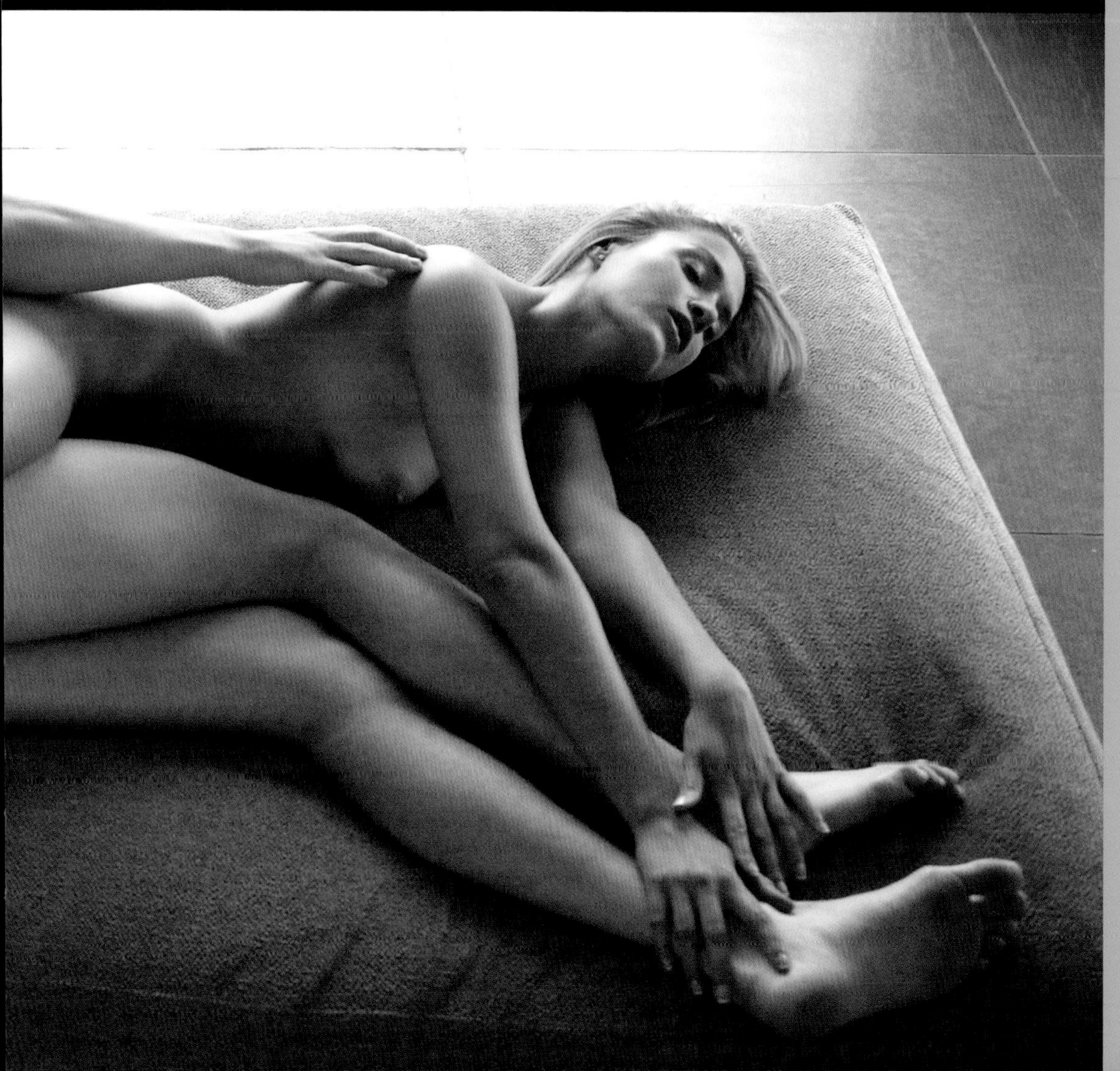

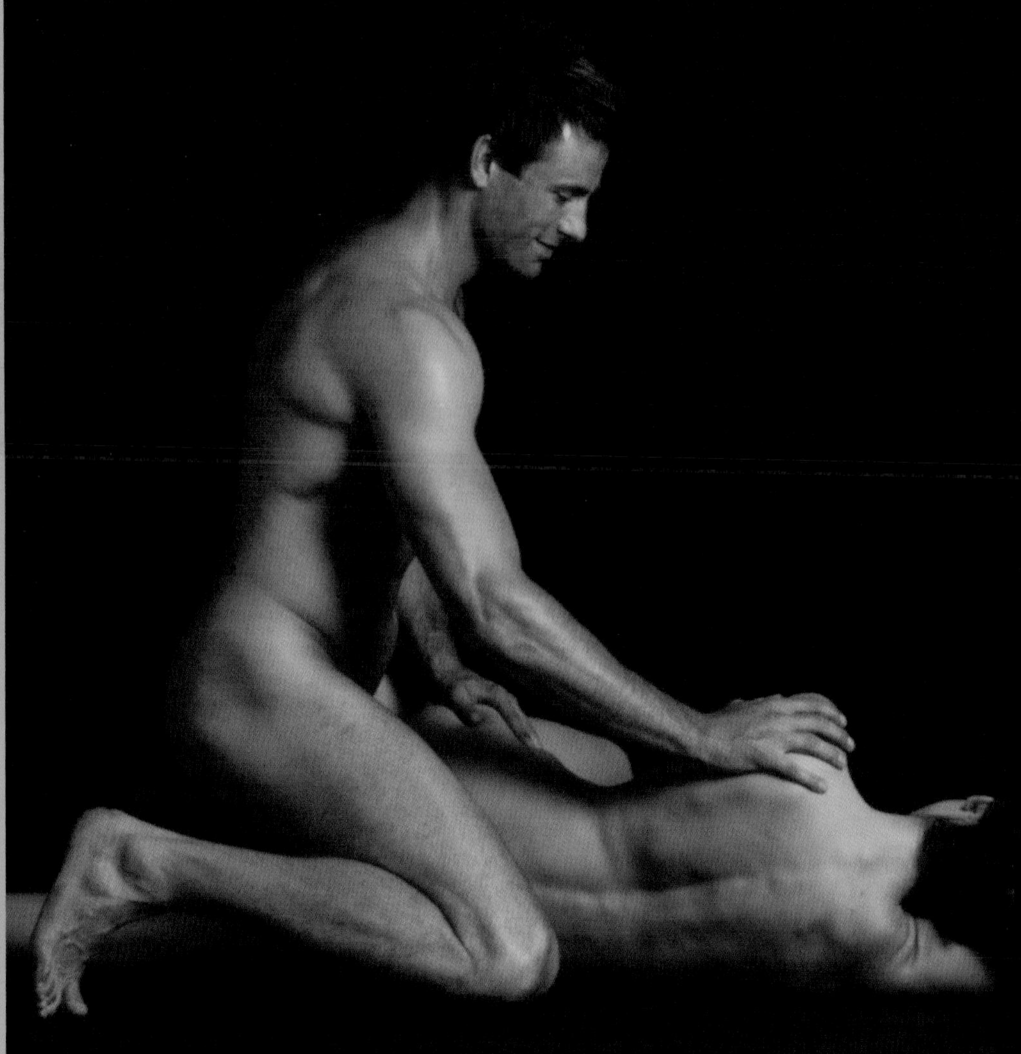

74 the straddle

A position with significance, the shape of this pose replicates a specific pattern the ancient Chinese used when fusing two pieces of jade together. She lies on her side, bending one leg at the knee and drawing it upward. He kneels behind her, straddling her side on, and entering her at a sideways angle, holding her shoulder to keep her in place. It's precise positioning, which gets you both in the mood for controlled, disciplined sex.

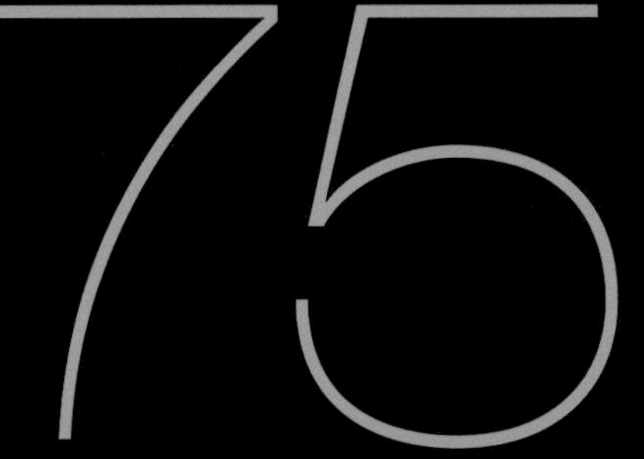

sexy starfish

Lie on the bed, heads in opposite directions. Scissor your legs so he can penetrate, then put your hands wherever it feels the most comfortable to get some leverage. Instead of moving apart, use a pushing, grinding motion that keeps pressure on the clitoris. It's a lazy Sunday-morning-style position (particularly suitable if neither of you have had time to brush your teeth!).

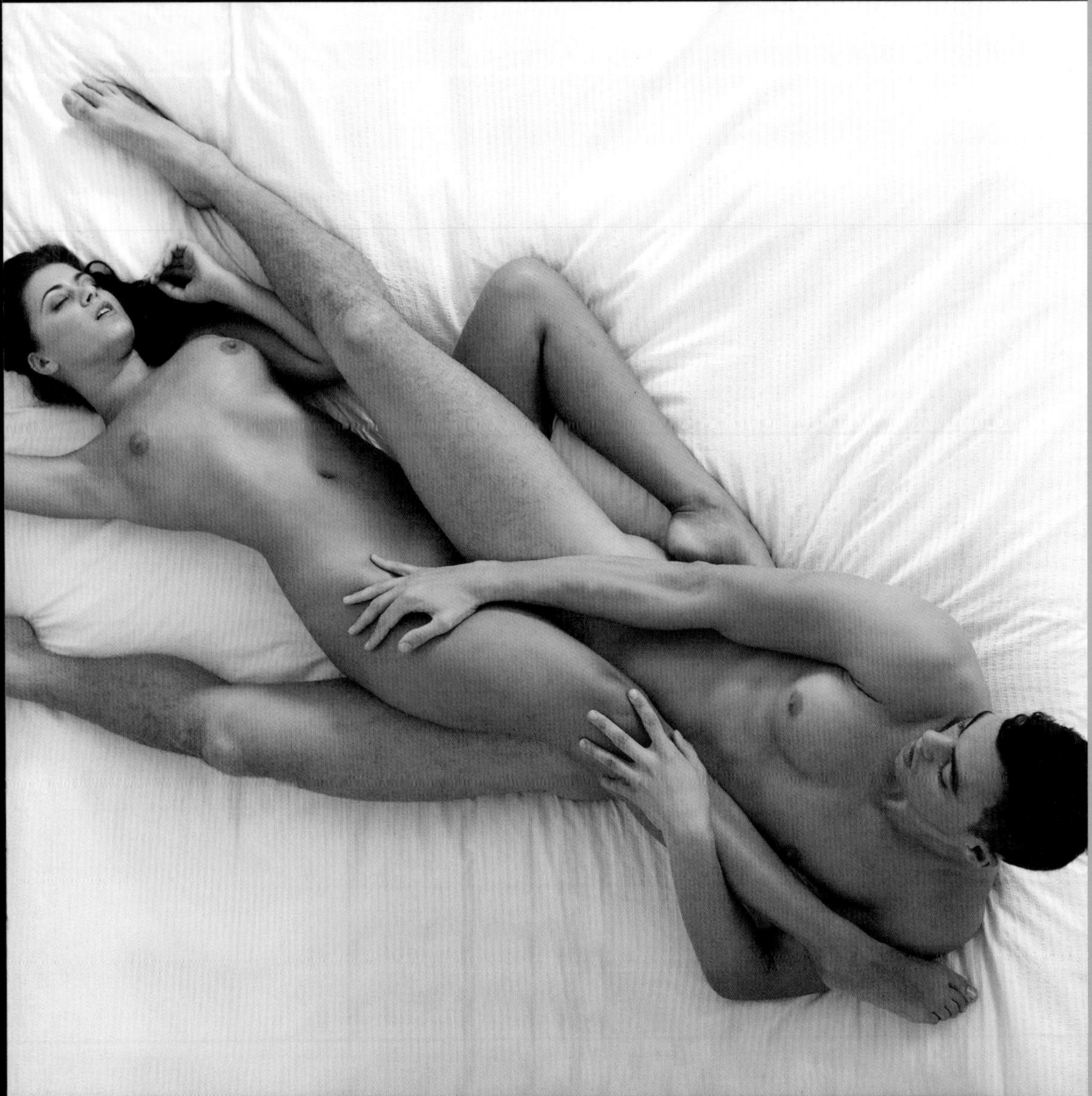

76 sensual squat

He squats with his legs apart and she climbs on board. This puts his head—conveniently—smack bang in between her breasts (what luck!), the perfect position to nuzzle or lick. She holds his shoulders and keeps her feet flat on the bed for balance. He holds her around the hips. Rather than thrusting, he moves in a gentle rocking motion, while she squeezes her pelvic-floor muscles. When his thigh muscles give out, he can roll backward and bounce her on his lap.

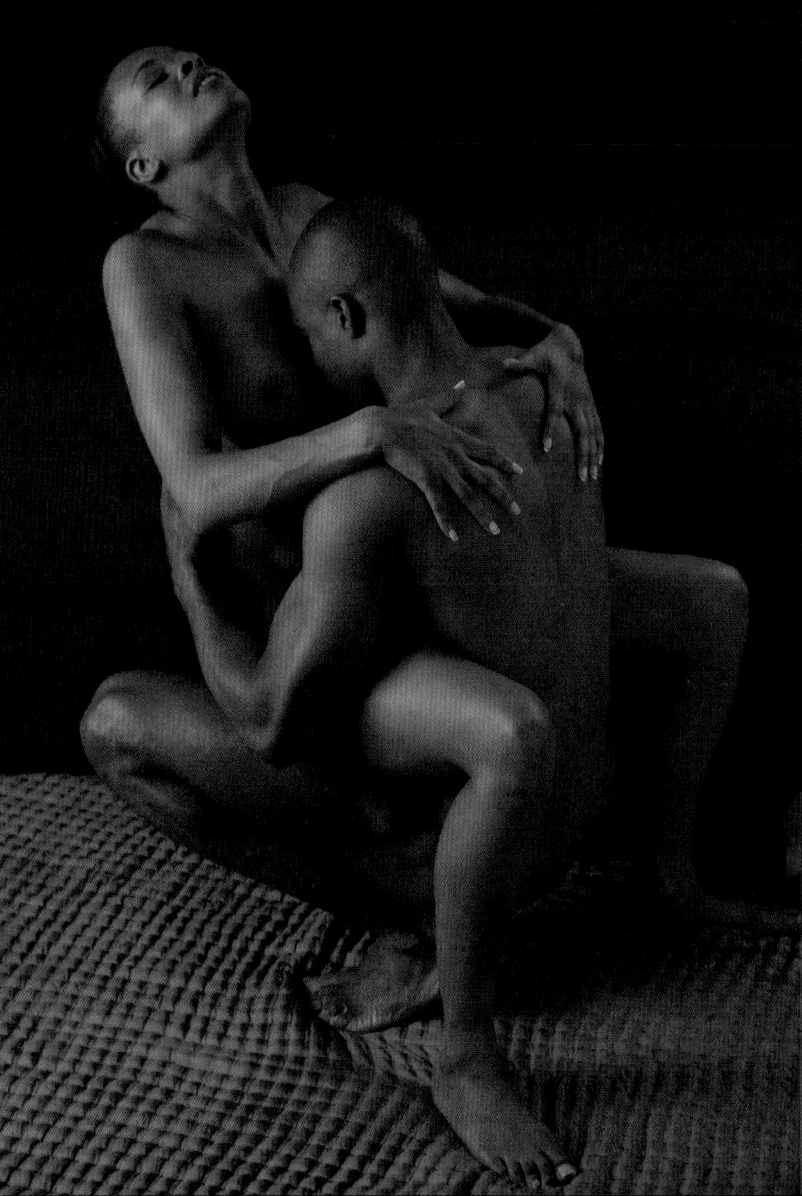

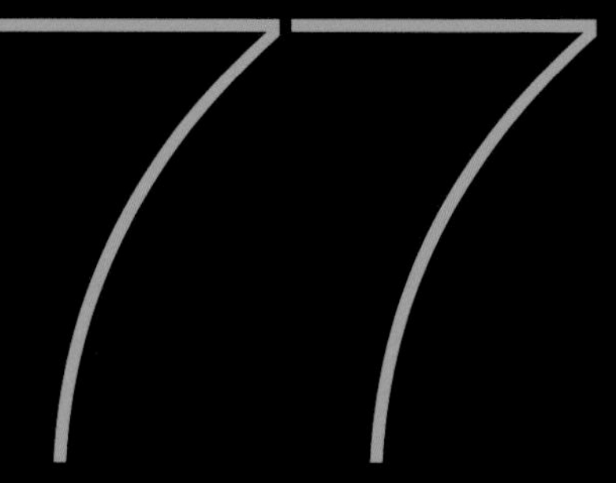

the deep

She lies on her back and he takes control. He needs good balance and you both need a relatively coordinated rhythm for this position, but it's worth making the effort because it puts both the penis and vagina in alignment. He usually enters with a downward thrust, so this is a deliciously different spin on penetration. Simple changes—such as him squatting instead of lying with legs outstretched—dramatically affect both the feel and style of thrusting.

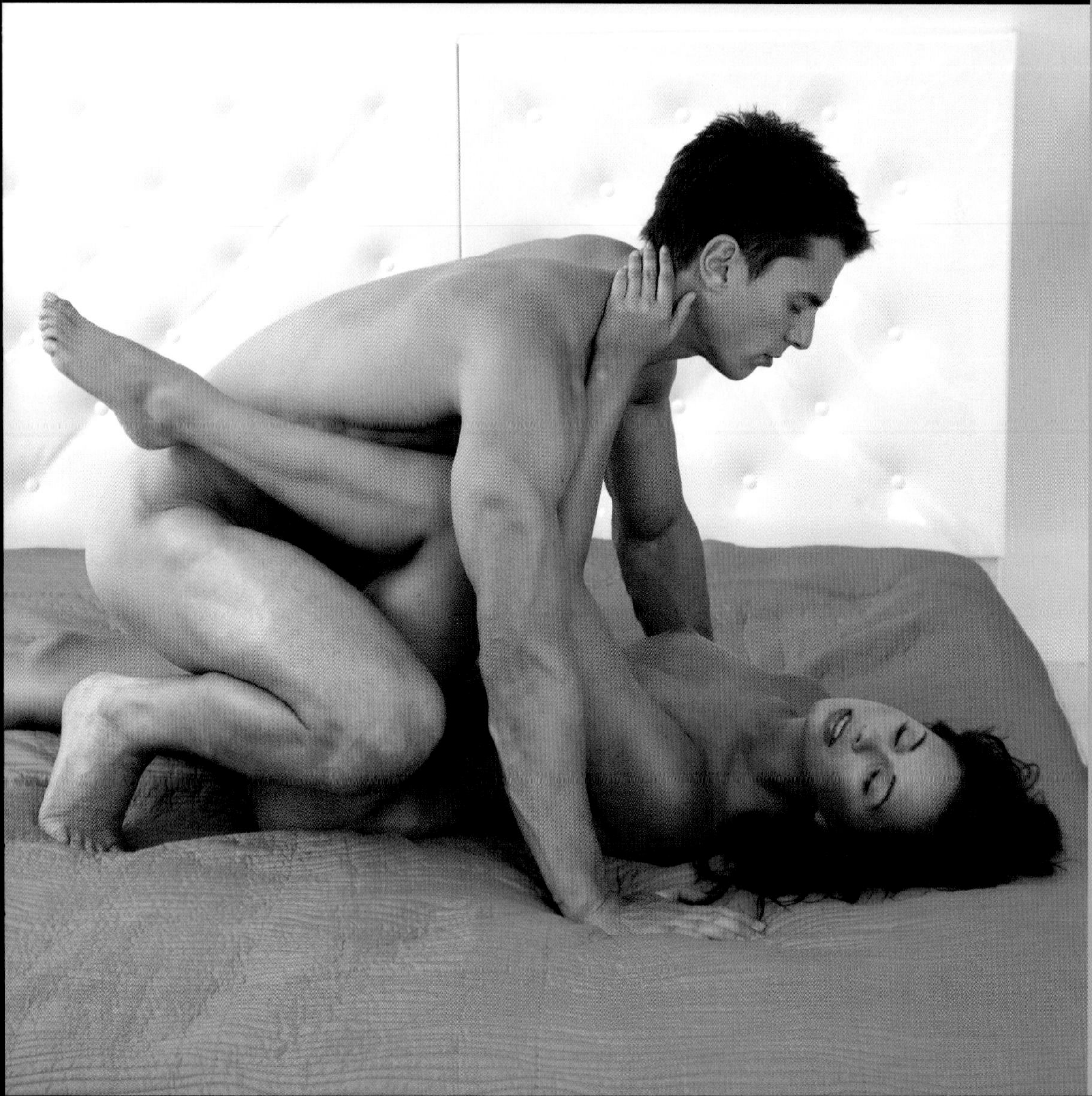

chapter 4

show off

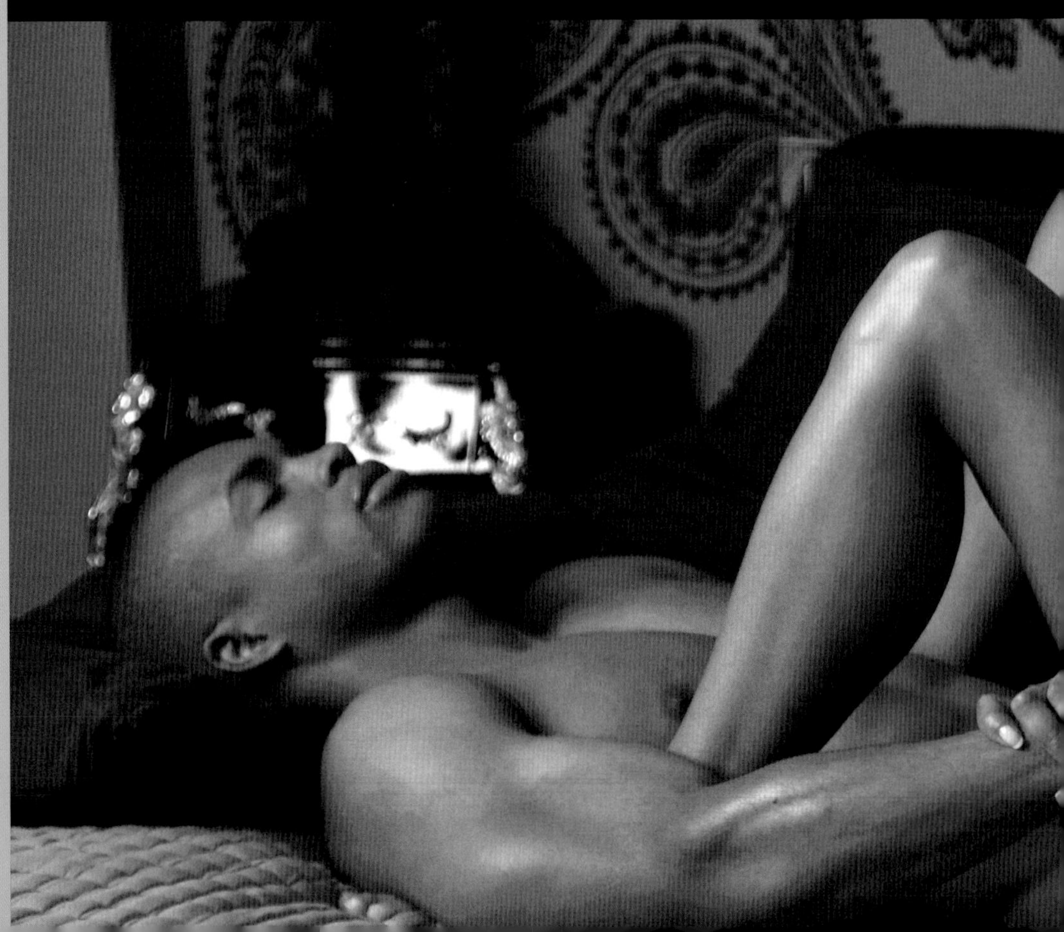

The positions you wish the neighbors would catch you in, if they happened to take a peek through the curtains.

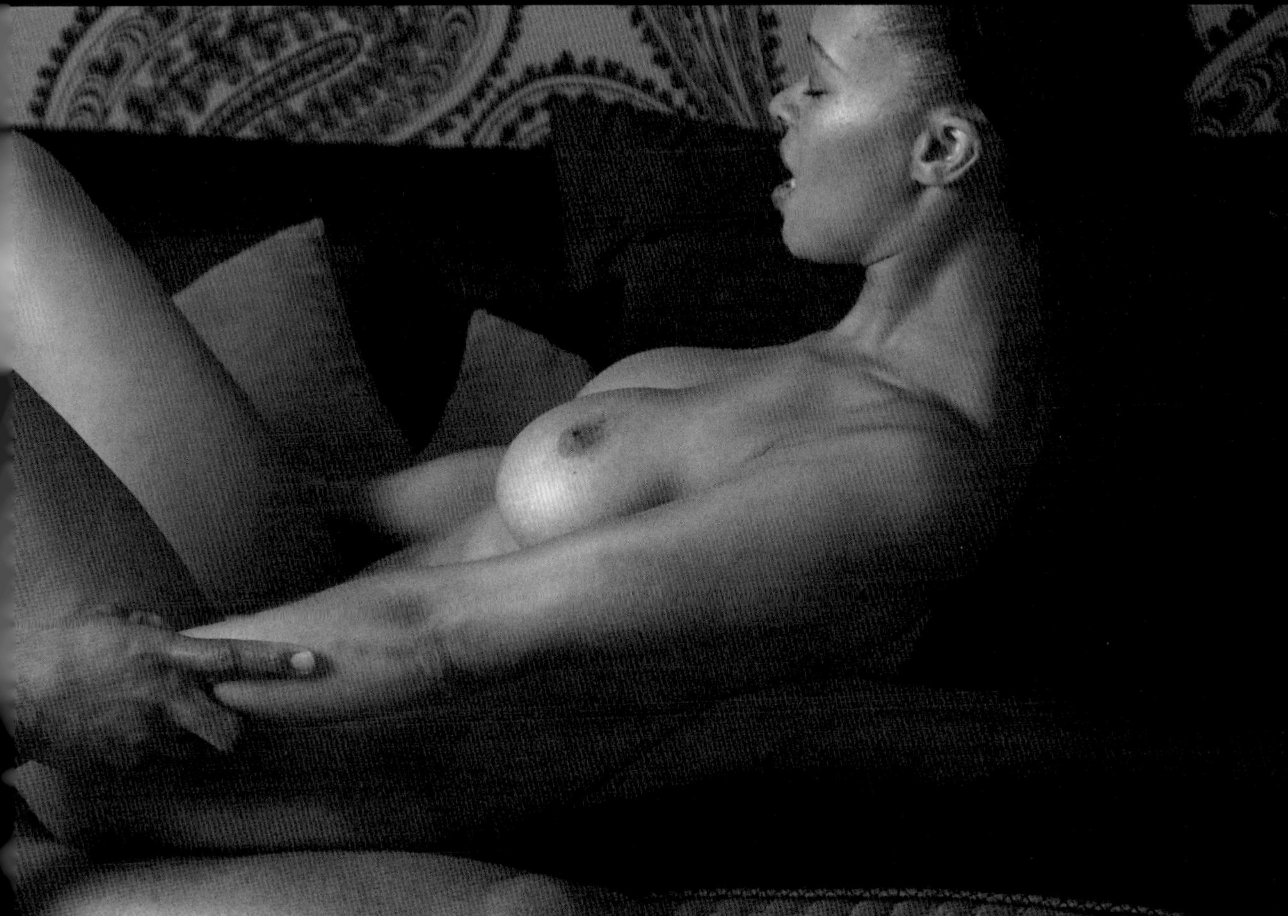

squeeze to please

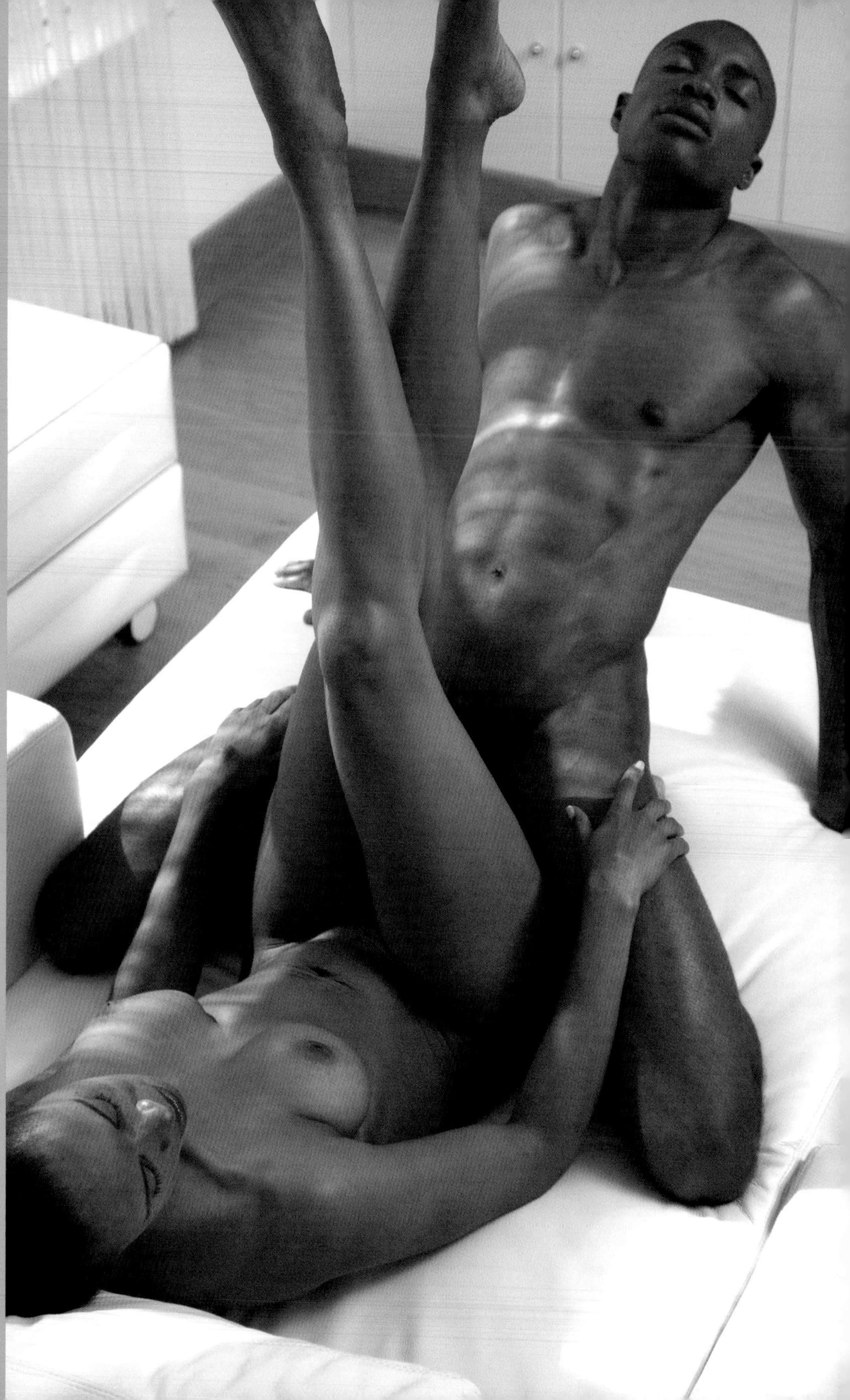

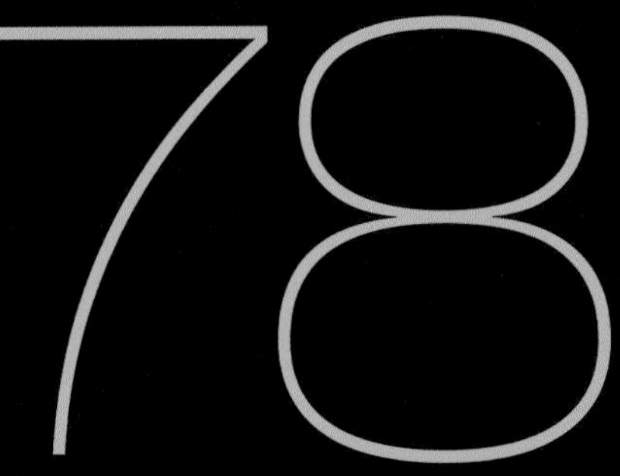

crossed lovers

She lies back and raises her legs straight in the air, and crosses one over the other. He penetrates and leans backward on his hands to support his weight. This is known as a "packed" position, which means her thighs are raised and placed one on top of the other.

It's purported to be the most intense way a woman can grip her partner's penis with her vagina, which is why it's on your must-do list. If she contracts her vaginal muscles at the same time, his penis feels a surprisingly fierce and sexy squeeze.

turn yourself on

It's a myth that the rampant desire that had you having a throw-down on the kitchen table in month one will continue to tap you on the shoulder six years in. It won't. The couples still enjoying great sex years into the relationship are those who've taken responsibility for turning themselves on, rather than relying on their partners to do it.

how to stay horny

* Research shows that people who have high libidos think about sex far more often than those with low desire, and you can teach yourself to be more sexual—and to want sex with your partner more often.
* Train your brain to turn yourself on every day, in every situation. A shower is far more sense-ational if you use scented gels, soaping yourself the way a lover would. On your daily commute, spot something you find attractive about everyone on the subway or at traffic lights (that's with subtle and stolen glances, rather than outright stares!).

sex up your senses

* Savor tastes on your tongue, dress in clothes you know flatter you; when you're chatting to a colleague, focus on their hands, and remember what your partner did with theirs the last time you had great sex.
* Read erotic books, hang sexy pictures in your bedroom, rent X-rated movies. The more you start thinking about sex, the more you keep thinking about sex. It's not your lover's job to keep you turned on, it's yours.

rock-a-boink baby

1 Stand facing each other. He then drops to one knee, as though he's about to propose. She lifts the same side leg as his high knee and places her foot, gently, on the top of his thigh, nestling into his hip bone. Her toes point out with her heel facing inward. This is the moment when you gaze intently into each other's eyes, connecting emotionally before you move on to the more physical stuff.

2 Enough gazing—you're now ready for some saucy stuff. She lowers herself onto his thigh, putting her arms around his neck for balance. He penetrates and you're both magically in position for some good, long erotic kissing. If you're feeling more sinful than spiritual, throw in some breast-fondling, too.

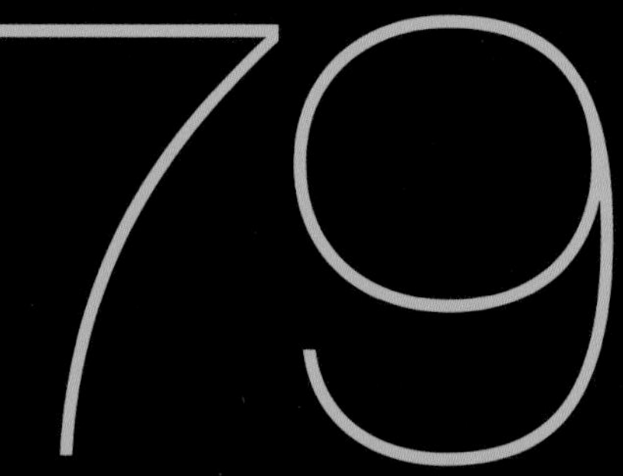

3 Just when you were starting to relax, it all gets very high energy—well, for him anyway. She leans back, he grips her around the waist, pulling her pelvis close, while she holds on to his shoulders for support. He pulls her backward and forward in small movements, but most of the work is done by her, as she internally squeezes and releases her vaginal muscles.

3

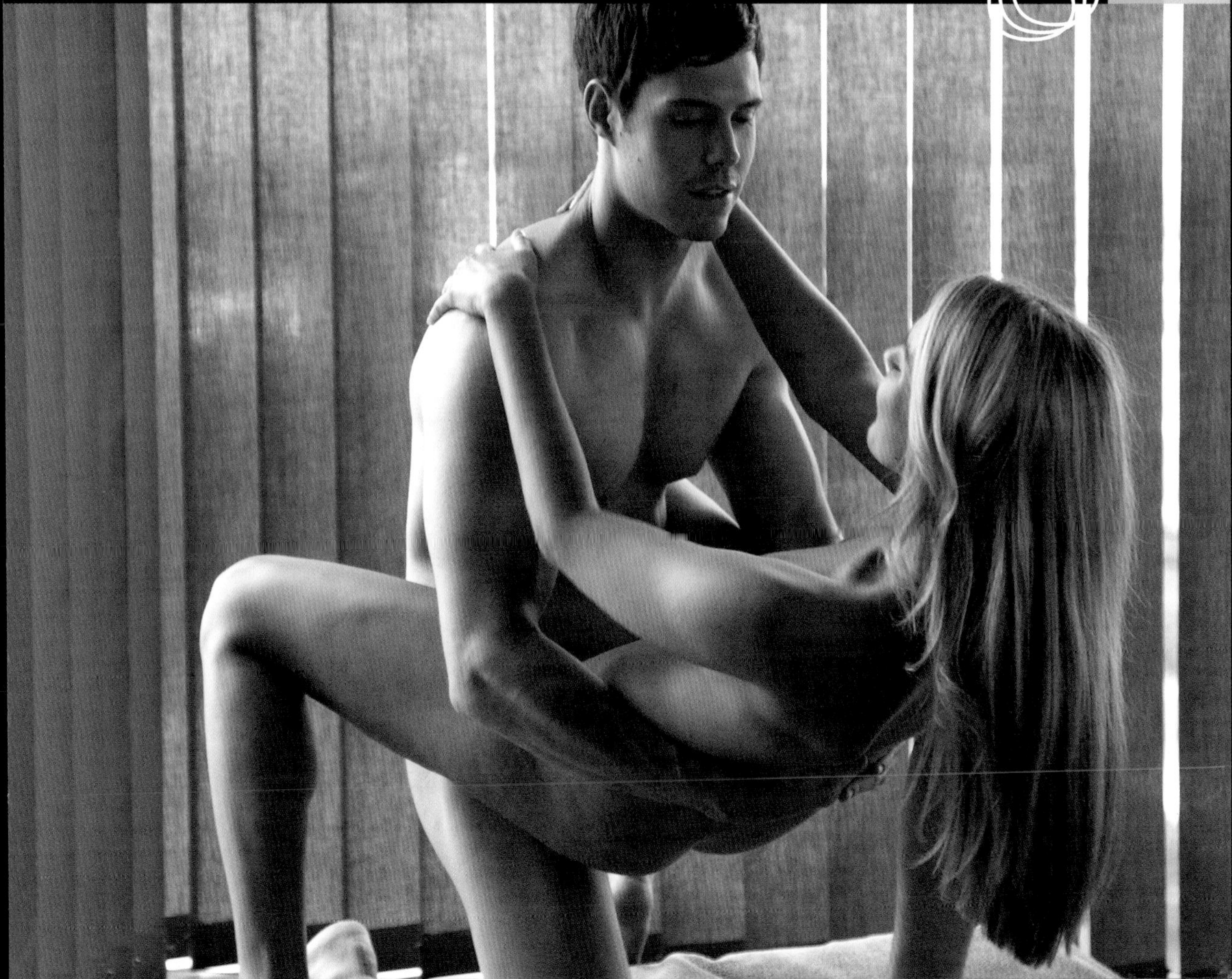

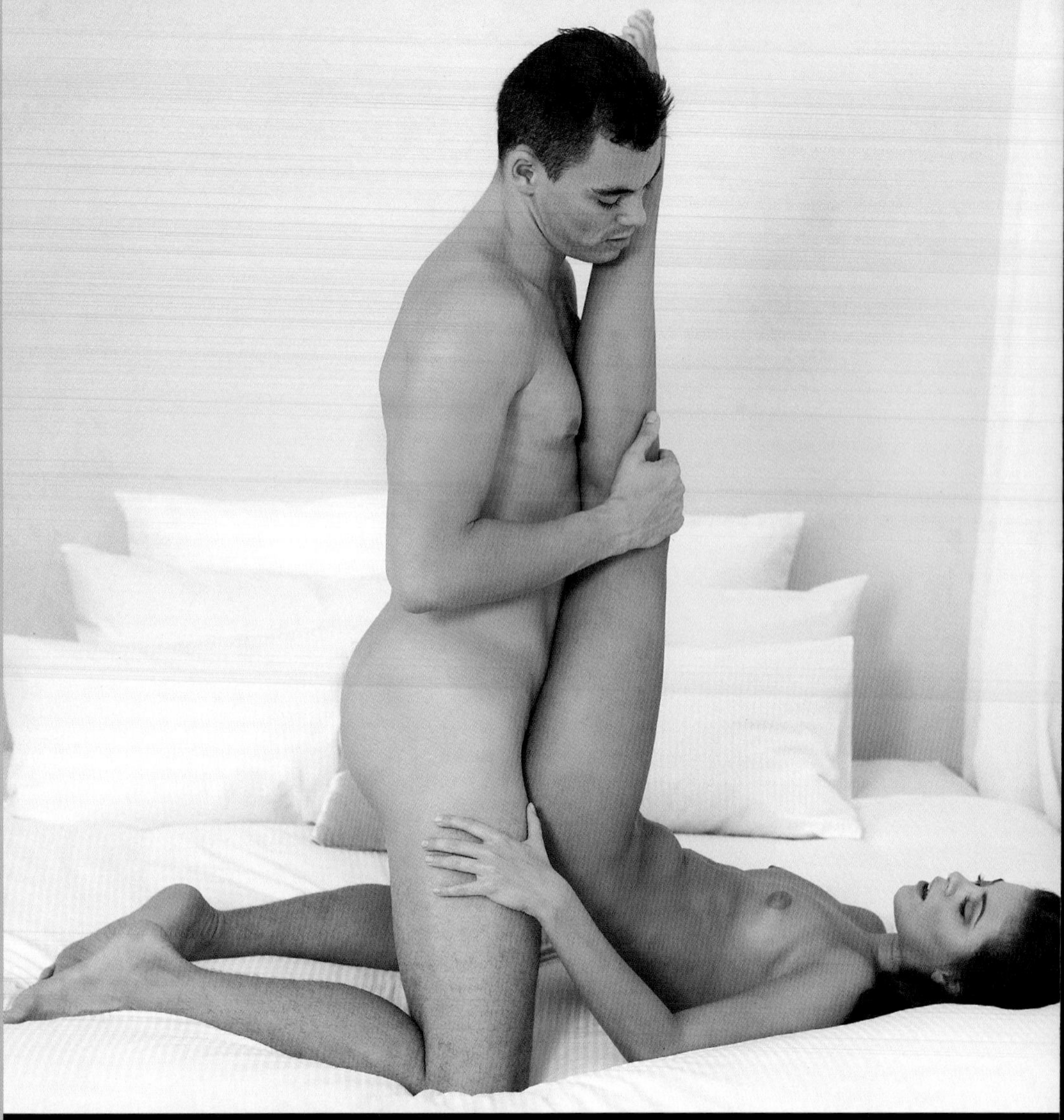

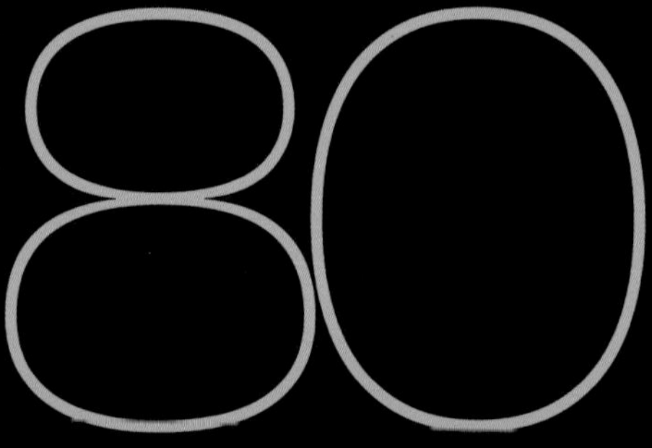

up, up, and away

This looks impressive and feels fantastic. The key to getting it right is to ensure he's reasonably well-endowed (it doesn't work for shorter penises) and to make sure his erection is nice and hard. He gets into position first and holds the base of his penis while she wiggles, also in position and using her hands, to allow him to penetrate. Once there, he varies the thrusting by lifting or lowering her body to alter the angle of penetration.

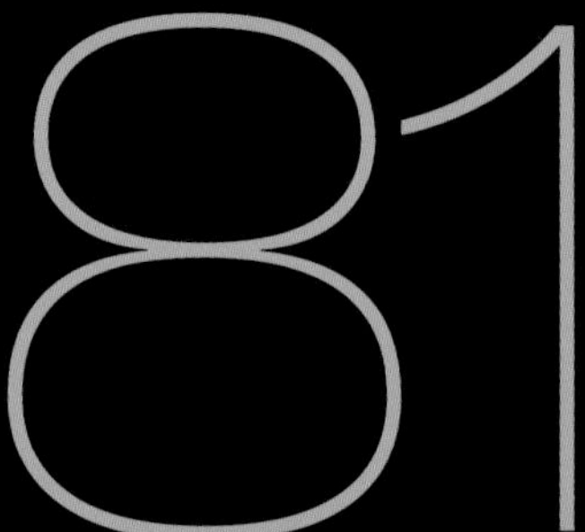

giddy-up

In this position, inspired by horseback riding, he lies on his back and draws his knees up, parting his thighs. She wiggles between them, using her hand to help insert his penis, then leans forward, using her knees to move up and down on his penis, "riding" him like he's a horse. (Hopefully he's just as well hung.) Putting pillows under his shoulders can make this easier. If her legs start to get tired (which is absolutely in the cards), you can move to a face-to-face sitting position.

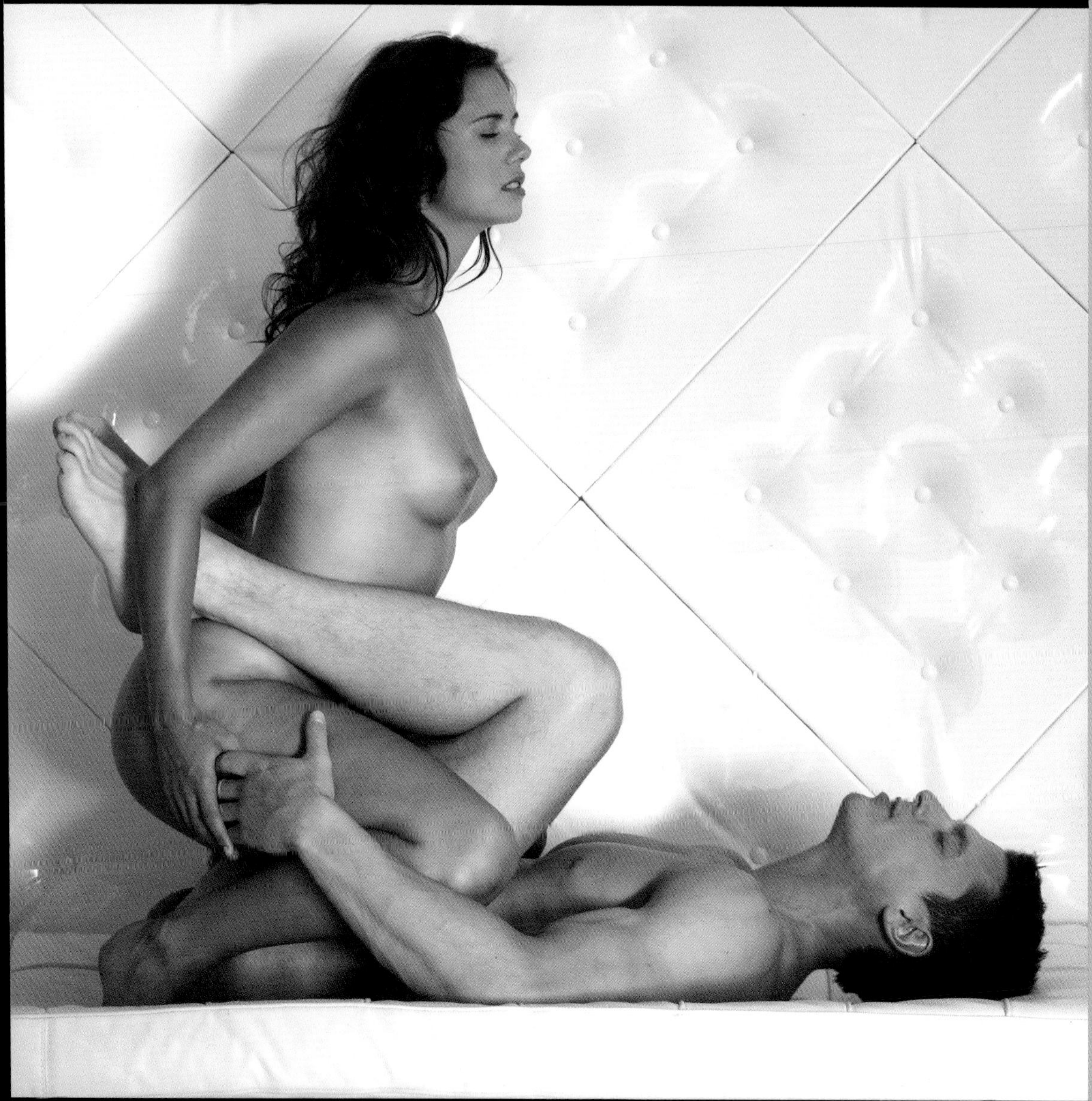

seesaw

1 He lies flat, thighs slightly parted. She plops herself on top (or delicately climbs astride, depending on her personality), sitting erect while each graps the other's arms. She balances by keeping her feet pressed to his sides, then slowly lets her head fall back. Stay there for a few minutes so she can get used to the feeling of blood rushing to her head during intercourse. Fans say it makes the feeling more intense; others feel slightly sick, in which case tip it back up again.

2 Pulling her tummy muscles tight (with silent thanks for sticking to that punishing sit-up routine!), she moves into position by wedging her feet into his armpits for support and leverage. You then hold each other's wrists firmly and pull each other up and down. This is easier to achieve if she uses her tummy muscles: keep them clenched for the "up" stroke and relax them to move backward. It takes a while, but you'll soon move into a gentle rhythm.

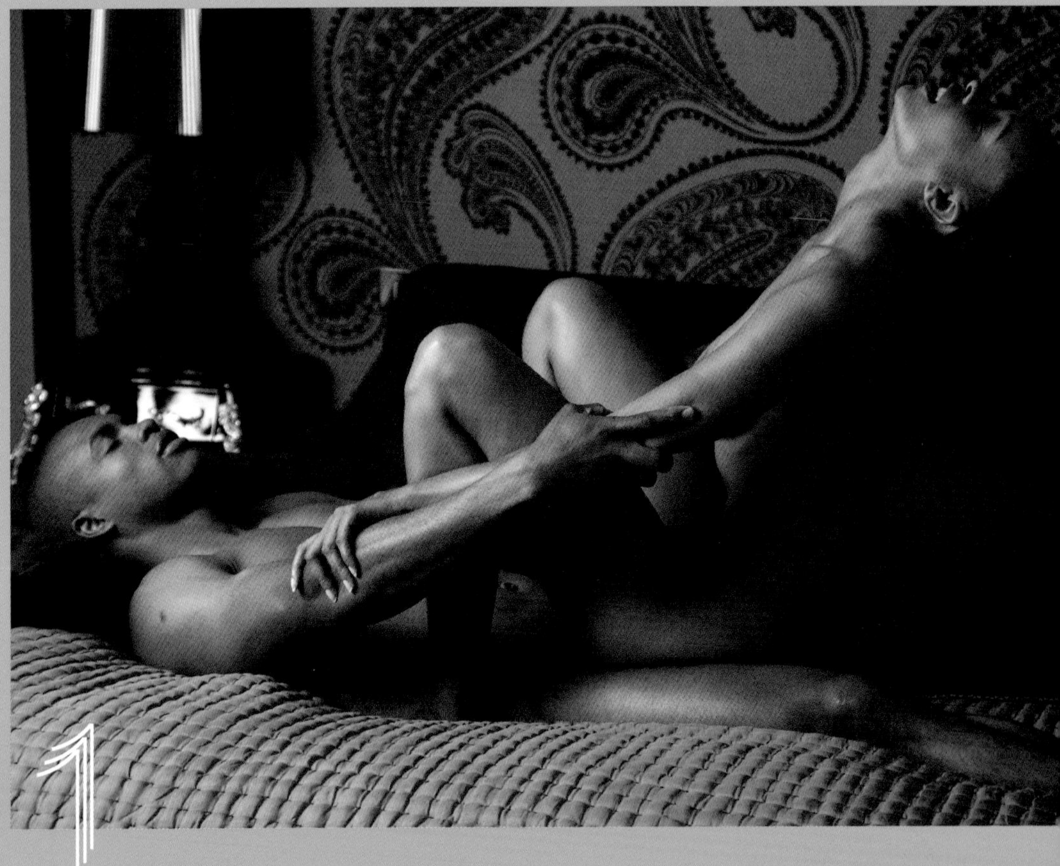
1

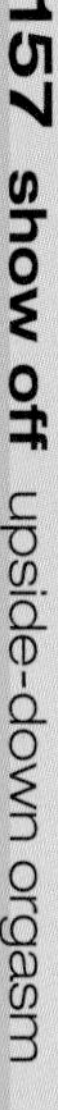

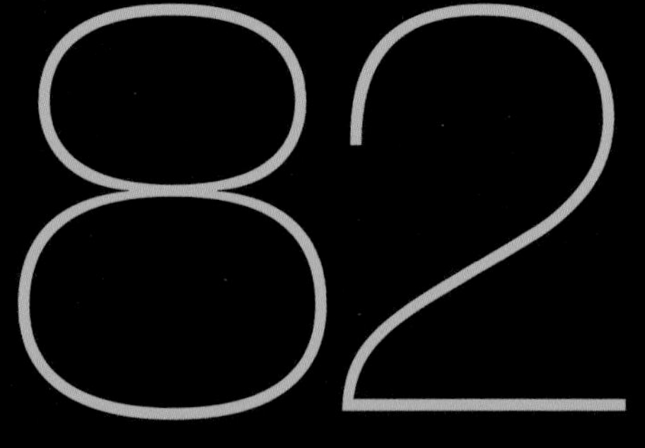

2

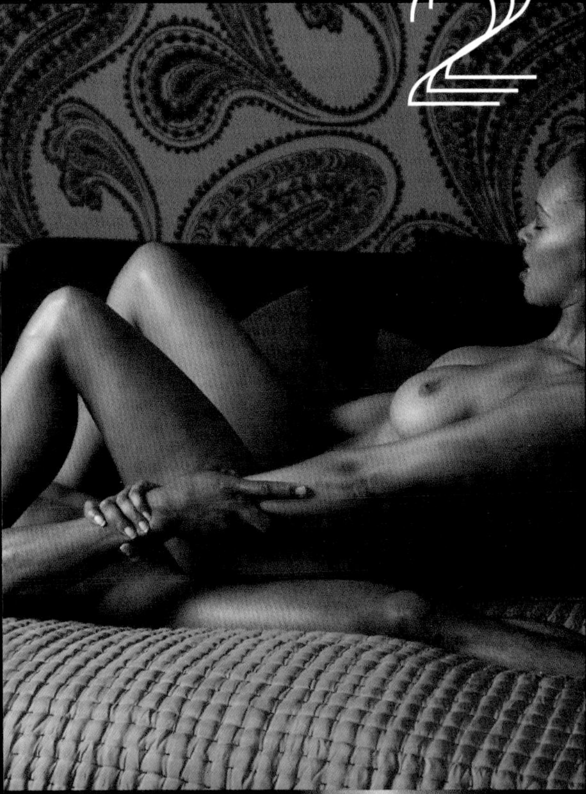

3 In the final stage, she leans completely back and you both move into a rocking motion. He's pulling her back and forth using his arms; she's using her tummy muscles and her arms. You work together rather than one leading, trying to find a natural balance point. Devotees claim "upside-down" orgasms feel wonderful because the rush of blood to the head makes everything more intense. Others just end up with a splitting headache.

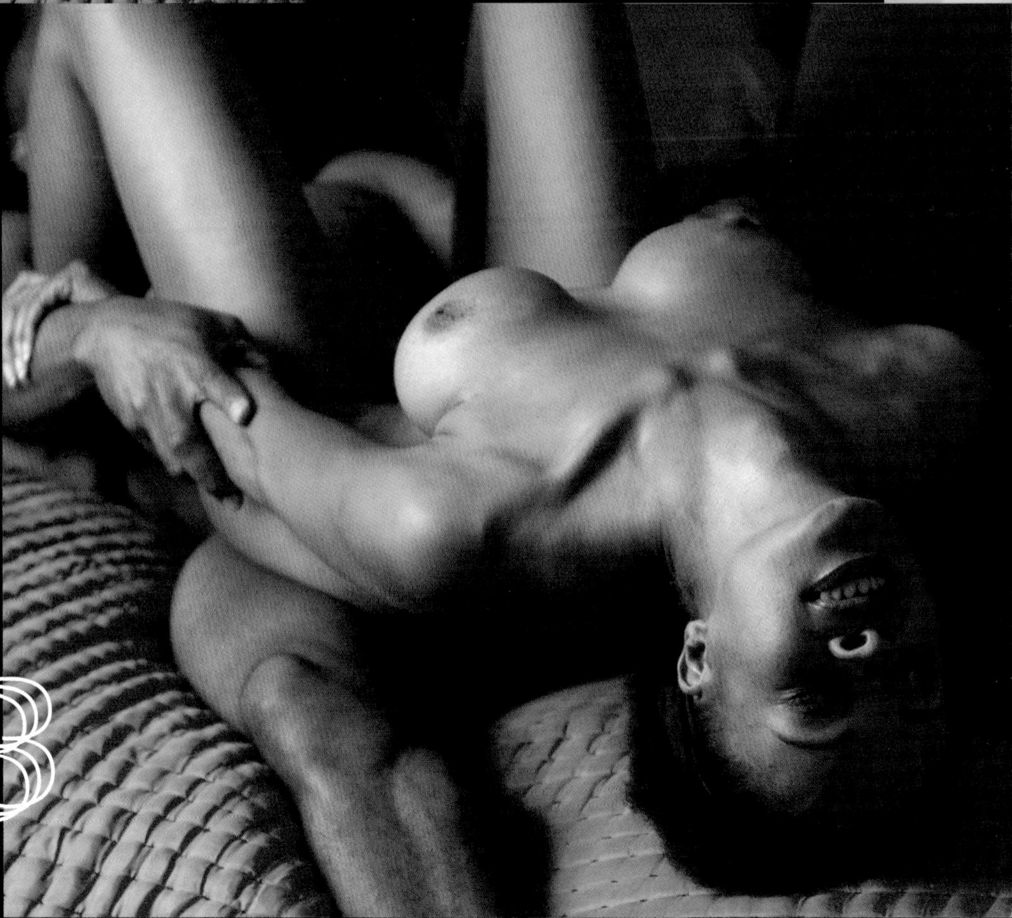

3

sex and the great outdoors

The fear of discovery, pounding heartbeats, that delicious jolt of adrenaline when you think someone's coming (and it's not either of you). Anyone who's ever had sex outside knows just how fantastic it can be. And as for that pesky problem of it being illegal to have sex in public (if you're caught, you could face a penalty), there are ways to indulge in al fresco sex on the sly. It's called being sensible. Give one or all of these a whirl...

on or in the car Yes, you could slip into the backseat and enjoy relative privacy but it's far, far sexier to do it on the car hood. She sits on the hood and he stands in front of her. She then wraps her legs around his waist to let him penetrate, then leans back on the hood, balancing herself with her arms.

Car sex is uber-erotic—not only do you risk getting caught, but it's also the sort of thing teenagers do. You both recapture the heady thrill of adolescence, feeling wild, free, and terribly ungrown-up.

against a tree She stands, leaning back against a tree, and he stands in front of her. She puts her arms around his neck and wraps her legs around his waist. For balance and support, she keeps her back firmly pressed against the tree and hangs on to any strong-looking branches. If that all sounds far too energetic, cheat! Get her to wrap one leg around his waist and keep the other on the floor. He should hold her thighs.

Penetration is deep, snug, and tight because most of her weight is bearing down on his penis and her vagina is angled. If she squeezes her thigh muscles, she gives him super-tight friction. It's primal sex at its very best, but probably not the position to use if you want to try out that new extend-an-orgasm technique. Standing positions tend to work only for quickies because his penis isn't the only thing that gets stiff.

"Recapture the heady thrill of adolescence—feeling wild and free."

on a picnic table Head to the park at dusk when everyone else is heading home. Take your dinner with you. Find a sturdy table provided in the picnic area, set it, have a feast, then clear it off, and lay each other! She lies back on the table and wraps her legs around his waist with him standing in front of her.

It's also the perfect position for oral sex—and nothing beats the feel of a hot tongue on your genitals in the fresh, open air. Believe me, it feels even naughtier than "doing it" because licking each other in public is just... well, super naughty!

know the rules Dress for sex (floaty skirts, no underwear, zipper rather than button-fly jeans, uncomplicated bras). Use props to hide behind (picnic blanket, sarong, beach umbrella). Be aware of the laws and customs of the country you're in. Have a code word that alerts you both to opportunities. Forget foreplay and instead use lube. Plan your escape and what to say if you get caught. And for goodness' sake, don't do it if being caught would be a nightmare!

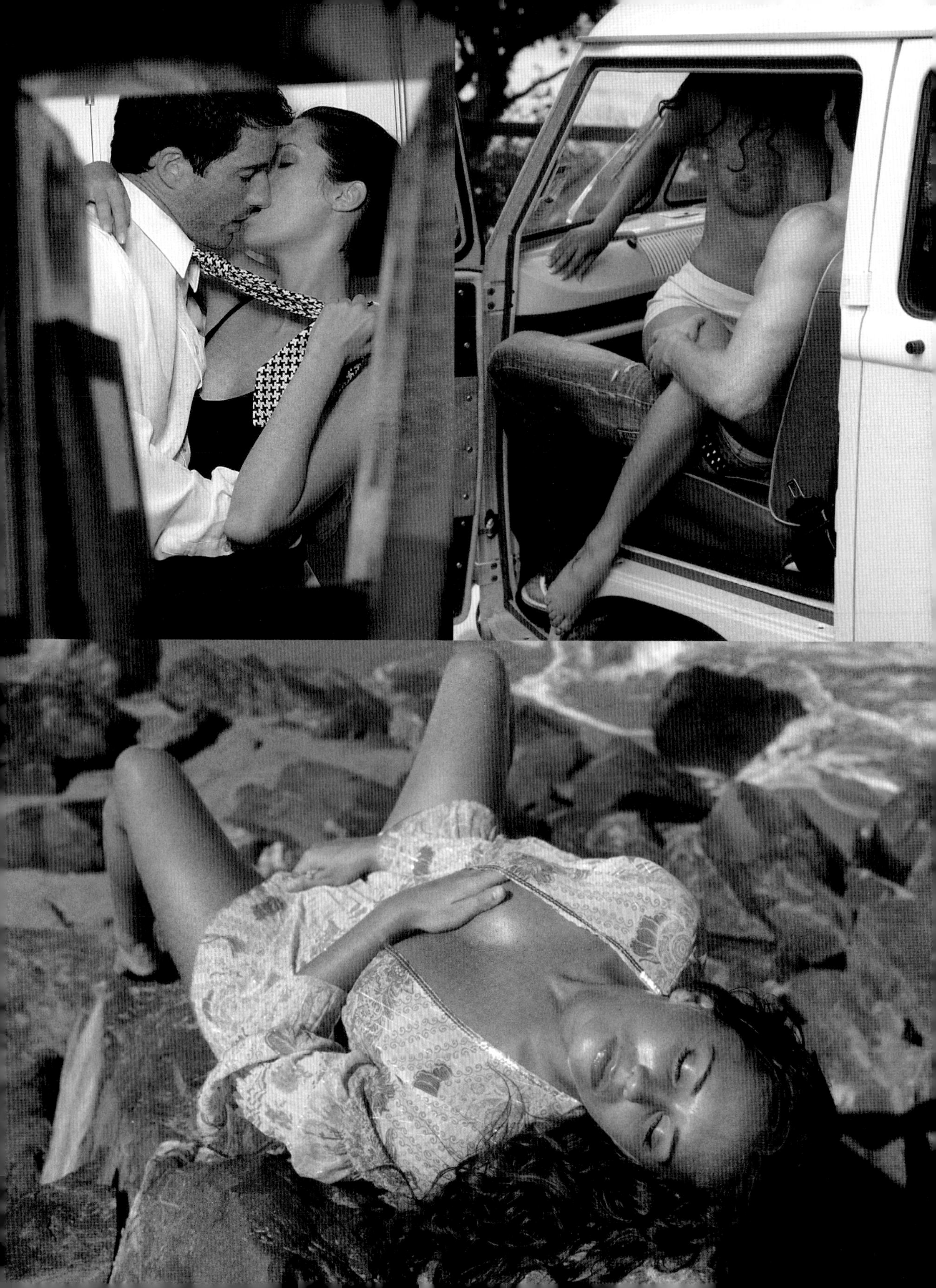

83

love lever

He sits on a high-backed chair; she straddles him then rests each ankle on his shoulders. If he's a fan of look-but-can't-do-anything lap-dancing, this will make his year. He cops a full view of her, while she squeezes her thighs together to increase pressure on his penis. Excellent for a man who needs extra friction (i.e., one who's older or who has had one too many drinks). Being precariously balanced means he can't stimulate her clitoris, so oral or hand work before or after wouldn't hurt.

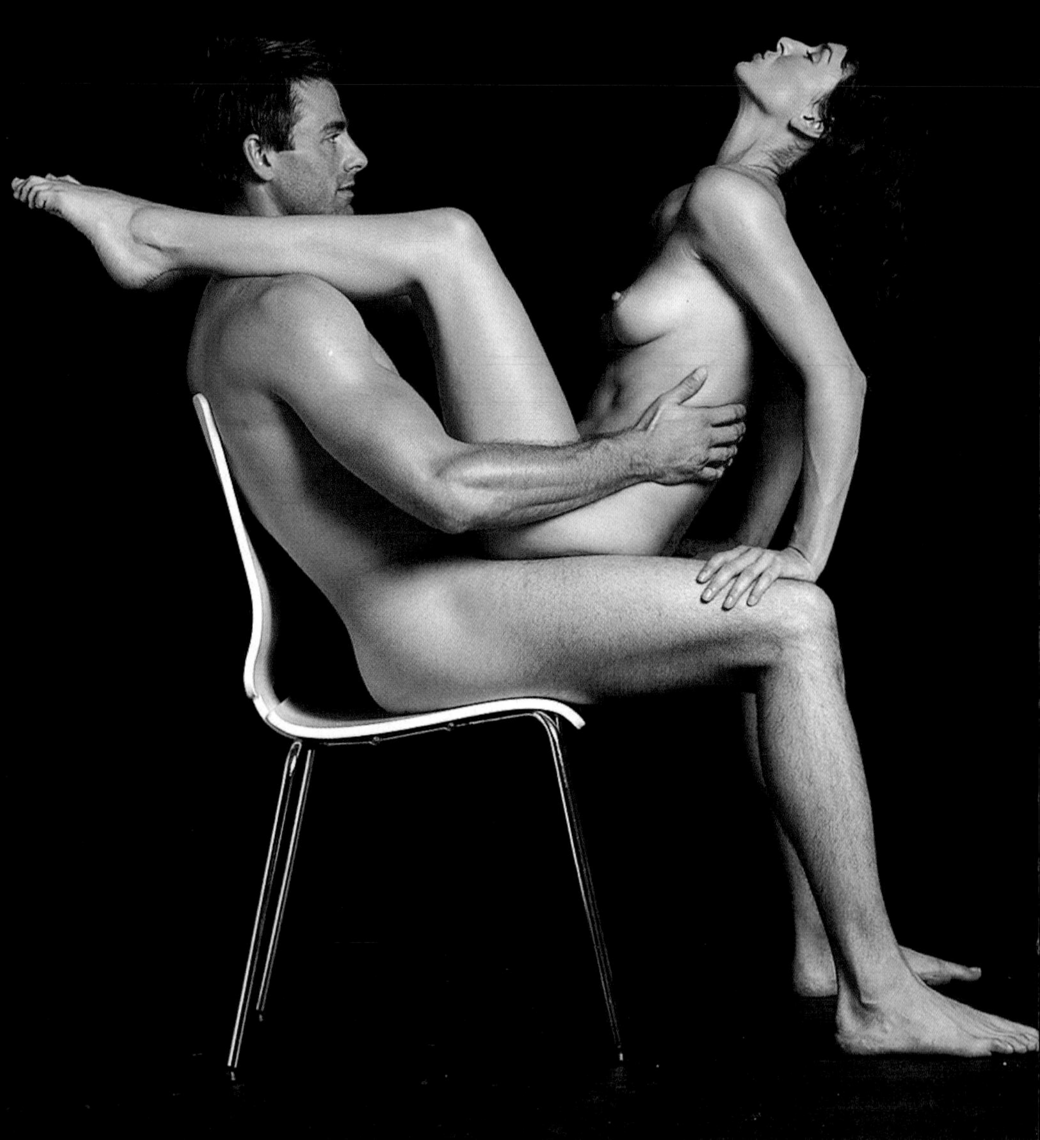

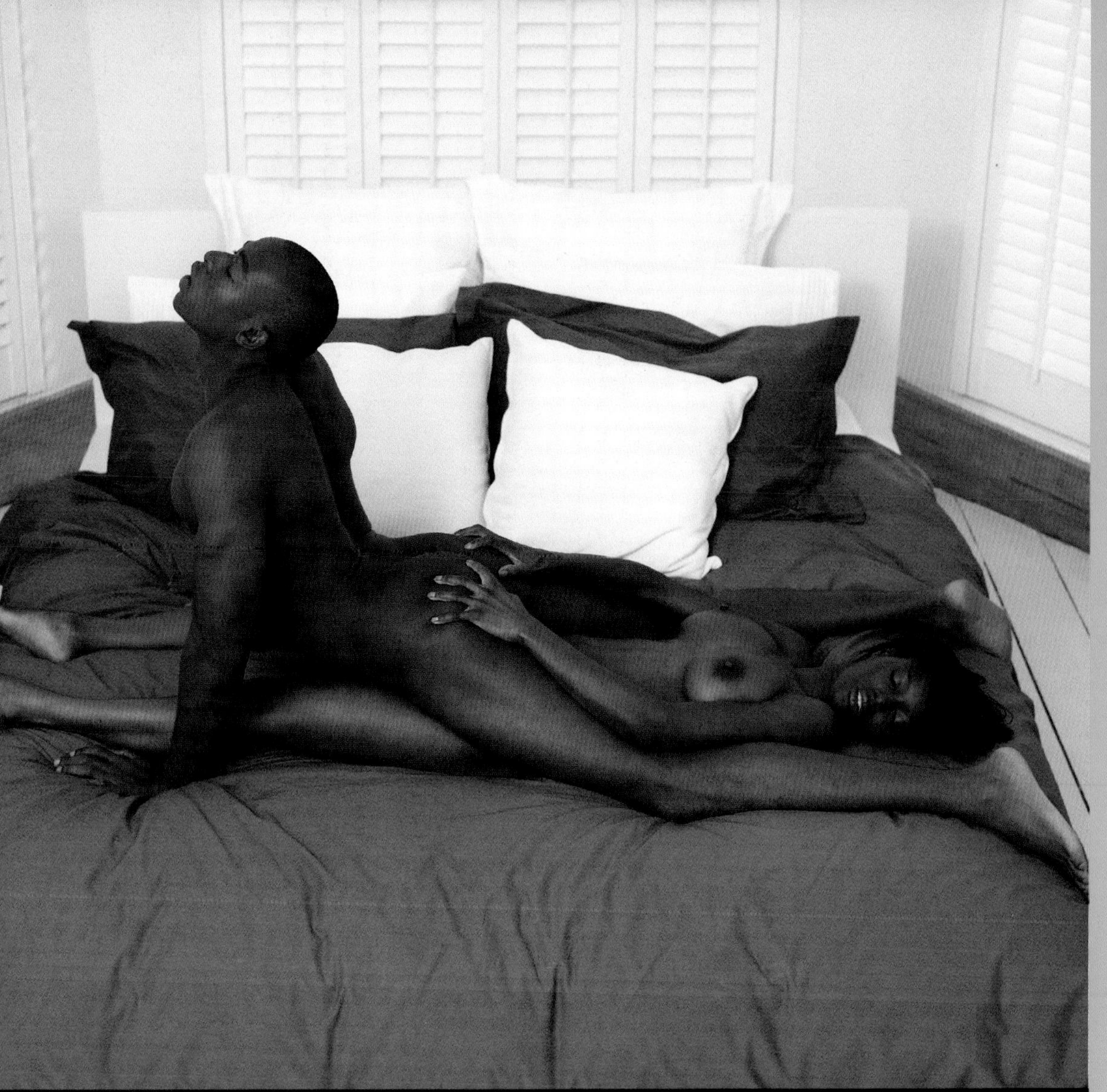

84

spin city

Who said the missionary position is boring? Spin it around for a sensational twist. If he's adventurous, he'll enter in the traditional position (heads the same end) and slowly spin around. (If you think this sounds difficult, try penetrating when he's in position!) This works best if he has a big penis and a not-so-hard erection. Some couples manage this one, lots don't. If you're in the latter category, put a big cross by this one on the Checklist page and write "good for analingus."

the fish

1 The *Kama Sutra* often looks to animals to get inspiration for positions and techniques. It claims that this position will make her feel like she's swimming. (Did people do drugs back then?) He kneels, rather sensibly, on a pillow with one leg raised. She takes a seat, lowering herself onto his penis. He enjoys a pitstop to play with her clitoris, fondle her breasts, kiss her neck, and generally ravish her!

2 She leans forward, resting her forearms on a piece of furniture. He holds her by the waist, pulling her back and forth to start thrusting gently. She's nicely supported by the (rather comfy looking) sofa, resting on his upper thigh, but not leaning too much to the side or he'll slip out.

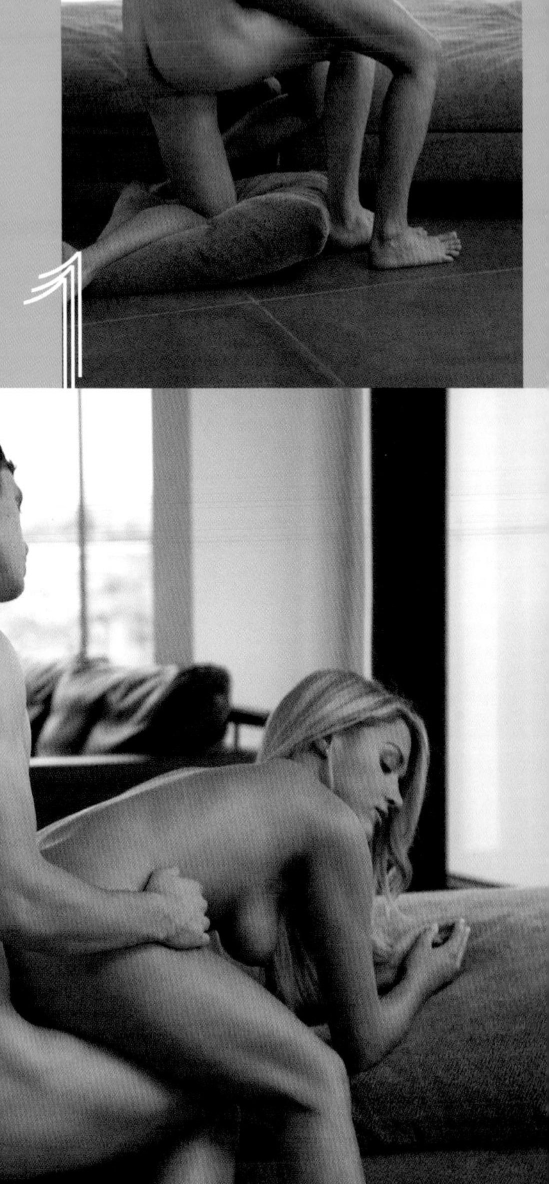

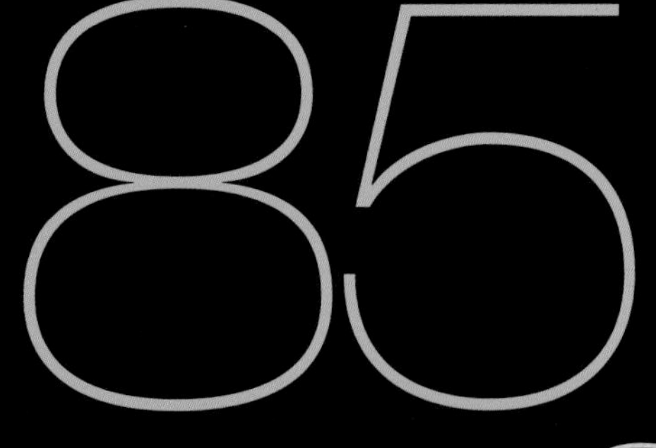

3 He stands up, not without some difficulty (if he didn't start with strong legs, he'll sure as hell sport bulging thigh muscles when we're finished!), and takes a firm hold of her upper thighs. She's now completely supporting her weight on her elbows and forearms, and braces herself as he moves into deep, passionate thrusting. Feel like a fish? Didn't think so.

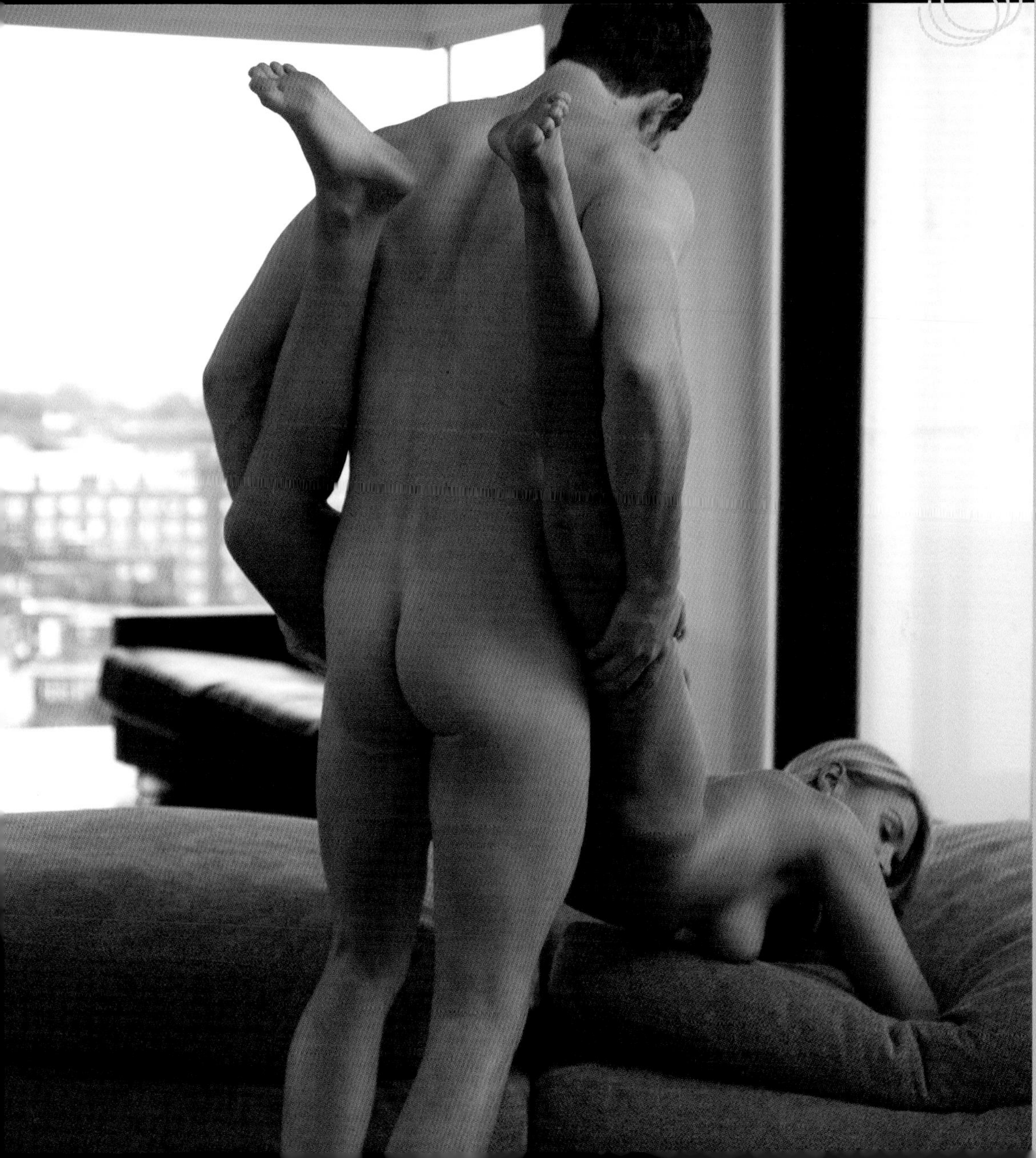

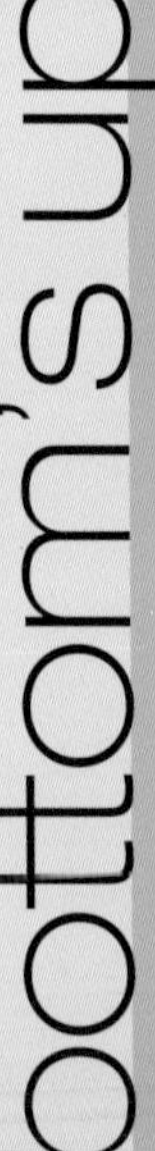
bottom's up

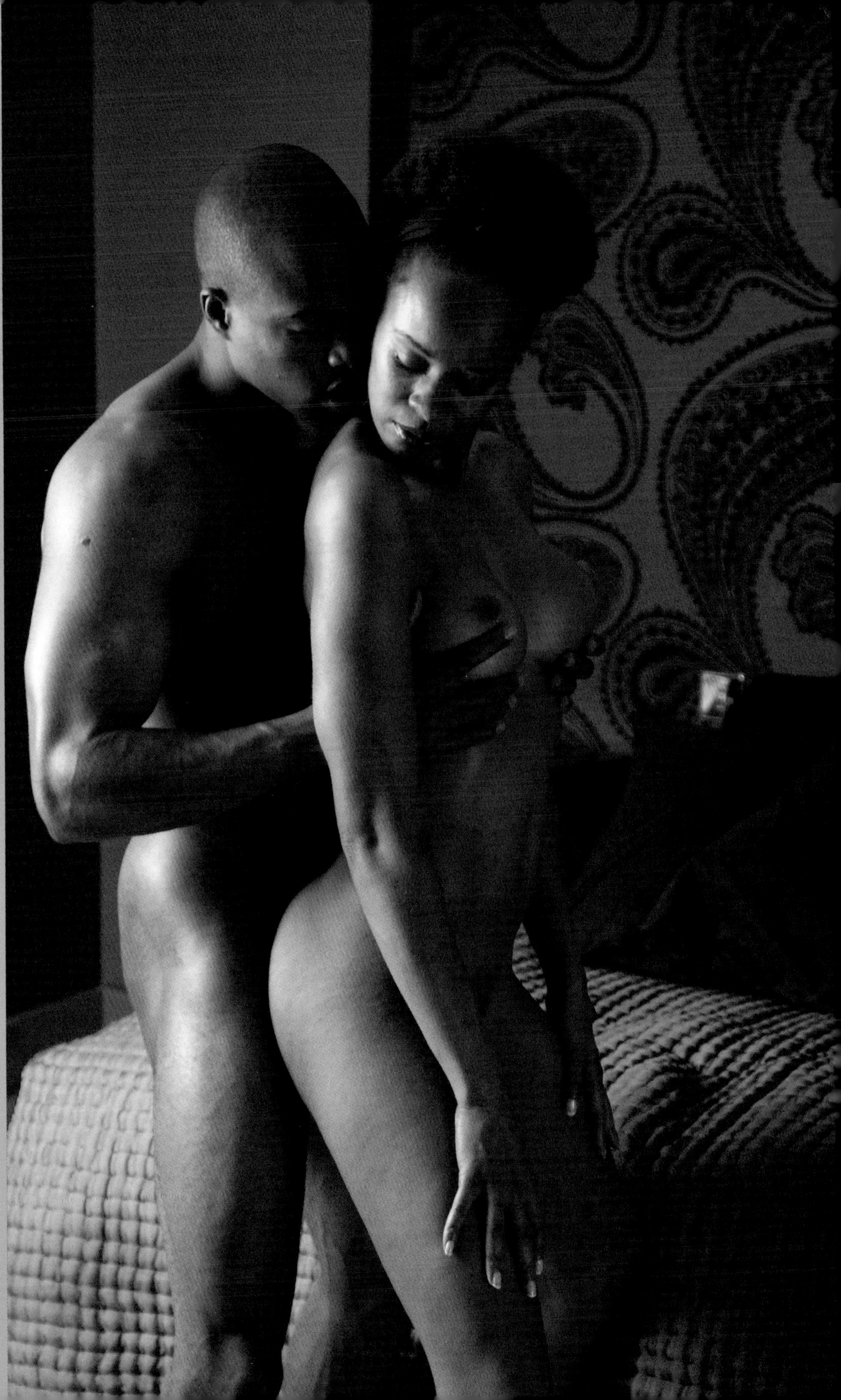

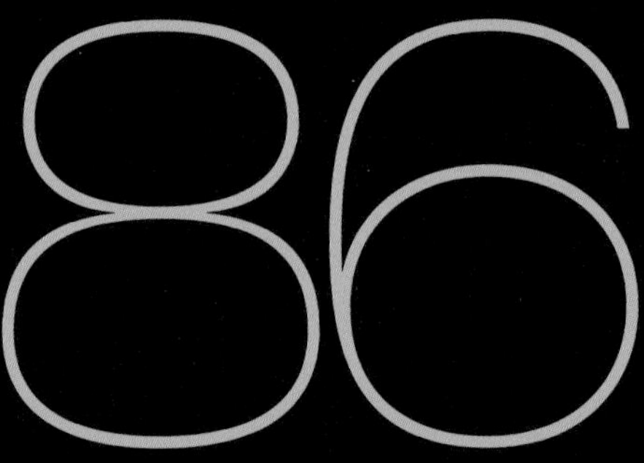

the tilt

Don't even attempt this one unless you're at least comparable in height. (Or wear high heels to even it up!) She also needs flexible hips because she has to tilt her bottom up and backward.

The wider she spreads her legs, the easier it becomes, but although placing her hands on her thighs gives some stability, if he's thrusting vigorously it's rather easy to topple over! So why bother? He can touch her breasts, clitoris, perineum—it's virtually all reachable—making all the effort on her part (almost) worth it.

timely turn-on

The position opposite is perfect for spontaneous sex. You both happen to be naked, you kiss and hug, and one thing leads to another. Snatch sex when you can, but also be aware of when your partner's most likely to be responsive.

no—or bad—timing

* Mismatched libidos—one person wanting more sex than the other—is often just bad timing. Some people like nothing more than to be woken by a hopeful prod in the back and/or a tongue snaking its way up their thigh. Others would cheerfully cut off the tongue and any other offending appendages for an extra five minutes of shut-eye.
* If you have a desire dysfunction, keep a chart of when you most feel like sex, then compromise. If you're a night person and he's most lively in the mornings, a little afternoon delight could solve your problems.

your natural high

* Our testosterone levels are highest when we first wake up.
* A woman's libido is highest just before ovulation, around 14 days after her period.
* When it comes to orgasms, men appear relatively unaffected month to month, but women are more likely to orgasm just before or during their periods, because increased blood flow adds pressure to the pelvic area and she has higher levels of progesterone.
* Don't be too smug boys: you might orgasm more regularly, but when women do, they climax harder, longer, and more often in one session than men do.

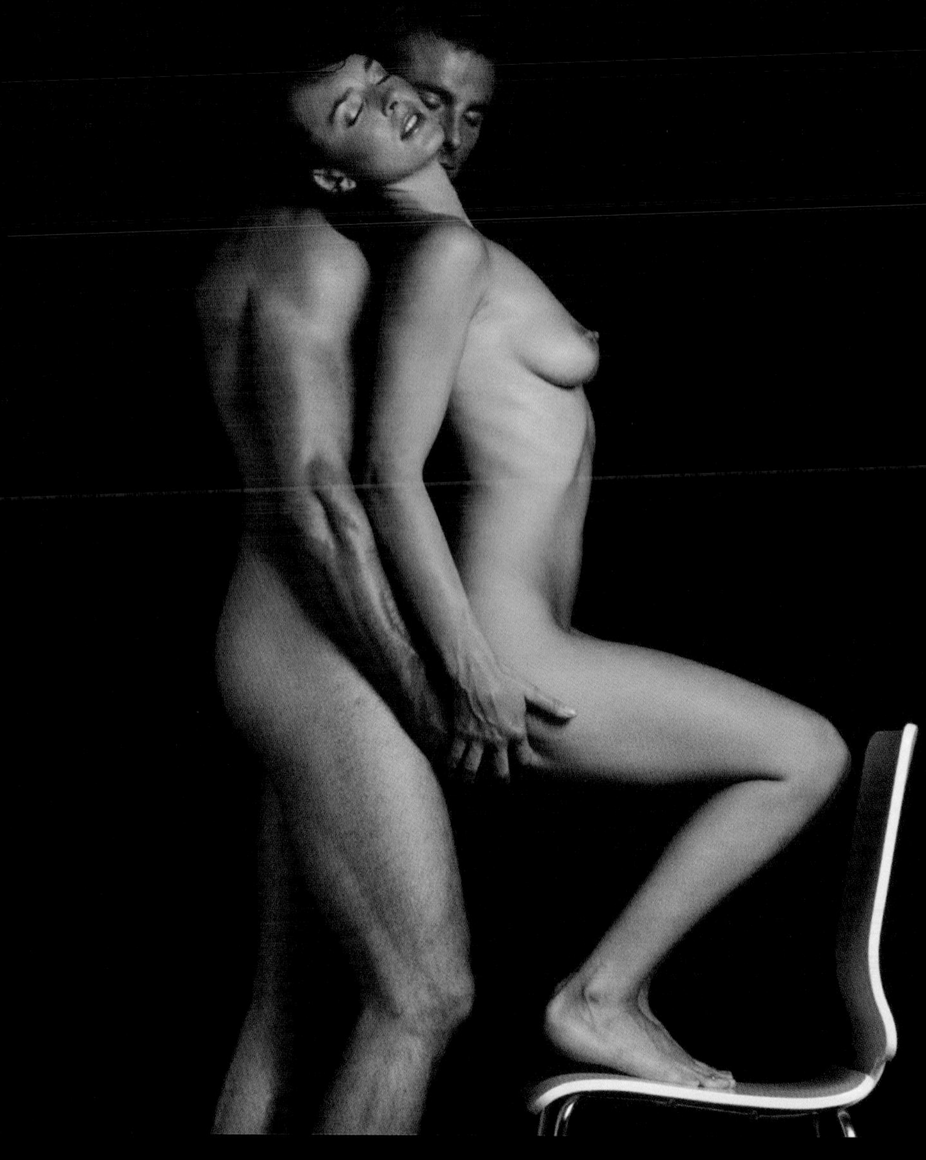

87

show-off sex

This is the position you'd love your partner's gorgeous ex to catch you in. Advanced isn't the word for it, bonkers probably is. Make sure the chair is wedged firmly up against a wall. (A very hard bed can also work.) She leans her shoulders back against his chest as he penetrates, tipping her bottom upward toward him. If he keeps slipping out (he will), she spreads her legs wider and tips her bottom even higher. If he's strong and she's supple, it's possible. Just.

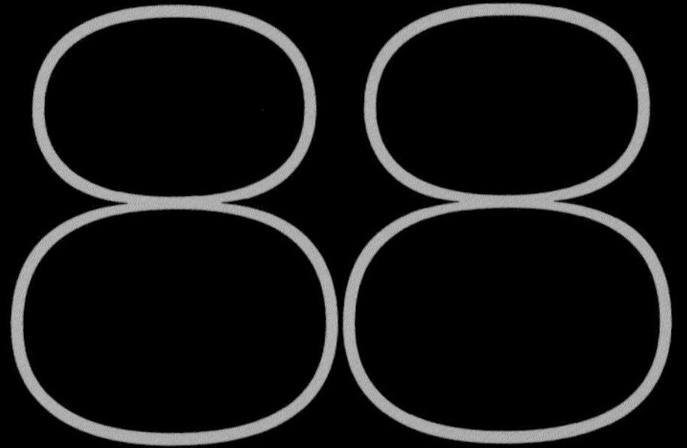

tight squeeze

The unusual entry angle here provides a feisty, fresh start for a sensational session. She lies on her back and lifts her legs up and back toward her head. He kneels in front and penetrates, leaning his hips against her bottom cheeks, while she rests her calves on his shoulders and hangs on to his bottom. Lifting her legs so high narrows her vagina and allows him to plunge incredibly deep. Vary the pace by switching between fast, shallow and deep, slow thrusts.

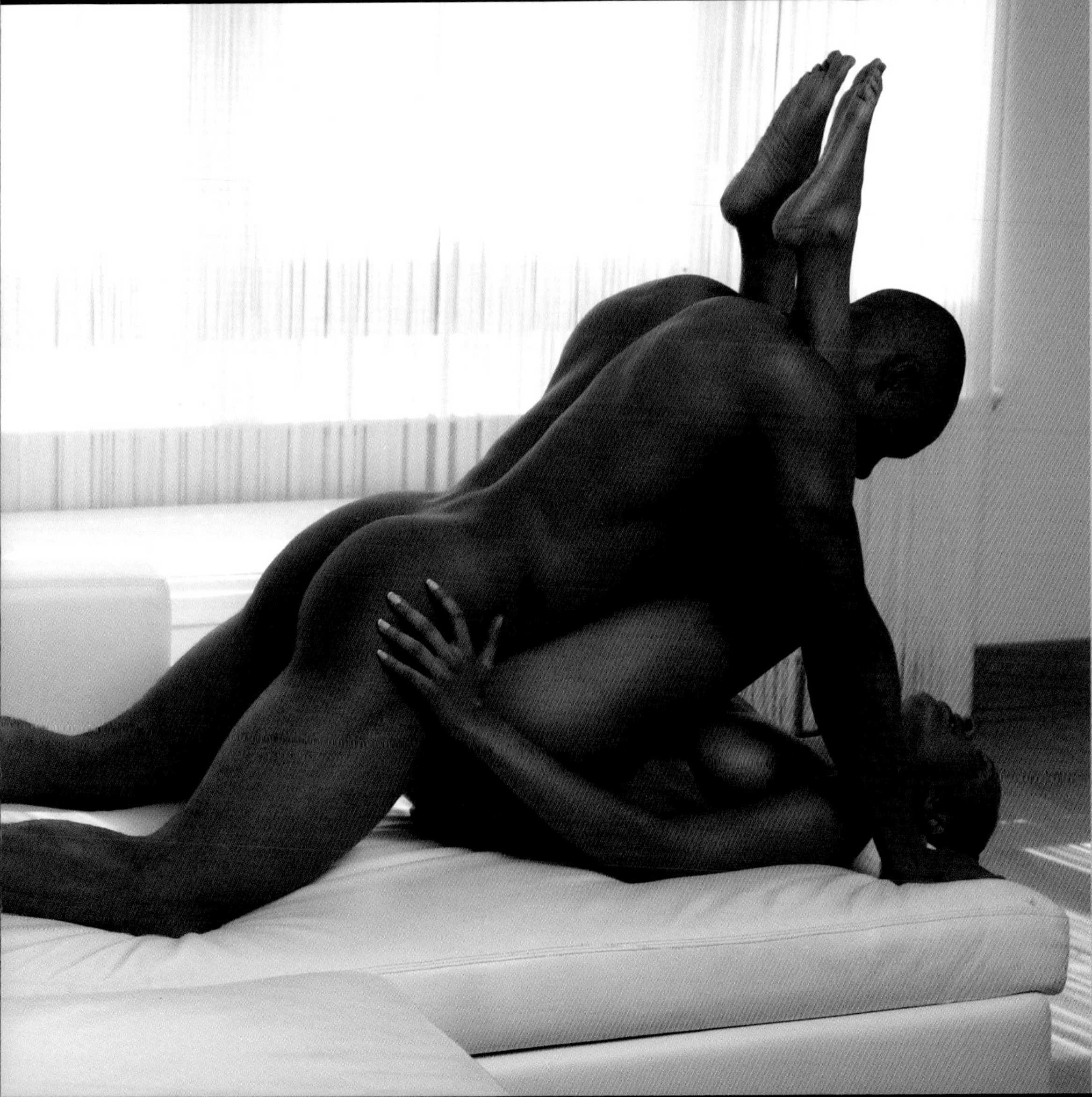

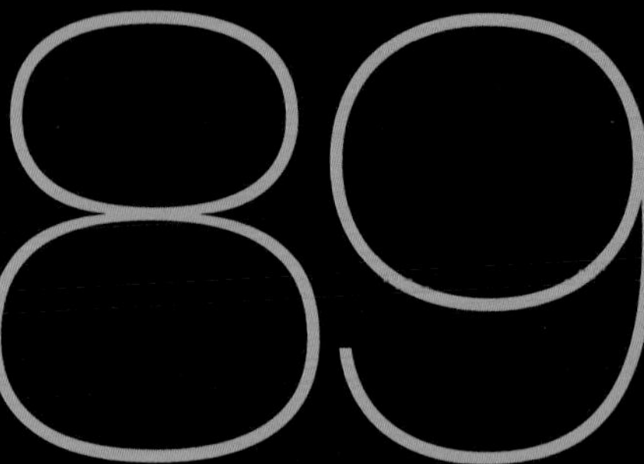

lounge lovers

This looks precarious—and it is. The trick to her not falling to the floor is him keeping his thighs firmly in place, positioned underneath her hips. Get too overexcited, let them fall apart and... well, let's hope an unhappy girlfriend is all you have to cope with!

He slouches back on the couch, she sits on his lap, then carefully leans backward, hands on his calves, and feet on the sofa by his side. In that position, you're both supposed to meditate about life, love, lust... how cool your new ceiling light is.

Again, the trick to mastering this one is to focus on what's happening internally, rather than relying on the traditional method of thrusting. She works her pelvic-floor muscles to squeeze his penis, he makes small movements by doing the same thing: pulling the muscles around his penis and anus tight, holding for a second or two, then releasing. We talk a lot about pelvic-muscle control for women, but it was the Chinese, more than 3,000 years ago, who first acknowledged that men can achieve multiple orgasms by delaying ejaculation via control of their PC (pubococcygeal) muscle. It pays for *both* of you to get a firm grip on yourselves!

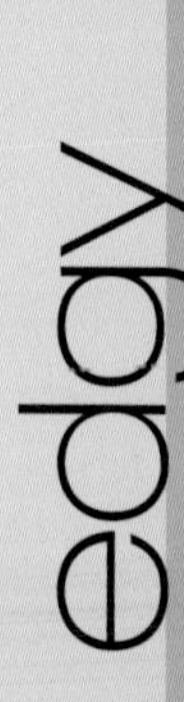

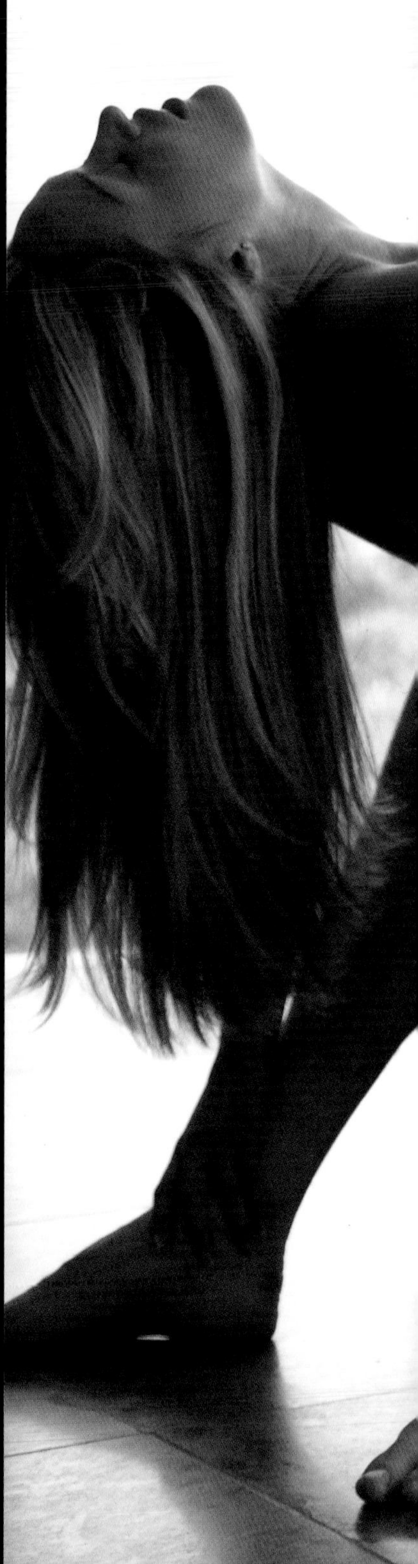

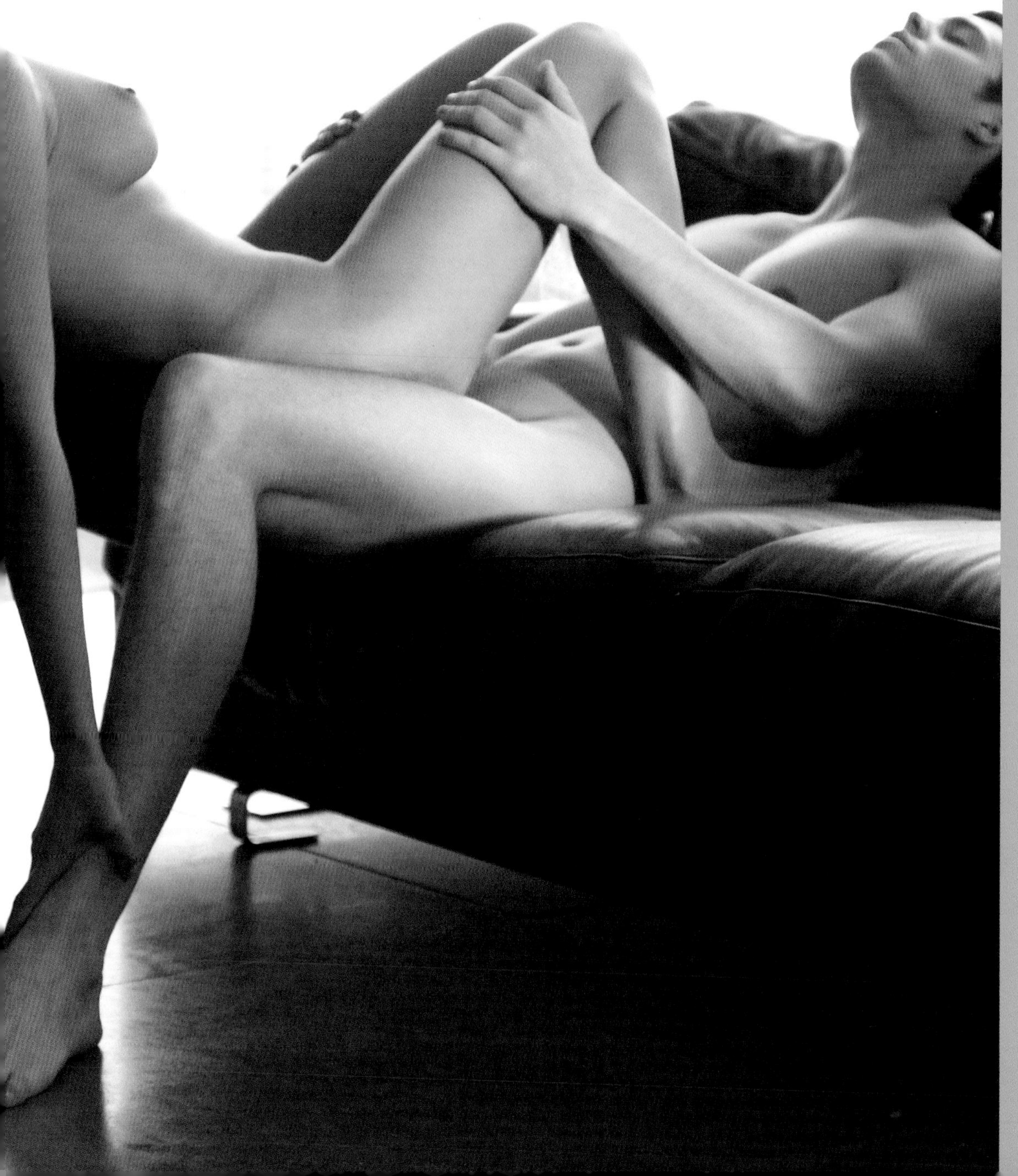

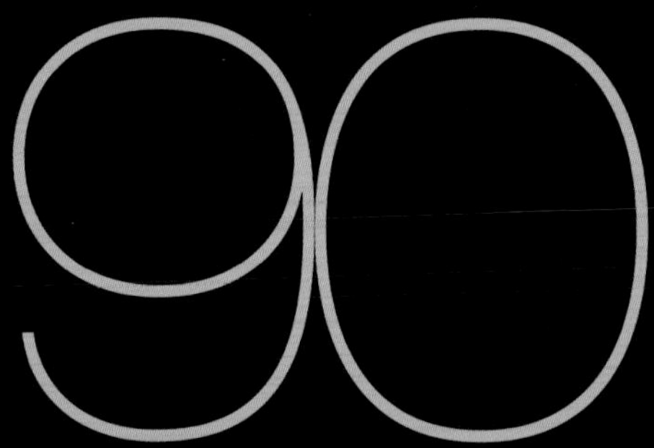

the wall thrust

This one looks deceptively easy until you stop to think about the angle at which he's penetrating her. Some men find it uncomfortable because the penis is bent at an awkward angle and unless she keeps her bottom well and truly tilted back and upward (if that makes sense!), it tends to pop out rather frequently. So why should you even try it? Because if you get it right, it's a fantastic position for one of those spur-of-the-moment boinks.

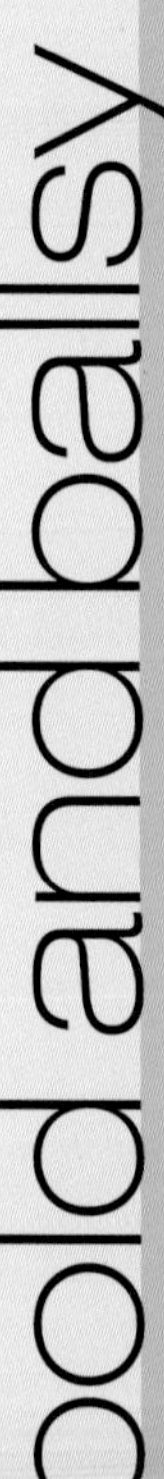

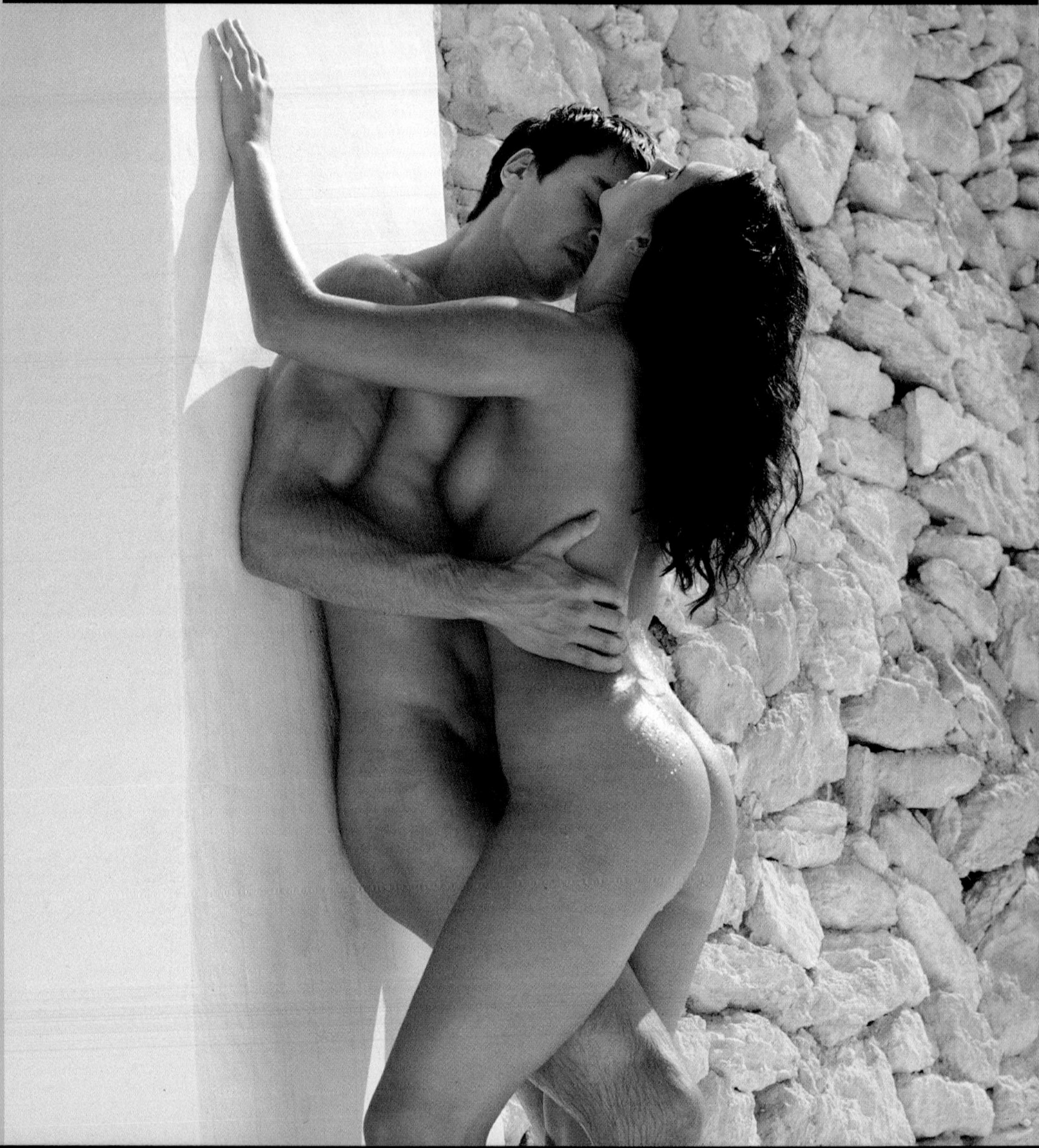

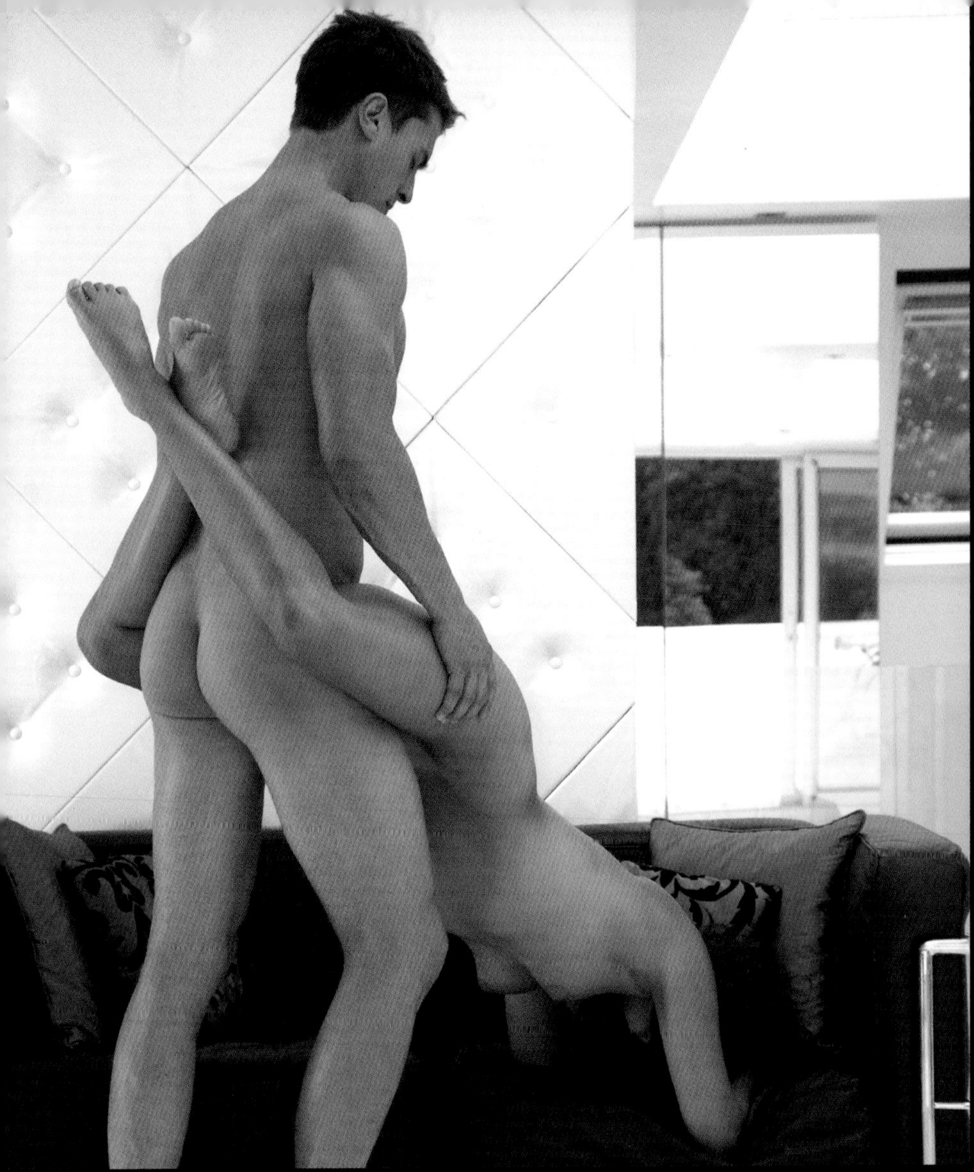

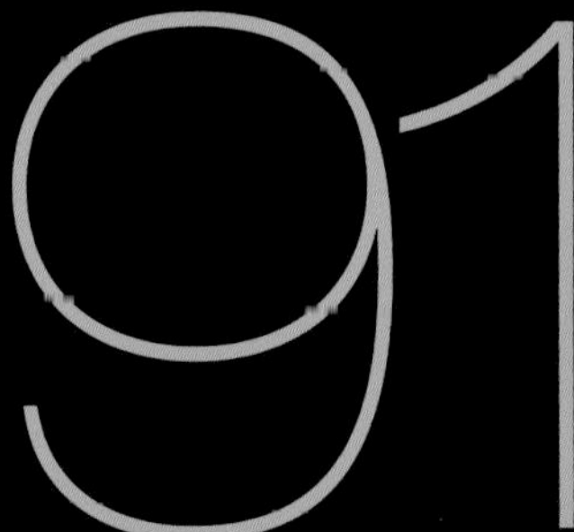

the tom cat

This was inspired by horny tom cats taking advantage of poor, defenseless (in heat) kitty cats. In other words, he has his wicked way and takes control. This clearly suits more athletic types, and he needs good upper-body strength. The payoff for all the effort is a deliciously tight vaginal canal, achieved by her clamping her legs around his back and locking her ankles. And we know what that means, don't we? More friction, which means better sex for everyone!

fast and furious

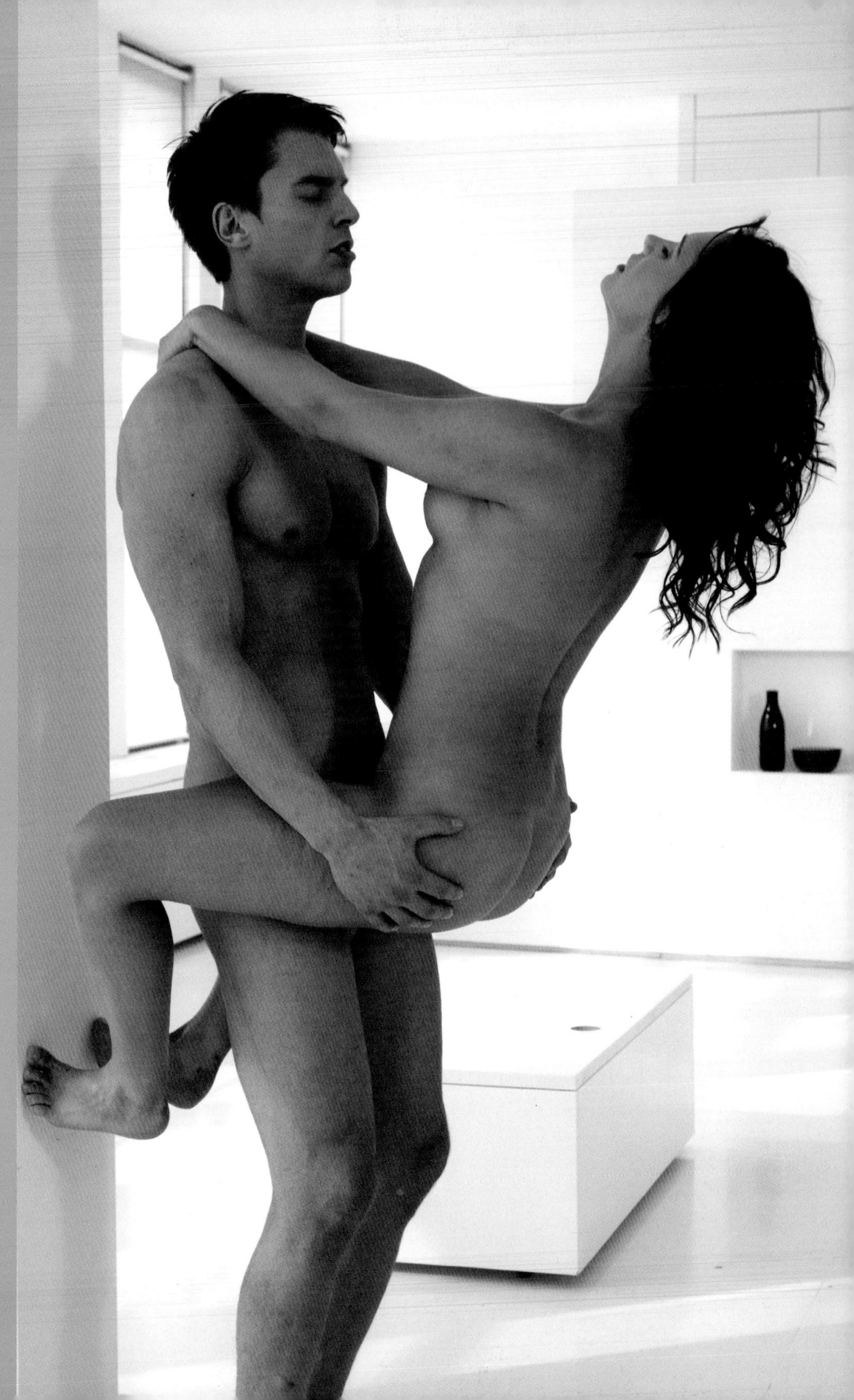

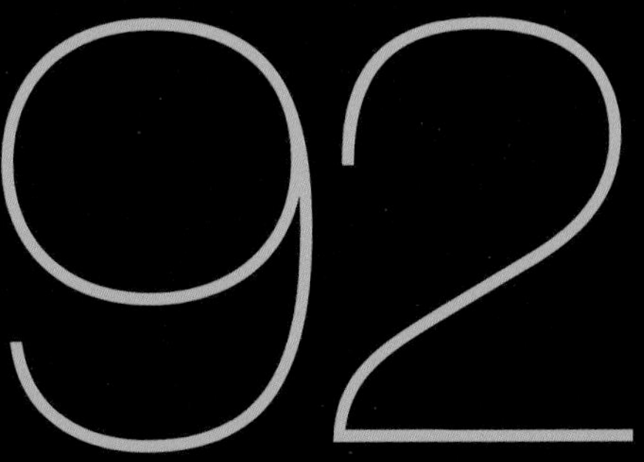

monkey

This is a pleasure pick-me-up, which feels as dynamic as it looks. Perfect for fast, passionate, impromptu sex, it's another one of those manly, caveman-type positions. Yes, it's a challenge—but so long as you don't expect it to last longer than a few minutes, it's totally do-able!

He leans against a wall and lifts her up by taking a firm grip of her bottom. She winds her arms around his neck, grips his thighs with hers, and puts her feet against the wall to give leverage and help him thrust. Thrusting becomes more of an up-and-down bobbing than an in-and-out motion. The closer you are in height, the easier it is.

thrust away

If you were to film most standard sex sessions, 95 percent of men would be thrusting the conventional way: in-out-in-out (yawn). Same speed, depth, hip motion, same everything. Thankfully, the *Kama Sutra* comes to the rescue...

new ways to thrust

* Churning: he grasps the base of his penis, then moves it in circles inside the vagina.
* Double-edged sword: he strikes sharply downward into the vagina. This is the opposite of modern thinking, which has brainwashed both of you always to aim for the front vaginal wall (the part under the belly) because that's where the G-spot is. This is a totally different sensation—rather nice, too!
* Rubbing: a pillow under her bottom raises her hips; he thrusts in an upward motion.
* Buffeting: he pulls out and then penetrates again with a fast, hard stroke. Some women (like me) wince at the thought of this one, so check before plunging right in there!
* Boar's blow: he puts continuous pressure on one side of the vagina. Recent evidence shows one side of the clitoris is nearly always more sensitive, so it's not wild conjecture to imagine that the same applies elsewhere!
* Bull's blow: he thrusts wildly in all directions like a bull tossing its horns. Reserve for long-time lovers or risk looking like an overenthusiastic loon.
* Sporting of a sparrow: he makes rapid, shallow, in-and-out strokes.
* Piercing: she lies on her back, keeping her pelvis low. He lies high up on her body and penetrates. The penis is *parallel* to the vulva, so his thrusting stimulates the clitoral area.

grown-up playtime

Some people love games, others loathe them. But even if you develop chronic diarrhea at the mere mention of the word "charades," you might find something to tickle your fancy here. As I say over and over: the couple that plays together, stays together. The reason I keep repeating myself is this: It's true! Stop playing and you'll fall out of love. Keep having fun and you'll stay together. Simple. Now, do as you're told. I order you to have fun!

make obscene calls One of you goes into another room, then dials the other, pretending they have no idea who they've just called—but with every intention of being shockingly vulgar. Ask questions: "What are you wearing?" Give instructions: "Pull your panties to one side," "Reach down and grab that big, lovely erection." At first, the other person may be outraged, but then oddly turned on...

be flashers Turn the lights off, then take turns lighting one area of your own body with a flashlight. Each lit body part must be touched, stroked, and/or licked for two minutes, then the flashlight gets passed on to the other person. (Note to boys: It gets very, very boring if the only thing ever under the spotlight is long and cylindrical.)

play "dress up" Nurse's outfits, baby-doll lingerie, all-in-one catsuits—they're straight out of the '80s and tons of fun. You pay through the nose for them in a sex shop and they're not terribly well made, but if you're flush and you like the look of them, why not! If the thought of you dressed up

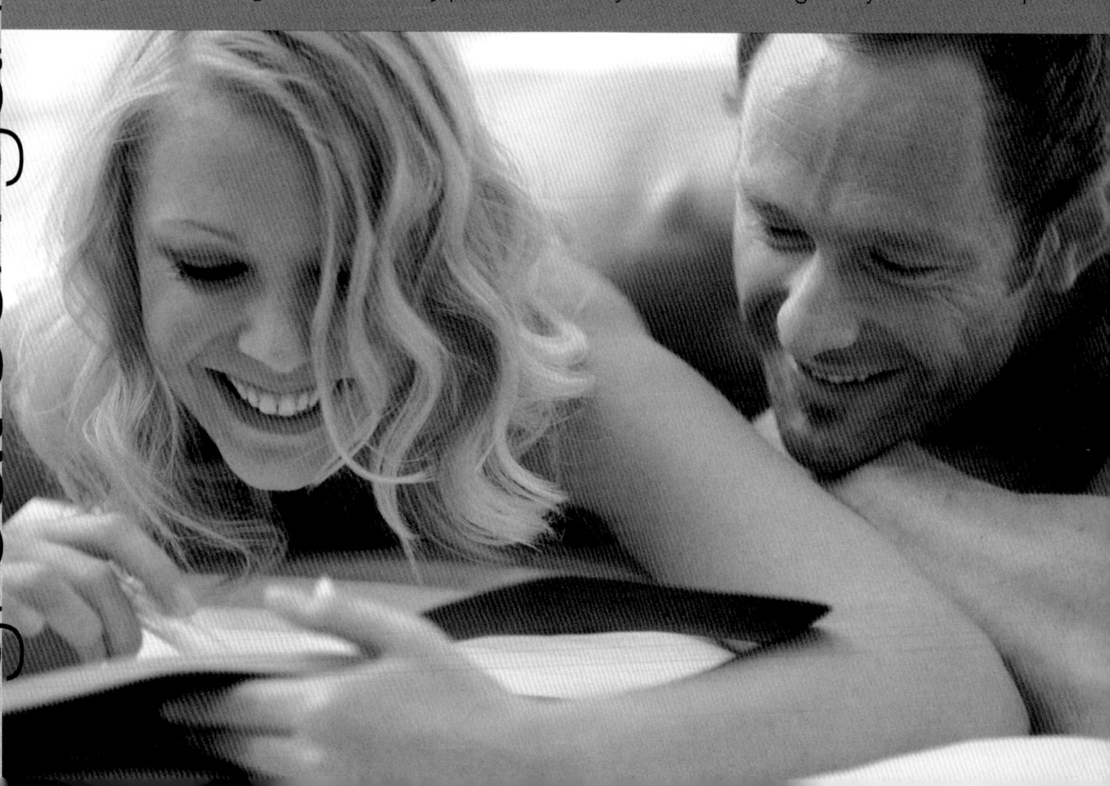

"We rarely make up a fantasy that doesn't appeal to us."

as Nurse Betty/Spiderman makes you want to scream with hilarity rather than lust, put together a less obvious home-spun creation.

give rewards Make up your own redeemable sex coupons and leave promises of treats around the house for your partner to discover. Their reward for being very, very good is you being very, very bad.

fantasy dice Write down and number the beginnings of six fantasies (something like "Suddenly I felt my girlfriend's mother put her hand on my knee under the table. Even worse, she was really attractive..." or "And there I was—in the middle of an orgy..."), then take turns throwing the dice. When the person lands on a number, they have to complete the corresponding fantasy out loud. It's a sneaky, not-too-embarrassing way to find out your partner's secret turn-ons because we rarely make up a fantasy that doesn't appeal to us.

be a sex therapist One of you goes somewhere private to take a call from a "patient," who pretends to ask for advice on how to please their partner. The therapist goes into lots of detail describing what would be a good way to do this. (All, of course, their personal idea of heaven!) If you like this, get the therapist to make an appointment for the patient, so the therapist can give "hands-on" demonstrations of each technique.

play guinea pig Grab all the sex toys you own (order some new ones if there's a lone vibrator lying forlornly in the drawer), then place them on a table in the bedroom, lined up in a formal fashion. Tell your partner they're needed as a "test dummy" for a project you're working on that night. Strip them naked and try out each and every toy on them. They have to rate them in order of pleasure.

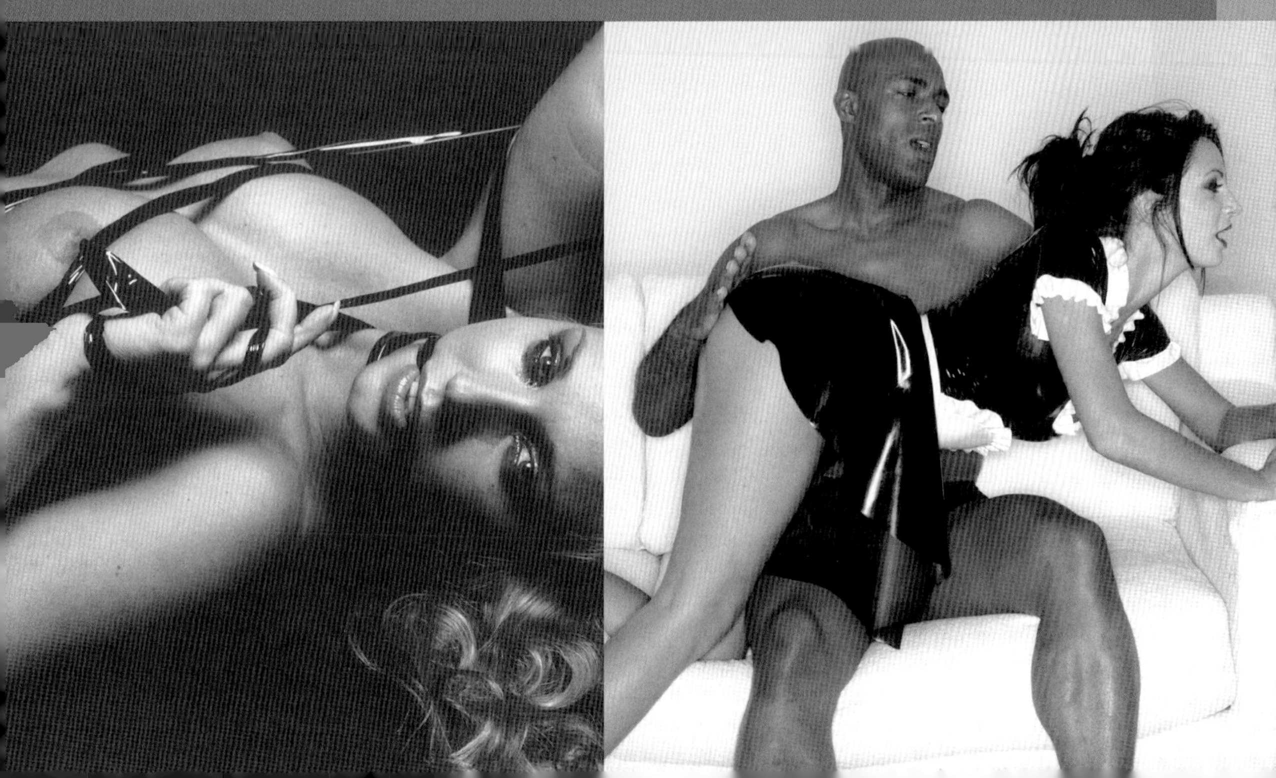

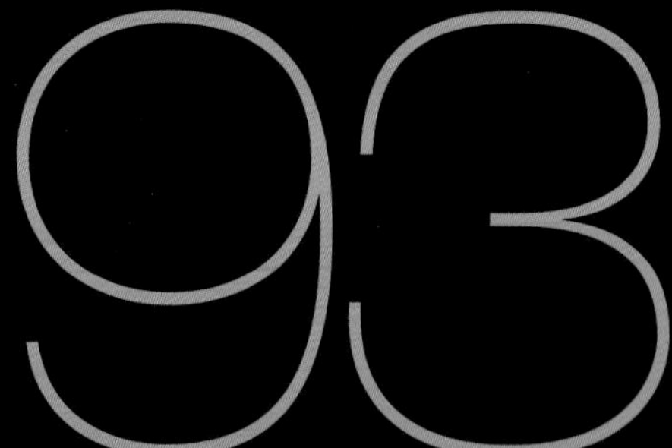

leap frog

Squatting doesn't feel that comfortable, but there are plenty of payoffs for the sore legs: he's got much more control over thrusting than if he were lying on top in the usual manner. She can lift one or both legs, depending on how deep she wants him. This one is definitely better suited to a short, saucy sex session than to a prolonged one, so try switching from the traditional missionary position to leap frog about five minutes before takeoff.

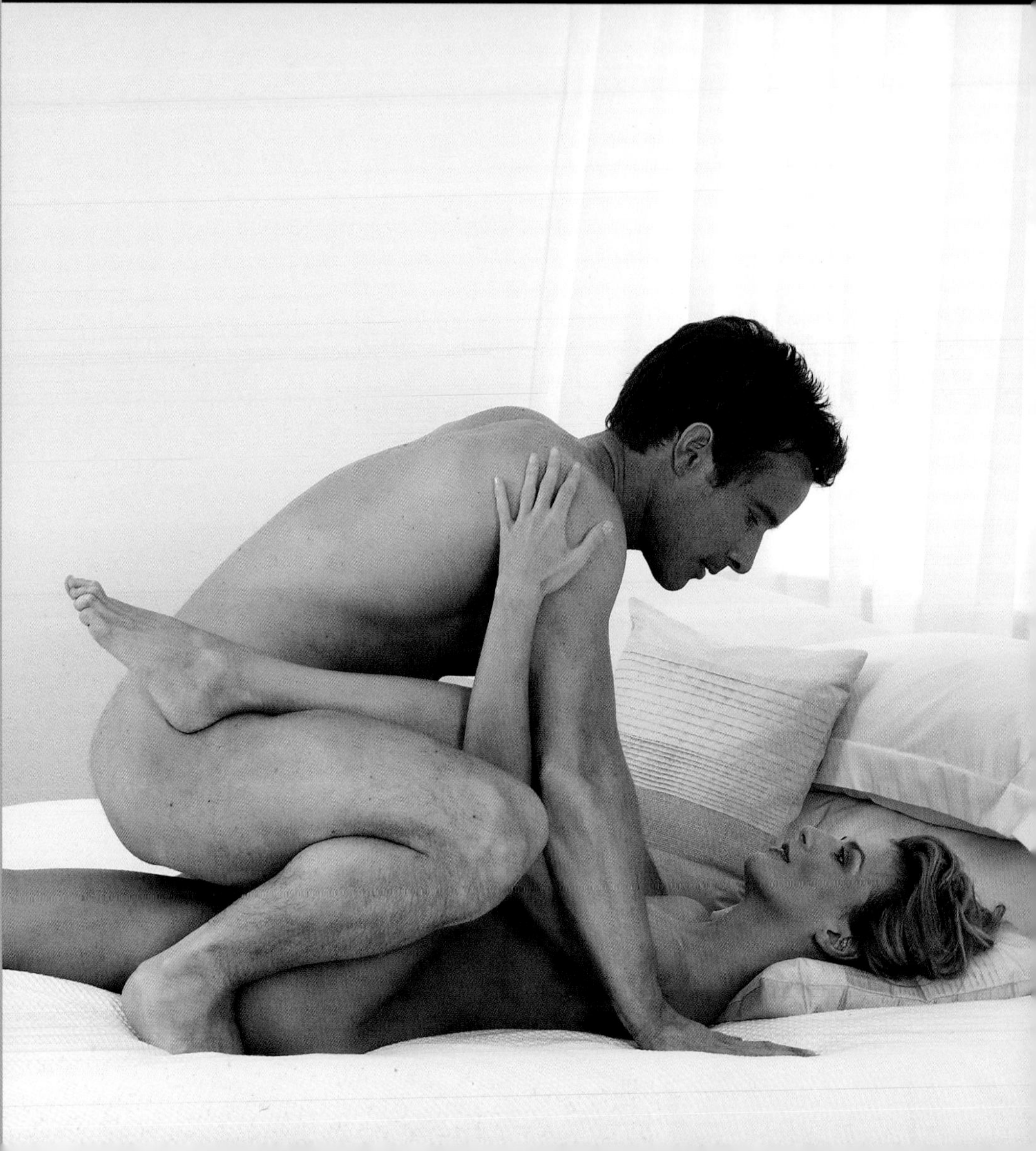

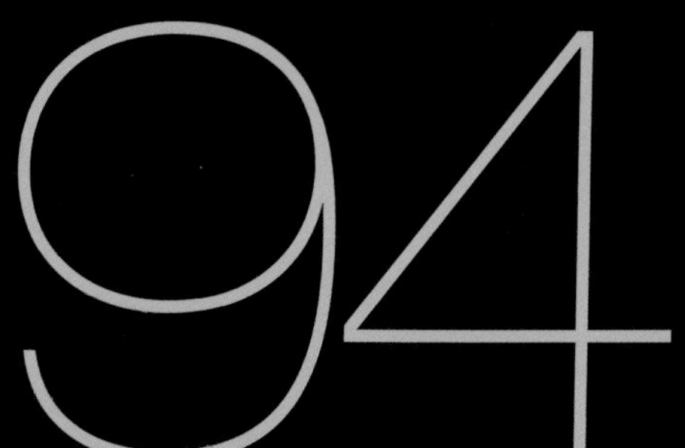

on target

Despite popular perception, the *Kama Sutra* only describes about 24 positions, with most involving the woman lying on her back with her legs at a variety of angles. But even subtle changes in position can make an enormous difference in the angle of penetration. A variation on the usual foot-to-chest positions, the man kneels instead of sits, and pulls her up, aiming for front-wall stimulation. G-spot fans will love it, but it's also ideal if he wants to work on her clitoris.

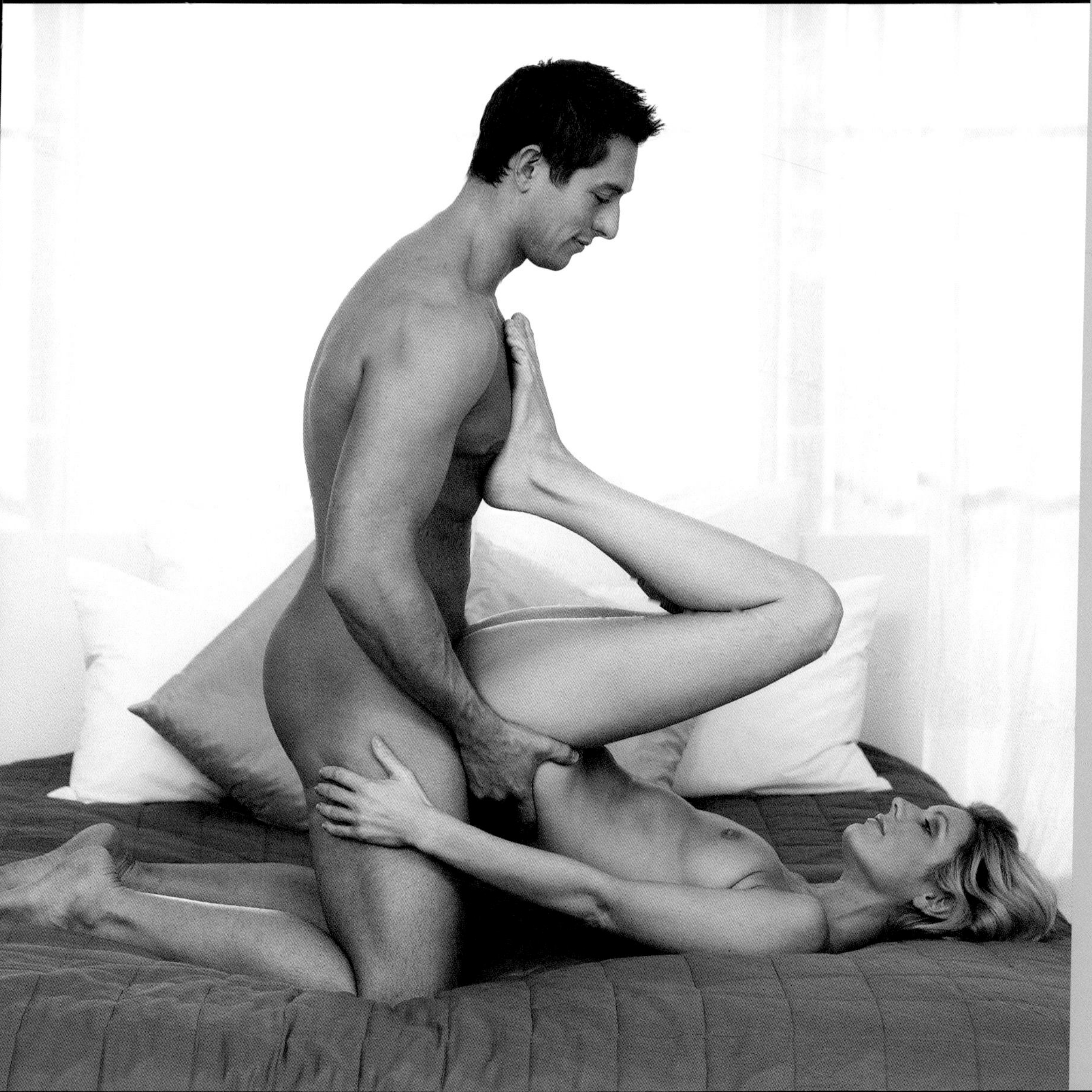

hang ten

1 If this position doesn't make him feel like King of the Jungle, nothing will! He kneels at her feet, worshiping her as the goddess she is (OK, I just made that part up, but he does need to kneel). She sits on his lap and you both get as close as possible, him relishing the feel of her breasts pressed in between, and both of you luxuriating in the feel of skin on skin.

2 She pulls back and raises herself slightly to allow him to penetrate. It's not cheating to use your hands to guide him in. Revert back to the same position you adopted in step one, except that this time he is inside. No thrusting at this point; instead, she contracts and releases her pelvic-floor muscles.

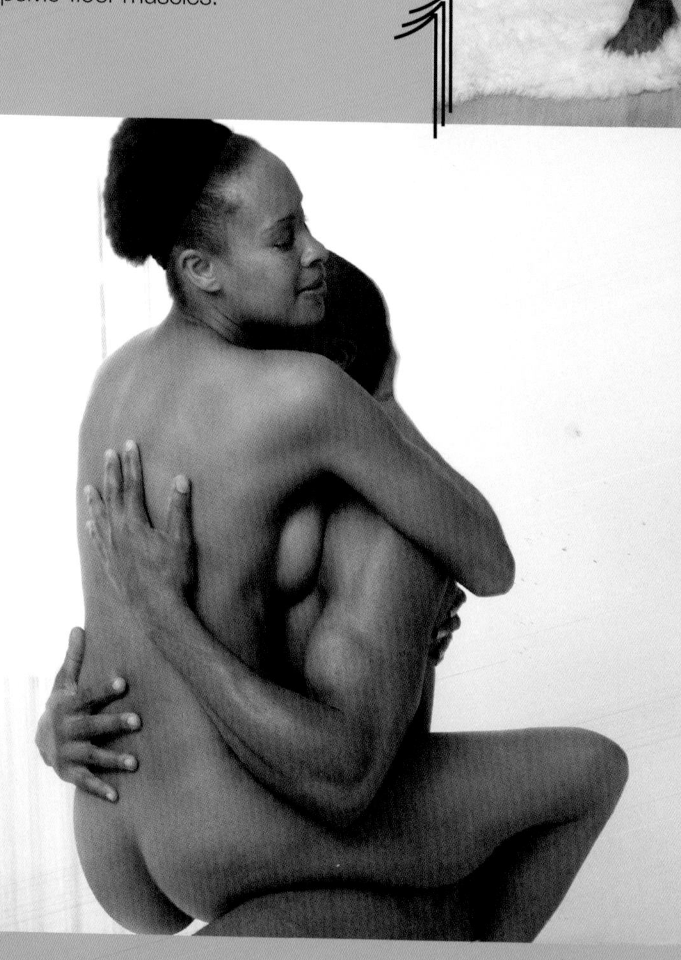

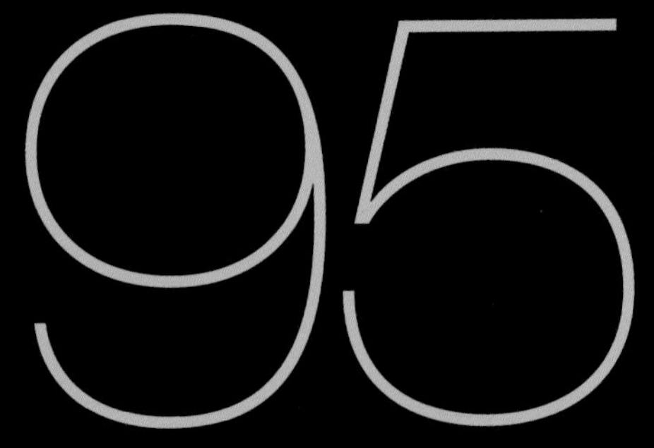

3 He stands as she holds on tight, keeping his knees bent. He then carefully lowers her so she's sitting as low as possible while still maintaining penetration. It's hard to do much more than simply bash against each other, so keep the pelvic floor "milking" motion going. If you want to finish with some good old-fashioned vigorous thrusting, it's relatively easy for him to plonk her down on a handy piece of furniture.

3

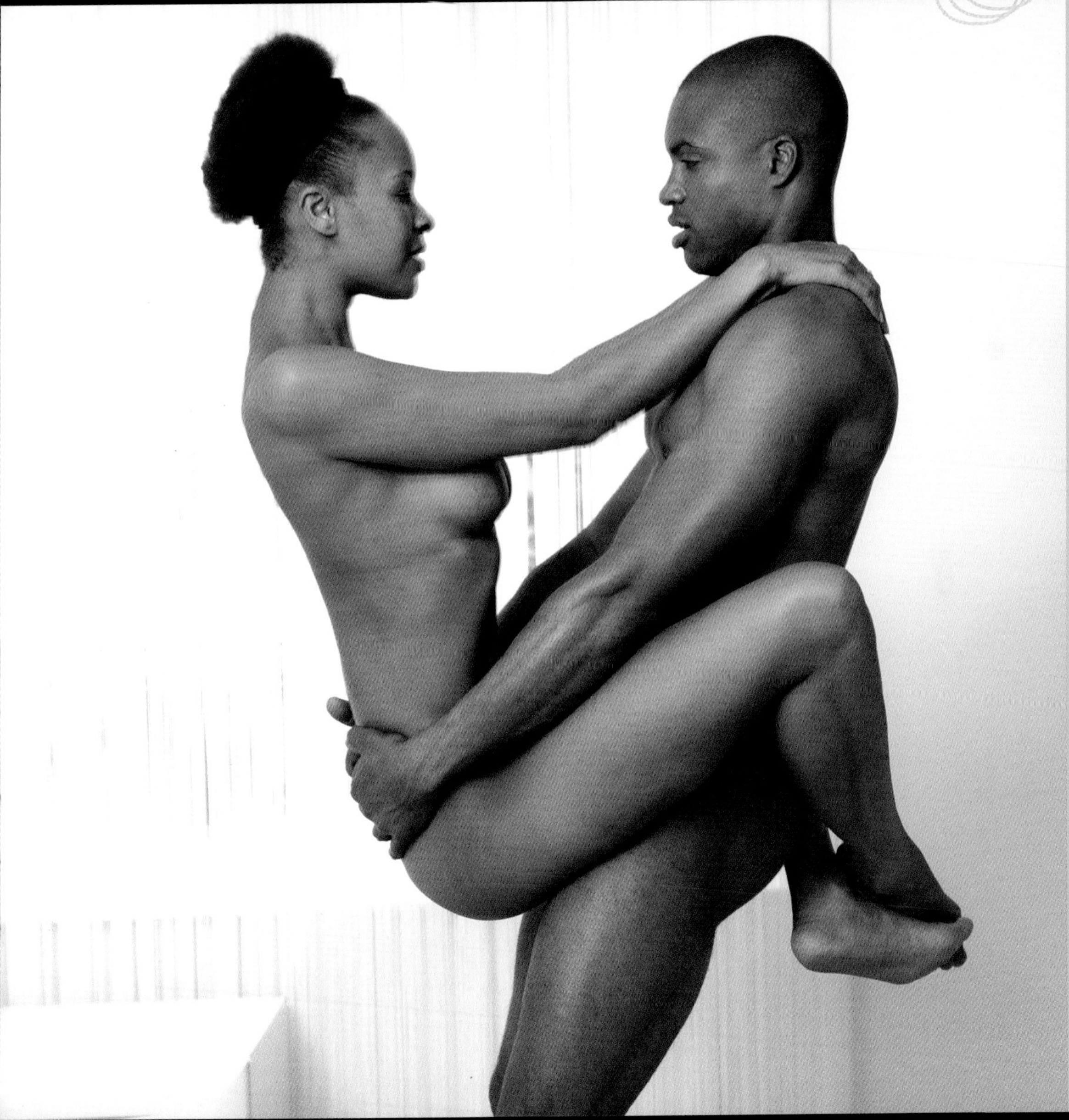

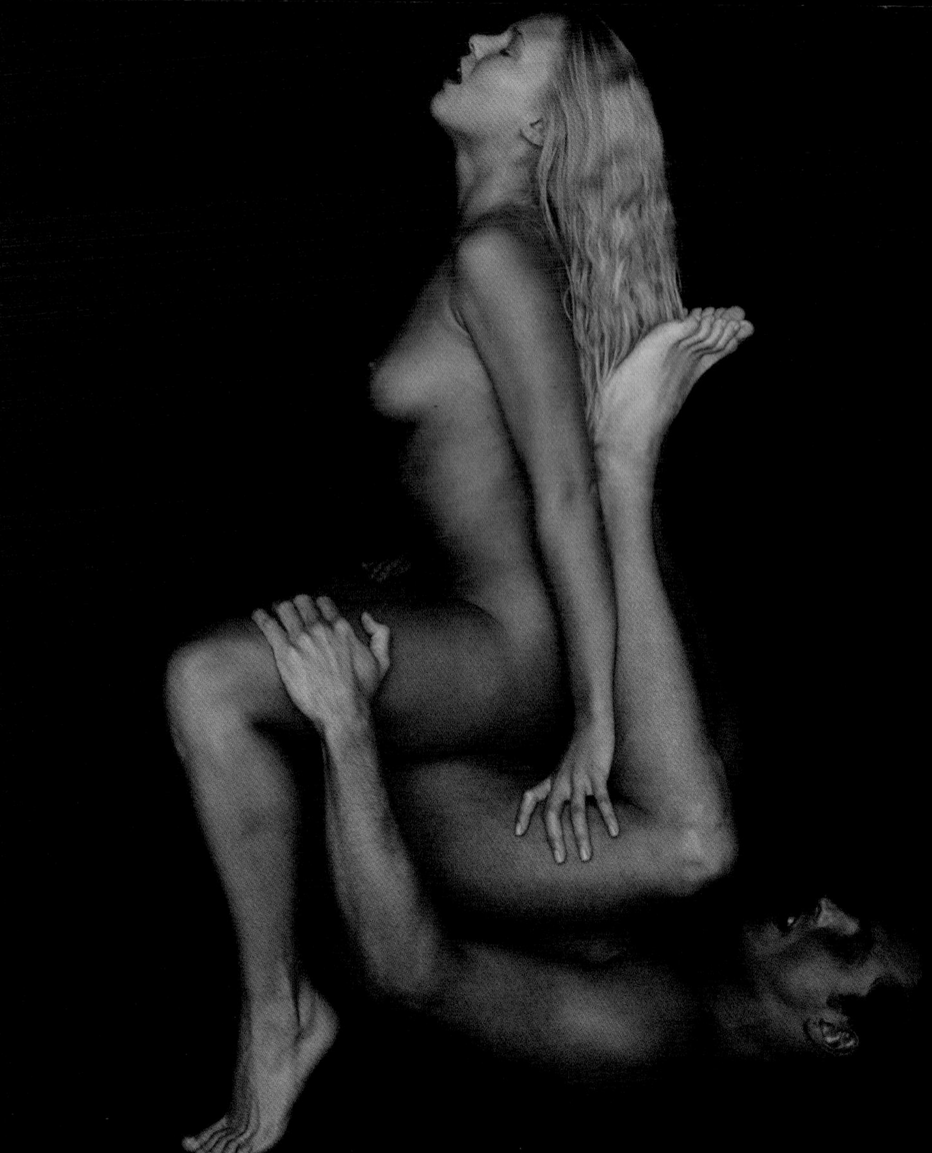

96

on your bike

He lies in the old "bicycle" exercise position. You face away and lower yourself onto his penis by sitting down on his bottom. His feet rest against your back; your fingers rest on his thighs for balance. Yes, this one may make you think: "Oh really?" His penis is bent back and through his legs, which is why a semi-erection works best. He might not love it, but you will. You're in the driver's seat (literally) so can custom-order your orgasm by controlling the depth and speed of thrusting.

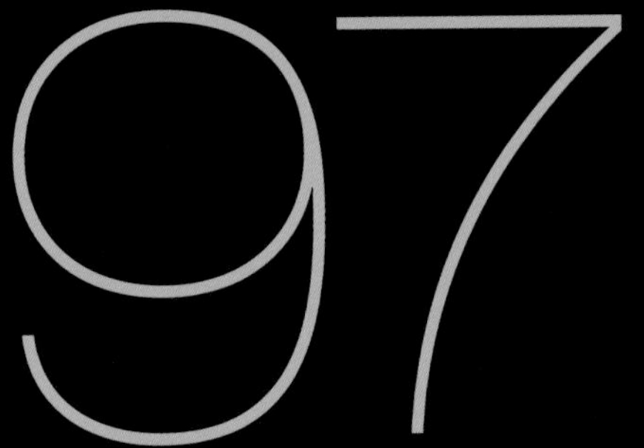

going down

He kneels on a hard surface, keeping his back straight. She lies in front of him with her legs on his shoulders. Holding his erection downward, he penetrates. Penetration is shallow, but this isn't a bad thing because most of the vaginal nerve endings are located within an inch or so of the entrance. Shallow means his penis targets her most responsive part with what also happens to be his most sensitive part—the head of the penis.

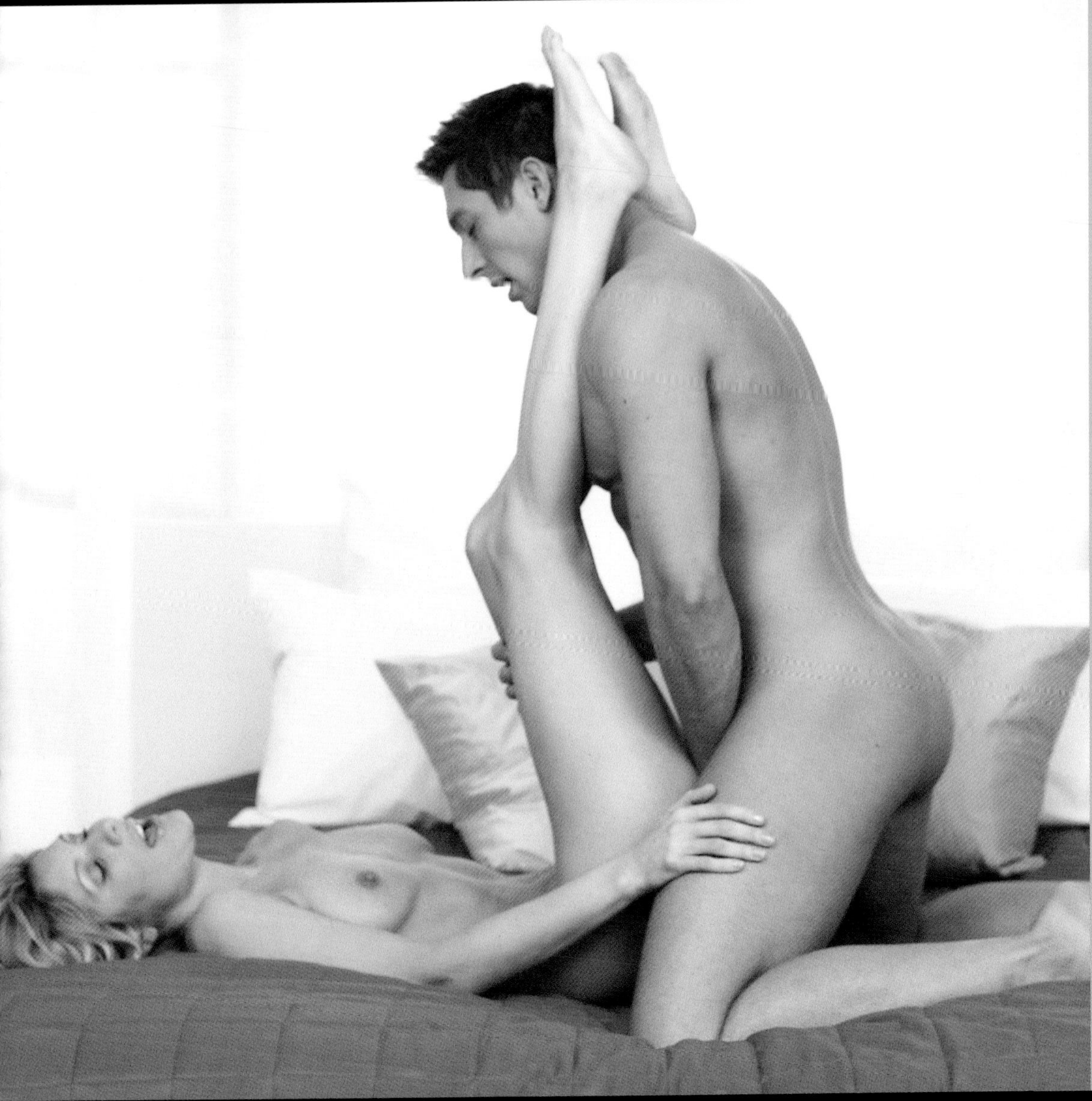

saucy sex tricks

Zap your love life from stale to salacious in seconds with these clever little tried-and-tested, raunch-rated sex tricks. Perfect for that fun-and-filthy weekend away or any time you have a notion to do something a little different.

give a hand job

for him Make him squirm in public by sucking his finger as though it's a small penis. Lean forward so no one else can see you (if you have long hair, hide behind it), maintain eye contact, hold his finger in your mouth, and swirl and lick and suck until he can't take it any longer. Unless you're lavishly licking up and down his finger like it's a lollipop, it's relatively easy to get away with it without being arrested. In other words, keep most of the action happening inside your mouth (even if there is rather a lot happening in his jeans).

for her Return the public humiliation by lifting her hand to your mouth as though you're going to kiss the back of it, then turning it over and burying your tongue in her palm. As with the above, do like you'd do if you were giving her oral sex. Again, if you hold her hand at the right angle and keep most of the tongue action close, Aunt Betty could be watching and simply think you're being romantic. Well, she will until your girlfriend slides off her chair!

drive him nuts

for him Get ballsy by taking control of his. It is a bit of a personal thing—some men hate having their testicles stimulated, others love it—but it's well worth giving it a try. So often, they're left shyly hanging back there while the star of the show, his penis, gets all the attention. Be a fan, perfect your ball game and you hold the key to his sexual heaven in your hot little hands. Think of his testicles in the same way he thinks of your breasts. You can cradle them, suck them, stroke them, knead them. What you can't and shouldn't do, though, is bite or pull them too hard.

Testicles are often sensitive all over, but take a good look the next time you're giving him oral. Search for a little ridge running up the middle, then follow it until you find the piece of skin that joins his testicles to his penis. This is usually the most sensitive part. It's best stimulated with your tongue, but use lubricant or your fingers (and saliva) and trace the area with your fingertips. Try circling the area where testicles and penis meet with the tip of your tongue, flicking it back and forth. Or use your tongue to lick swirling patterns around each testicle. Later, when you fellate him, use one hand to lightly cup his testicles and gently "juggle" them.

do it standing up

for both of you We can thank Alex "Joy of Sex" Comfort for this inspired oral position, done standing up to give her the unique sensation of an orgasm in the air. She lays face-up on the bed, he straddles her, then picks up her legs, putting them around his neck. He can then nuzzle in and lick her. It sounds uncomfortable, but her shoulders and head are supported by the bed. Not only can she see what's going on, he's perfectly positioned for thorough clitoral stimulation.

This doesn't appeal? Then let yourself be tempted by some Tantric: "The Crow" is the rather exotic name for the classic sixty-nine position turned on its side: you both lie on your sides, head to toe, facing each other. Each of you draws your inner thigh

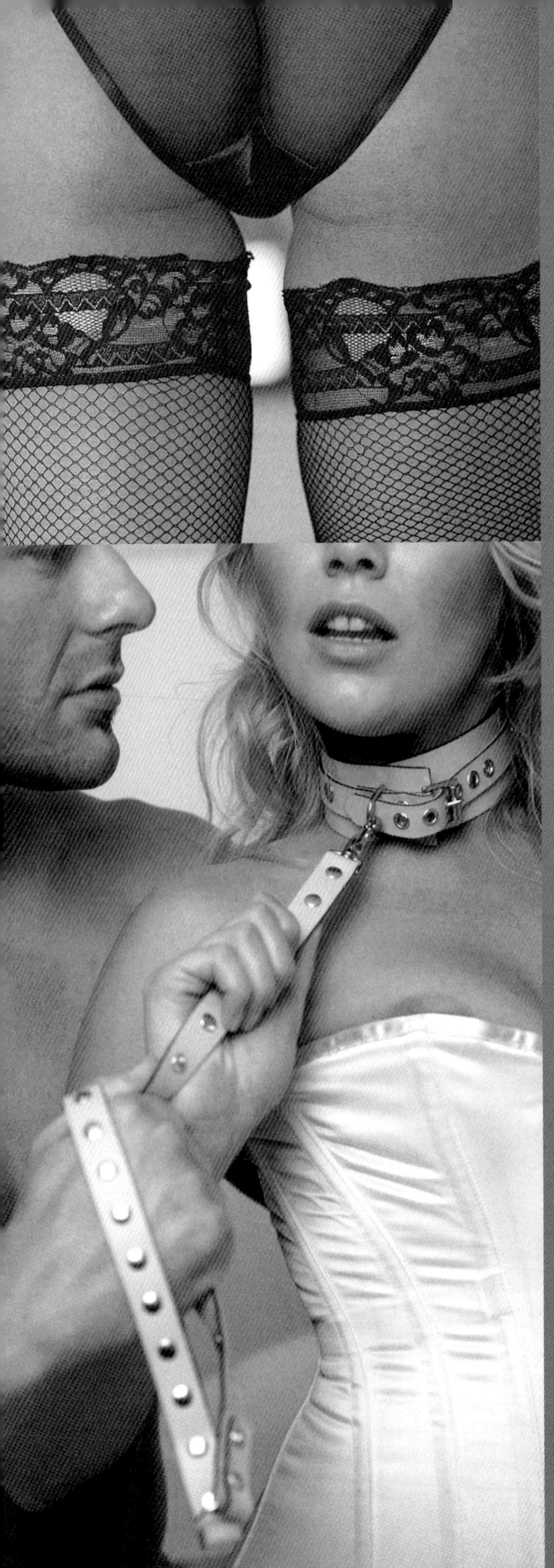

"Perfect your ball game and you hold the key to his sexual heaven."

up so it can be used as a pillow for your partner's head. It's a simple variation on the norm but a lot more comfortable.

startle the senses

for both of you They do it in movies (usually ones starring Sharon Stone), but few of us use ice cubes anywhere but in drinks. It's a shame really, because an ice-cold mouth pressed against hot genitals feels exquisite! Put a glass full of small ice cubes nearby when you're having sex and pop some in your mouth before you fellate him; insert one into her vagina before performing oral sex (not too big, though—you want to chill, not numb). If ice cubes feel too startling, try chilled champagne or ice cream.

Next, raise the temperature by adding a hot drink and alternating the sensations—stimulation by a cool mouth followed by a hot mouth. Varying the temperature and taste activates two sets of nerve endings to serve up a sensory smorgasbord.

take a detour

Can't have penetrative sex because you've got your period? Just "pretend" by lubricating his penis, keeping your thighs firmly together, and letting him thrust between them. Position yourself so his penis is sliding through the lips of your vagina, stimulating the clitoris, but not penetrating.

Alternatively, try gluteal sex: he applies lots of lubricant to his penis, you lie on your stomach and put a pillow under your hips. He then thrusts between your buttocks. Or oil your breasts and hold them firmly together while he thrusts in between.

the interlock

1 You're either flexing those well-toned and honed muscles of yours or rolling around laughing after taking a look at this one. You need to be strong, supple, and yoga fit to last longer than a few minutes. But hey, big points for trying! It starts off simply: he sits with straight legs and she climbs on top.

2 He holds on to her waist, and she leans back, taking her weight on her hands. She then puts one foot on the floor and rests the other leg on his shoulder. Don't attempt to take this to superhuman lengths by attempting to place *both* legs on his shoulders. He either collapses under your weight (not great for the ego) or you end up being awkwardly bounced around and feeling like a sack of potatoes (ditto).

1

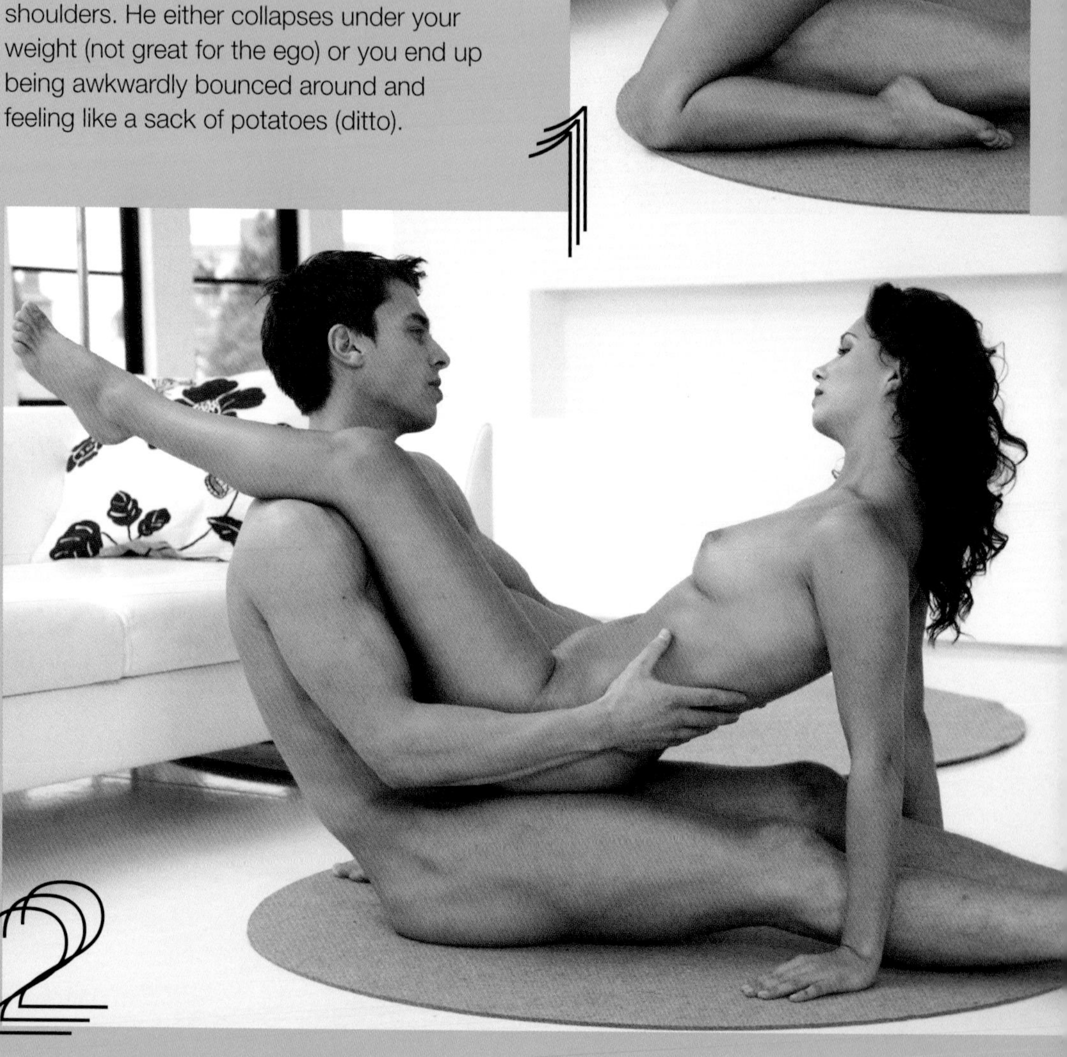

2

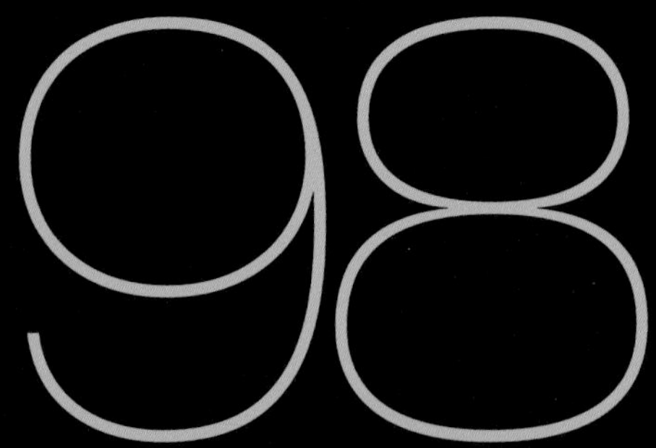

3 In the final move, he lets her go so she's totally supporting her own weight, and moves his hands into a mirror position. Keeping both feet on the ground, he pushes up on his arms and thrusts his hips upward to create movement. It's a novel sensation, and you both feel terribly smug for a bit, having managed it. Then your arms hurt. Then you notice your belly jiggling. Then you collapse, quickly moving into an old favorite to finish the job.

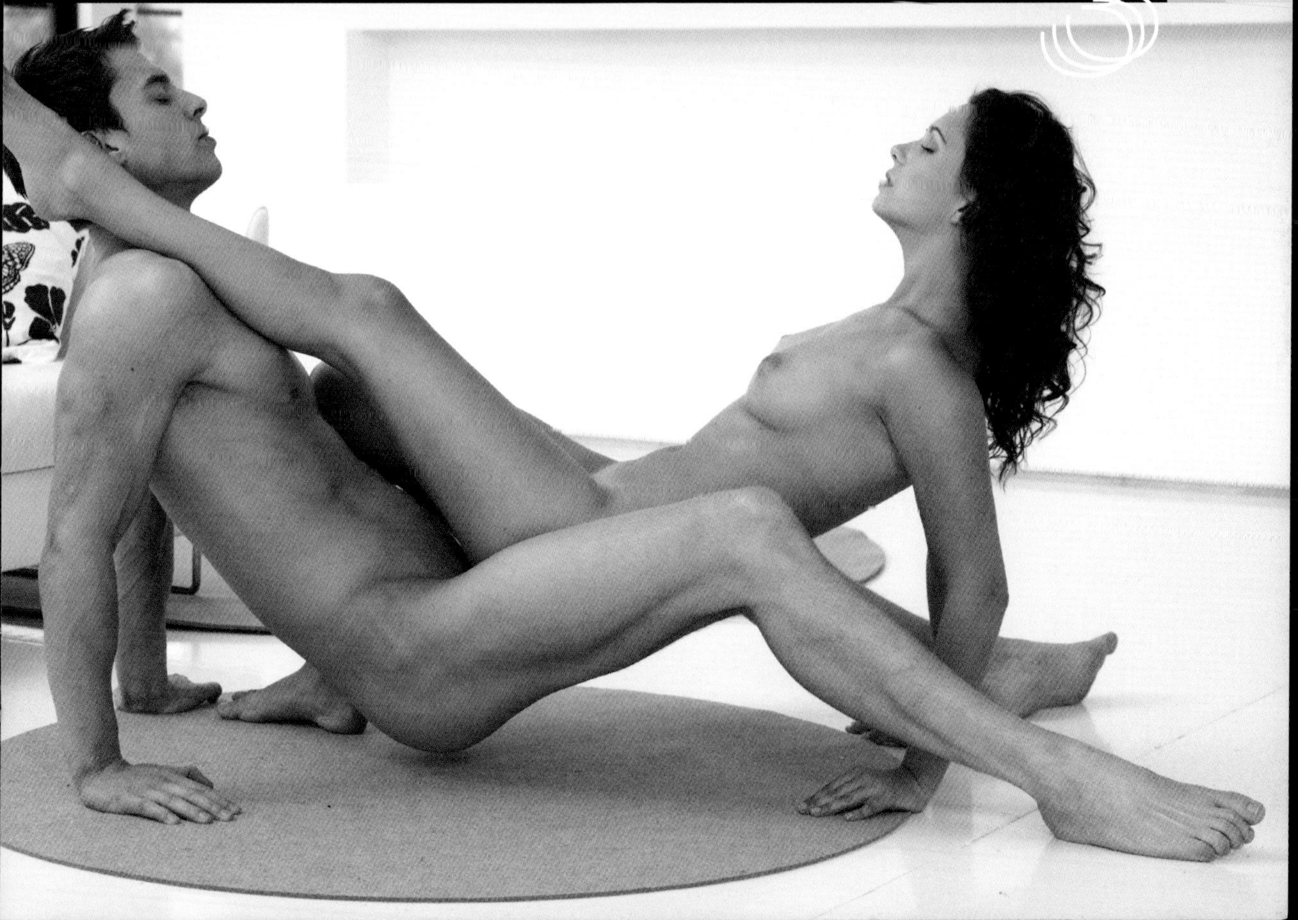

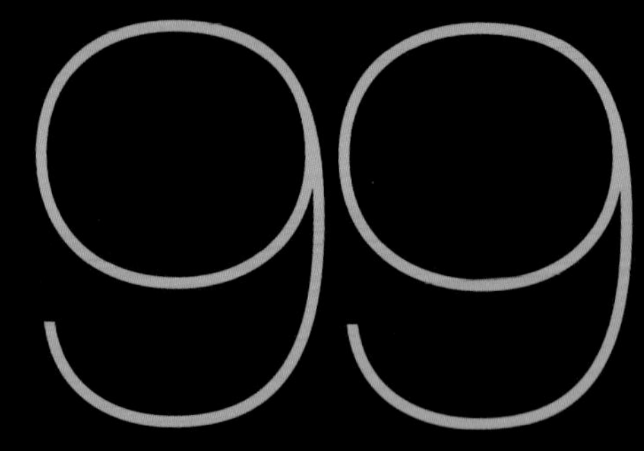

the corkscrew

She's on top, then through a series of moves, she turns around while he's still inside her and ends up facing the opposite way. So she starts by riding him, rodeo-style. Then, using her hands to steady herself, lifts one leg over her body and begins to turn sideways. She continues rotating, stopping at intervals for a few thrusts, until she's facing away. He gets a unique "corkscrew" feeling on his penis, and is simultaneously treated to a revolving-restaurant-type view of her body.

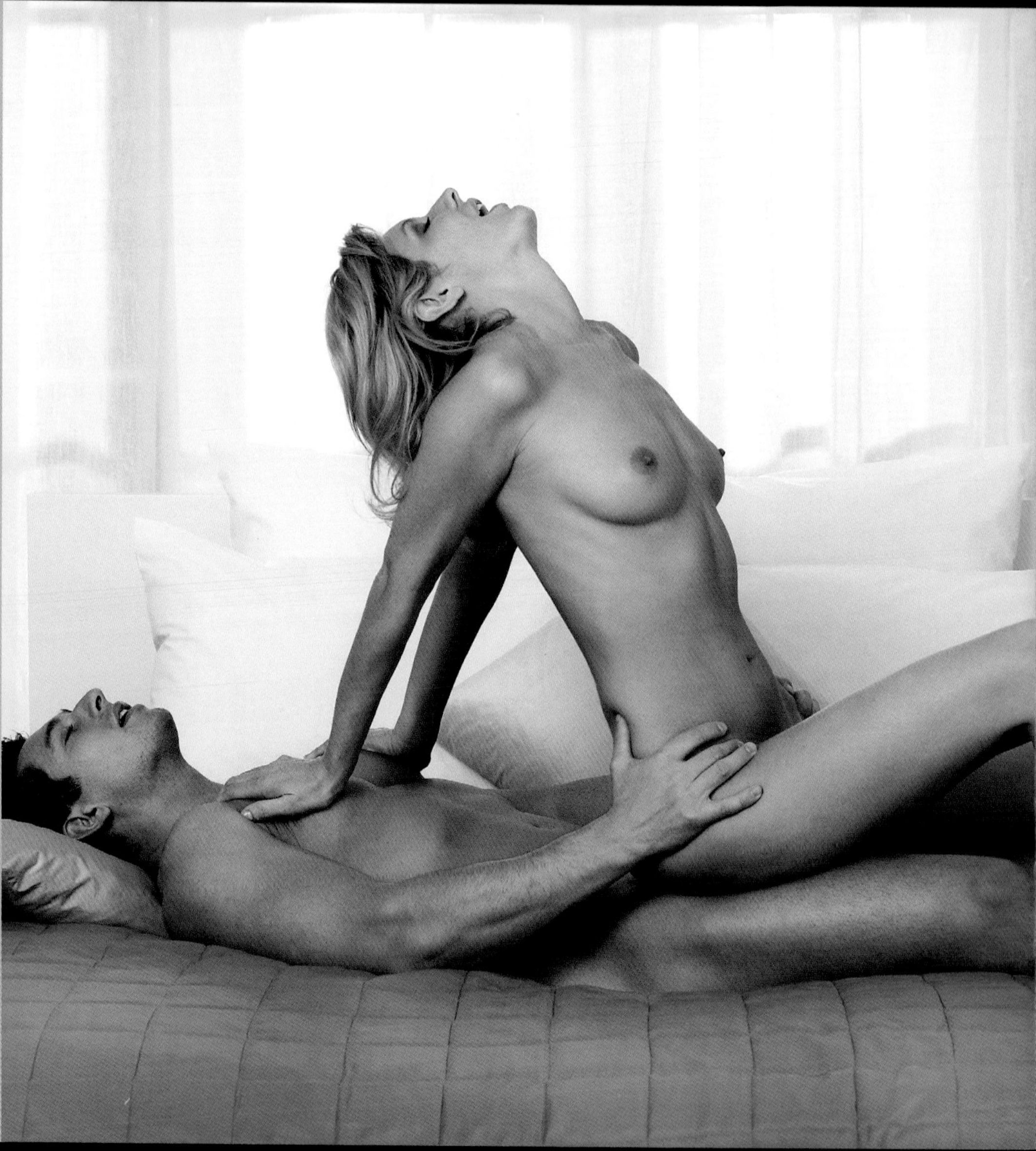

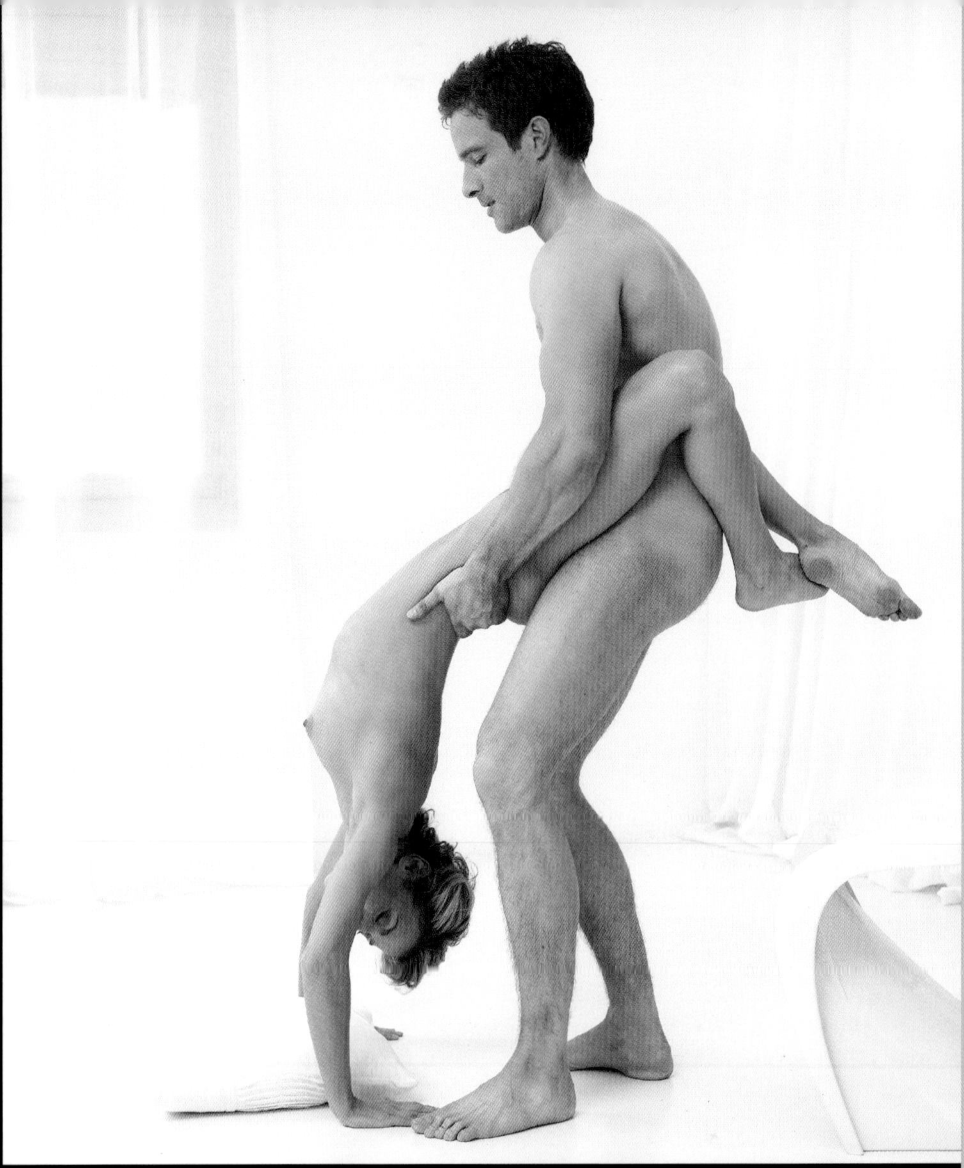

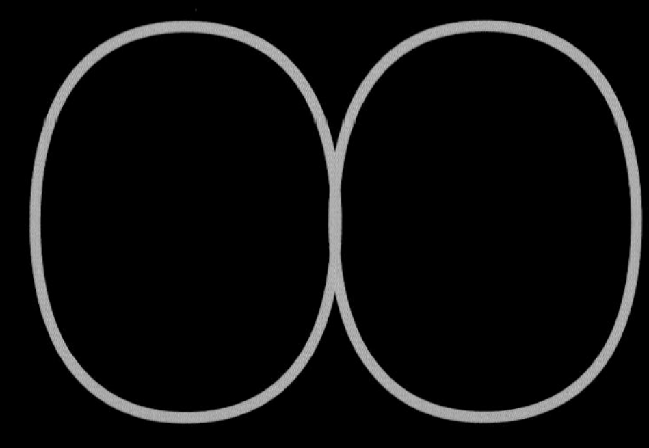

head rush

Stand facing each other. She jumps up and wraps her legs around his waist, and her arms around his neck. She lets him penetrate, then very slowly and carefully lets go and allows her body to fall backward until she's in a handstand position with her palms on the floor, facing away from him. He supports her by holding her waist and buttocks. Yes, you need to be flexible, but it's actually not as difficult as it sounds (and you've got to admit, it looks so impressive!).

checklist

Found some new favorites?

01	02	03	04	05
11	12	13	14	
	22	23	24	25
31	32	33	34	35
41	42	43	44	
51		53	54	55
61	62	63	64	65
71	72	73	74	75
81		83	84	
91	92	93	94	95

Check the numbers of the positions you loved.

06	07	08		10
16	17	18	19	20
26	27	28	29	30
36	37		39	40
46	47	48	49	50
56	57	58		60
	67	68	69	70
76	77	78	79	80
86	87	88	89	90
96	97	98		100

acknowledgments

DK would like to thank the following people: Charlotte Seymour for design assistance; Kate Meeker for editorial assistance; Marie Lorimer for indexing; Angela Baynham for proofreading; and John Davis, Andrew G. Hobbs, John Ross, and John Rowley for photography